NANOTECHNOLOGY SCIENCE AND TECHNOLOGY

ELECTROSPINNING AND ELECTROPLATING

FUNDAMENTALS, METHODS AND APPLICATIONS

NANOTECHNOLOGY SCIENCE AND TECHNOLOGY

Additional books in this series can be found on Nova's website under the Series tab.

Additional e-books in this series can be found on Nova's website under the eBooks tab.

NANOTECHNOLOGY SCIENCE AND TECHNOLOGY

ELECTROSPINNING AND ELECTROPLATING

FUNDAMENTALS, METHODS AND APPLICATIONS

TOBY JACOBS
EDITOR

nova
science publishers
New York

Library of Congress Cataloging-in-Publication Data

ISBN: 978-1-53612-363-0

Published by Nova Science Publishers, Inc. † New York

CONTENTS

PREFACE

Electrospinning is a simple and efficient process in producing nanofibers. The use of an electrospinning process in fabricating tissue engineering scaffolds has received great attention in recent years due to its simplicity and ability to fabricate ultrafine nanofibers. Chapter One investigates the process of formation of ultrafine fibers and nonwoven membranes by electrospinning from natural degradable polymers – polyhydroxyalkanoates (PHAs); physical, mechanical, and biological properties of the products have been included. Chapter Two aims to give an insight into the use of this interesting class of polymers in electrospinning as well as to explore the wide range of possible applications. Chapter Three reveals the fundamental working principles of electrospinning process and the effect of electrospinning process parameters towards the nanofibers morphology. Chapter Four provides detailed information on the background of electrospinning, fundamental principles and theory, investigation on parameters involved in nanofibers' structural/ biological/mechanical characteristics, advantages of superb properties and biomedical applications of electrospun nanofibers, particularly in tissue engineering heart valves. Chapter Five focuses on the fabrication and characterization of electrospun PVDF, PVDF/PLA (50/50 wt %) and PVDF/G (99.5/0.5 wt %) membranes. Chapter Six presents the main results of recent experimental investigation of the electrodeposition and characterization of Fe/TiO2 composite coatings obtained from an environmentally friendly methanesulfonate iron plating bath containing colloidal TiO2 particles.

Chapter 1 - An integrated study has been performed to investigate the process of formation of ultrafine fibers and nonwoven membranes by electrospinning from natural degradable polymers – polyhydroxyalkanoates (PHAs); physical, mechanical, and biological properties of the products have been studied. Then, electrospinning was used to prepare ultrafine fibers from PHAs with different compositions: P(3HB) and its copolymers P(3HB-*co*-4HB), P(3HB-*co*-3HV), and P(3HB-*co*-3HHx). The main process parameters, that influence UF-fiber diameter and properties of fibrous non-woven membranes) (polymer concentration, solution feeding rate, working distance, and applied voltage), were investigated and their effects evaluated. This study was the first to compare biological and physical/mechanical parameters of PHAs with different chemical compositions as dependent upon the fractions of monomers, constituting the polymers and fiber orientation.

Electrospun polymer membranes, prepared from the [P(3HB-co-4HB)], were tested as wound dressings. The developed nonwoven membranes can be used as the equivalent of collagen skine dressings in the treatment of burns of degree II. Experiments on laboratory animals with model skin defects showed, that the membranes fitted the wound shape good, protected the wound from external influences, and facilitated wound healing, promoting fast repair. The successful experiments on laboratory animals were followed by pilot clinical trials of nanomembranes, comprised of PHA membranes as wound dressings in the treatment of septic wounds. During the regeneration phase, PHA membranes served as a scaffold for the new tissue on the skin and filled out soft tissue defects. The formation of the uniform and sufficiently vascularized tissue is a prerequisite for quicker wound healing and can serve as a basis for the subsequent skin grafting and spontaneous re-epithelialization of superficial wounds. The wound dressing, tested in this clinical trial, performs important physiological functions of natural skin, provides a barrier against secondary infection, reduces fluid loss, and, at the same time, does not keep the air out.

Chapter 2 - With the increasing dominance of the electrospinning process, the diversity of materials that have already been tested in this area increases, so an interesting group of polymers is highlighted due to its solubility in water. A great advantage in the use of these polymers is that they have low indices of toxicity and biocompatible features, what give to them a wide range of applications. Among the water-soluble polymers most commonly used in electrospinning, the authors can mention PVA, PVP, PEG, PEO, collagen, chitosan, alginate among others, with applications in industry, commerce, medical and food. A highly exploited application of water-soluble polymer nanofibers is in the field of medicine, including tissue engineering, drug delivery vehicles, cell growth, curatives, etc. A new area that has been highlighted is the use of these polymers as sacrificial polymers, helping in the production of ceramic nanofibers. Ceramic nanofibers have been gaining attention because of their good mechanical properties, thermal and corrosion resistance. They have been studied as agents for the release of drugs in the health area, but also as components for photoelectrodes, such as sensors, catalysts, filtering agents, among others.

This chapter aims to give an insight into the use of this interesting class of polymers in electrospinning as well as to explore the wide range of possible applications.

Chapter 3 - Electrospinning is a simple and efficient process in producing nanofibers. The use of an electrospinning process in fabricating tissue engineering scaffolds has received great attention in recent years due to its simplicity and ability to fabricate ultrafine nanofibers. Most of the recent progress in tissue engineering has embarked on the use of nanofibers as tissue engineering scaffolds. This is because nanofibers can replicate the structural design of natural human tissue at the nano-scale thus shortening the healing time. Although electrospinning is a simple process, there are still several parameters which need to be controlled or optimised in order to produce nanofibers with different characteristics. Different applications might require nanofibers with specific criteria to be produced. Hence, this review will reveal the fundamental working principles of electrospinning process and the effect of electrospinning process parameters towards the nanofibers morphology. Various polymeric materials and their composites/blends have been successfully electrospun for tissue engineering (TE) scaffolds and they have been tabulated. In many cases, secondary processes are also integrated with the electrospinning process so as to develop 3D TE scaffolds and overcome limitations in term of the nanofiber thickness.

Chapter 4 - In recent years, the application of natural/synthetic based nanofibers in different industries such as textile, environmental engineering, biomedical engineering, energy and electronics have been the subject of many researches. This is particularly due to their unique properties (particularly high surface-to-volume ratio that is approximately 1,000 times more than that of human hair). Electrospinning is a straightforward and promising technique used to fabricate ultrafine quality of continuous nanofibers within a diameter range of 20-1000 nm. As a customary setup for electrospinning, a high potential electrical field is applied to the emerging solution at the spinneret nozzle tip for transforming the jet into the nanofibers. Electrospinning can be employed in a laboratory as well as in industries when expanded. Obviously, the process/system parameters involved influence the structural and mechanical properties of electrospun nanofibers. The microstructure of nanofibers and subsequently the macro-properties of electrospun mats can be modified by varying the parameters involved in electrospinning process. The fabricated electrospun mats are interconnected, non-woven nanofibers deposited over the collector surface. High porosity, remarkable mechanical properties such as an elastic modulus within the MPa/GPa range and capacity to be formed into a variety of shapes are the other properties of electrospun nanofibers. Co-axial electrospinning is an advanced method of electrospinning where a dual nozzle spinneret is used for fabricating a core/shell structure of nanofibers. Any conductive polymer solution can be used as the shell for any other conductive polymer solution or nanoparticles depending on the application. This review of an electrospinning technique provides detailed information on the background of electrospinning, fundamental principles and theory, investigation on parameters involved in nanofibers' structural/ biological/mechanical characteristics, advantages of superb properties and biomedical applications of electrospun nanofibers, particularly in tissue engineering heart valves. In addition, the reasons for common instabilities, which result in the failure of Taylor cone formation and subsequently the failure of fiber production, are also explained.

Chapter 5 - Electrospinning is a versatile technique for generating ultrathin fibers from a rich variety of materials, including polymers and ceramics. Polyvinylidene difluoride (PVDF) is a smart polymer which exhibits piezoelectricity and it is often combined with other materials in order to improve or modify its properties. This work was focused in the fabrication and characterization of electrospun PVDF, PVDF/PLA (50/50 wt %) and PVDF/G (99.5/0.5 wt %) membranes. Analyses of PVDF, PVDF/PLA and PVDF/G membranes were performed by scanning electron microscopy (SEM) and energy-dispersive x-ray micro-analysis. As a result, low porous flexible membranes were obtained with fiber diameters in a range from 50 nm to 700 nm. These membranes are a promising tool in fields such as biomedical engineering, robotics and electronics as scaffolds, sensors or actuators due to their ferroelectric nature.

Chapter 6 - The chapter presents the main results of recent experimental investigation of the electrodeposition and characterization of Fe/TiO_2 composite coatings obtained from an environmentally friendly methanesulfonate iron plating bath containing colloidal TiO_2 particles. The effect of plating bath composition and electrolysis conditions on the content of titania particles in coatings has been investigated. The content of the TiO_2 particles in the electrodeposited composite coatings increases with an increase in titania concentrations in the suspension electrolyte and with a decrease in the current density. The kinetics of Fe/TiO_2 composites electrochemical deposition is shown to obey the improved Guglielmi's model. The inclusion of titania particles in the iron matrix results in an increase in microhardness of electrodeposits due to dispersion strengthening effect. The electrocatalytic properties of Fe/TiO_2 composites are studied by means of voltammetry, electrochemical impedance spectroscopy (EIS) and chronoamperometry methods. Iron/titania electrodeposited composite coatings exhibit enhanced electrocatalytic activity towards hydrogen and oxygen evolution reactions (HER and OER) in an alkaline solution. The electrocatalytic activity increases with an increase in TiO_2 content in iron matrix. The kinetic parameters are calculated on the basis of Tafel plots and EIS measurements and possible mechanisms of the HER and OER are considered. The chapter also reports the performance of Fe/TiO_2 electrodeposited composite coatings as heterogeneous photocatalysts for the decomposition of some organic contaminants. Although iron electrodeposited matrix is a cheap, available, nontoxic and easily repairable support for TiO_2 photocatalysts, it is not corrosion-resisting enough. In order to improve the corrosion stability, as-deposited Fe/TiO_2 composite coatings obtained from a methanesulfonate iron plating bath are modified by cathodic treatment in a solution containing cerium (III) methanesulfonate. As a result, a very thin layer of cerium oxides is formed on the surface of Fe matrix. The corrosion resistance of iron/titania coatings after their modification by ceria film is studied by means of voltammetry and electrochemical impedance spectroscopy. The surface modification of Fe/TiO_2 composites by ceria layer results in a marked improvement in their corrosion stability which allows their application as photocatalysts for wastewater treatment. The photocatalytic properties of TiO_2 particles immobilized on Fe/TiO_2 composite electrodeposits modified by ceria layers are tested in the reaction of photochemical degradation of methyl orange and methylene blue dyes in water under the action of UV radiation.

In: Electrospinning and Electroplating
Editor: Toby Jacobs
ISBN: 978-1-53612-363-0

Chapter 1

ELECTROSPINNING OF DEGRADABLE PHAS: PROCESS, PROPERTIES, APPLICATIONS

Tatiana G. Volova[1,2,*], Dmitriy B. Goncharov[1], Elena D. Nikolaeva[1] and Ekaterina I. Shishatskaya[1,2]
[1]Institute of Biophysics of Siberian Branch of Russian Academy of Sciences, Akademgorodok, Krasnoyarsk, Russia
[2]Siberian Federal University, Krasnoyarsk, Russia

ABSTRACT

An integrated study has been performed to investigate the process of formation of ultrafine fibers and nonwoven membranes by electrospinning from natural degradable polymers – polyhydroxyalkanoates (PHAs); physical, mechanical, and biological properties of the products have been studied. Then, electrospinning was used to prepare ultrafine fibers from PHAs with different compositions: P(3HB) and its copolymers P(3HB-*co*-4HB), P(3HB-*co*-3HV), and P(3HB-*co*-3HHx). The main process parameters, that influence UF-fiber diameter and properties of fibrous non-woven membranes) (polymer concentration, solution feeding rate, working distance, and applied voltage), were investigated and their effects evaluated. This study was the first to compare biological and physical/mechanical parameters of PHAs with different chemical compositions as dependent upon the fractions of monomers, constituting the polymers and fiber orientation.

Electrospun polymer membranes, prepared from the [P(3HB-co-4HB)], were tested as wound dressings. The developed nonwoven membranes can be used as the equivalent of collagen skine dressings in the treatment of burns of degree II. Experiments on laboratory animals with model skin defects showed, that the membranes fitted the wound

* Corresponding Author: volova45@mail.ru.

shape good, protected the wound from external influences, and facilitated wound healing, promoting fast repair. The successful experiments on laboratory animals were followed by pilot clinical trials of nanomembranes, comprised of PHA membranes as wound dressings in the treatment of septic wounds. During the regeneration phase, PHA membranes served as a scaffold for the new tissue on the skin and filled out soft tissue defects. The formation of the uniform and sufficiently vascularized tissue is a prerequisite for quicker wound healing and can serve as a basis for the subsequent skin grafting and spontaneous re-epithelialization of superficial wounds. The wound dressing, tested in this clinical trial, performs important physiological functions of natural skin, provides a barrier against secondary infection, reduces fluid loss, and, at the same time, does not keep the air out.

Keywords: electrospinning, ultrafine fibers, nonwoven membranes, PHA, biological and physical/mechanical properties, scaffolds, cell proliferation, wound dressings, skin regeneration

INTRODUCTION

Electrospinning (electrostatic spinning) is a promising technique, that can be used for fabricating micro- and ultrafine fibers and fibrous scaffolds (mats) and membranes. This technique was introduced in the 20th century to fabricate synthetic fibers. Several variants of production of fibers and devices, using electrostatic force, were patented in the 1930s-1940s. "Electrospinning" has become a widely used term quite recently (1994), but theoretical underpinning of electrospinning was produced by Taylor in the 1960s (Taylor, 1969). In the electrospinning process, ultrafine fibers are formed between two oppositely charged electrodes: one is placed in a polymer solution or melt and the counter electrode is a collecting metal screen. Electrospinning is used to produce ultra- and nano-fine fibers and other porous fibers-based structures, from solutions and melts of polymers with different structures. Electrospun products have been used in various applications, such as filtration and protective apparel, tissue scaffolding and drug delivery, nanocomposites, and sensor applications. Fiber constructions, prepared from various materials by electrospinning, are promising candidates to be used as scaffolds for *in vitro* cell cultures and as medical devices for surgical reconstruction (wound dressings, barrier membranes for guided tissue regeneration in maxillofacial surgery, etc.). The process of electrospinning has been found to have great potential in cell technologies and tissue engineering. Several types of electrospinning process have been described, which are used to produce fibers and membranes from both synthetic and natural polymers such as gelatin, carboxymethyl cellulose, polyethylene oxide, polylactide, polyurethanes, polyvinyl alcohol, polytrimethyl terephthalate, dimethylformamide, etc. A number of processing parameters, such as applied voltage, polymer solution feeding rate, solution density, working distance, capillary diameter, etc., can greatly affect fiber formation and

3D-structure of non-woven. In order to be able to tailor the properties of the resulting products, one needs to determine the processing parameters for each particular type of polymer material.

Electrospinning studies, using PHAs, have not been conducted until quite recently. The first papers, reporting the employment of this technique to produce ultrafine fibers from poly-3-hydroxybutyrate and copolymers of 3-hydroxybutyrate with 3-hydroxyvalerate, were published in 2006 (Volova et al., 2006a; Tong, Wang, 2007). By now, the method has been tested to prepare electrospun products of PHA copolymers (Tong et al., 2012; Wang et al., 2012; Yu et al., 2012).

The purpose of this study was to electrospin ultrafine fibers from PHAs with different chemical composition [P(3HB) and copolymers P(3HB-*co*-4HB), P(3HB-*co*-3HV), and P(3HB-*co*-3HHx)], and compare their structures and physical-mechanical and biological properties. In the present investigation, the main focus is to construct experimental dressings from degradable PHAs, intended for skin wound repair, and evaluate their effectiveness in experiments on laboratory animals, as well as results of pilot clinical trials of ultrafine PHA fibers as wound dressings in the treatment of septic wounds.

1. Polyhydroxyalkanoates – Natural Degradable Biopolymers

Polyhydroxyalkanoates (PHAs) – biopolymers of microbial origin – have very many attractive properties that make them promising materials for various applications, including biomedical ones. PHAs have significant advantages over other biomaterials, including these, based on polylactides:

- the high biocompatibility of PHAs, poly-3-hydroxybutyrate in particular, is accounted for by the fact, that the monomers constituting this polymer – 3-hydroxybutyric acid – are natural metabolites of body cells and tissues;
- PHAs are not hydrolyzed in aqueous media, as they undergo true biological degradation, which occurs via the cellular and the humoral pathways; the resulting monomers of hydroxybutyric acid do not cause abrupt acidification of tissues and, hence, do not give rise to any pronounced inflammatory reaction;
- PHAs bioresorption rates are much slower than those of polylactides and polyglycolides; PHA-based implants can function *in vivo* for between several months and 2-3 years, depending on their form and implantation site; moreover, PHA degradation can be controlled timely;

- PHAs are produced by direct microbial fermentation; no multistage technology is needed, such as monomer synthesis, polymerization, addition of plasticizers and modifying components;
- PHAs can be synthesized from feedstocks like as saccharides, organic acids, alcohols, mixtures of CO_2 and H_2, products of plant biomass hydrolysis, industrial wastes of sugar and palm oil production, hydrogen-containing products of processing of brown coals and lignin of hydrolysis;
- PHAs constitute a family of polymers of various chemical structures, consisting of monomers, containing between 4 and 12 or more carbon units, including high-crystallinity thermoplastic materials and construction elastomers;
- PHAs properties - crystallinity, mechanical strength, temperature characteristics, and biodegradation rates, - can be controlled by varying the composition of the culture medium and tailoring the chemical structure of the polymer; and
- PHAs can be obtained and processed from various phase states (powder, solution, gel, melt), using conventional techniques.

PHAs are very promising polymers as, being thermoplastic, like polypropylene and polyethylene, they also have antioxidant and optical properties, as well as piezoelectricity. PHAs are highly biocompatible and can be biodegraded in biological media. In addition to poly-3-hydroxybutyrate (P3HB), there are various PHA copolymers, which, depending on their monomeric composition, have different basic properties - degree of crystallinity, melting point, ductility, mechanical strength, biodegradation rate, etc.

The first of the discovered polyhydroxyalkanoates (PHAs) was poly-3-hydroxybutyrate P(3HB).

However, pure poly-3-hydroxybutyrate is brittle and has a low extension to break. The lack of flexibility and thermal stability limits its range of applications. The discovery of the ability of microorganisms to synthesize PHA copolymers gave an impetus to extensive investigations of these biopolymers. It was found, that the presence of 3-hydroxyvalerate in PHA copolymers was a factor, that significantly affected material properties, decreasing its melting point and crystallinity and making it more ductile, elastic, and processable, than poly-3-hydroxybutyrate (Luizier, 1992). Variations in monomer proportions of the PHA lead to considerable changes in its thermomechanical and fibrous properties. An extensive search for microorganisms, capable of synthesizing PHA copolymers, was conducted in many countries. Rather soon, it was found, that some microorganisms under certain growth conditions were able to synthesize not only homogenous poly-3-hydroxybutyrate, but also various PHAs, containing monomer units of 3-hydroxybutyrate and other hydroxy derivatives of hydrocarbon acids. By now, over 150 various of PHAs have been described, but the PHAs that are practically produced and investigated are the homogenous poly-3-hydroxybutyrate (3HB) and copolymers of

3-hydroxybutyrate and 3-hydroxyvalerate, P(3HB/3HV), and 3-hydroxybutyrate and 3-hydroxyoctanoate, P(3HB/3HO). PHAs of different chemical composition differ in their structure and basic physicochemical properties. This line of research has attracted much attention because even a slight variation in the proportions of monomer units in a PHA can lead to a fundamental change in its properties, including thermomechanical ones, which is very important for practical purposes.

The main PHA structures are:

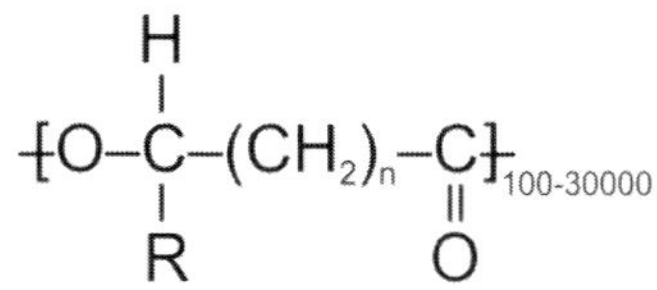

n = 1 R = hydrogen–poly(3-hydroxypropionate),
R = methyl–poly(3-hydroxybutyrate),
R = ethyl–poly(3-hydroxyvalerate),
R = propyl–poly(3-hydroxyhexanoate),
R = pentyl–poly(3-hydroxyoctanoate),
R = nonyl–poly(3-hydroxydodecanoate),
n = 2 R = hydrogen–poly(4-hydroxybutyrate),
n = 3 R = hydrogen–poly(5-hydroxyvalerate).

Most of the known hydroxyalkanoic acids have been detected as constituents of biosynthetic PHAs. Analysis of the diversity of polyhydroxyalkanoates showed, that biosynthetic polymers contain Has, exhibiting the R-configuration, but no HAs exhibiting the L-configuration. PHAs can be divided into three groups, depending on the number of carbon atoms in the monomer units:

1) short-chain-length (SCL) PHAs, which consist of 3–5 carbon atoms;
2) medium-chain-length (MCL) PHAs, which consist of 6–14 carbon atoms; and
3) long-chain-length (LCL) PHAs, which consist of 17 and 18 carbon atoms.

The best-known representative of short-chain-length PHAs is poly-(R)-3-hydroxybutyrate, P3HB. Short-chain-length PHAs consist of poly-(R)-hydroxyalkanoates, containing 3 to 5 carbon units. Medium-chain-length PHAs consist of aliphatic (R)-monomers of hydroxy acids, containing 6 to 14 carbon units. They are synthesized when the PHA producing strain is cultivated on the medium containing n-alkanoates or their precursors. Long-chain-length PHAs consist of more than 14 carbon atoms. This division of polymers into groups was based on the notion of high substrate specificity of PHA synthases, which were supposed to be able to accept only certain hydroxyalkanoic acids in the course of intracellular polymerization of monomers into PHAs.

PHAs that contain a single type of repeat unit, are known as homopolymers, while PHAs, containing a mixture of repeat units are known as copolymers (Olivera et al., 2001 a, b; Luengo et al., 2003). PHA characteristics, including physical and mechanical properties, are determined by the molar fractions of monomers in the polymer. The properties of PHA homopolymers are significantly different from those of PHA copolymers (Chen et al., 2006; Laycock et al., 2013). Short-chain-length PHAs are thermoplastics that have a high degree of crystallinity; they are rigid and brittle crystalline materials, that have low elongation-to-break. Medium-chain-length PHAs are elastomers with low crystallinity and a low melting point (Lenz and Marchessault, 2005).

PHAs are synthesized by microorganisms from various carbon sources. The cost of the carbon source contributes significantly to the overall production cost of a PHA. Thus, one of the main objectives of PHA investigations is to find inexpensive substrates for PHA production. This objective can be attained by finding new substrates for the already known PHA-producing organisms, discovering new PHA-producing strains, and engineering recombinant strains, which can utilize various substrates, including new ones. In principle, PHAs can be produced on various substrates. Among the best known, ones are individual compounds, such as carbon dioxide and hydrogen, saccharides, alcohols, and organic acids; byproducts of alcohol, sugar, and hydrolysis industries of olive and palm oil production; and unusual substrates, including toxic ones.

The choice of the substrate used for PHA production is determined by physiological-biochemical properties of PHA-producing microorganisms, economic efficiency of the production strategy, and the field of application of the ready produce.

Since PHAs can be used in medicine, pharmacology, food industry, agriculture, and municipal engineering, the scale of their production may vary from dozens of kilograms (for medical and pharmacological applications) to several thousand tons per year. The quality and cost of the substrates for different production scales and applications may vary, too.

A virtually inexhaustible supply of feedstocks for large-scale PHA production can be provided by plant biomass generated in great quantities every year. Residues of agricultural crops, contain polysaccharides of various structures and compositions; they can be hydrolyzed to yield a wide range of water-soluble sugars, including maize and soy hydrolysates, cotton plant vegetative biomass hydrolysates, etc. High cell concentrations and PHA yields can be obtained by growing various bacterial species on hydrolyzed hemicellulose, containing xylose.

Polyhydroxyalkanoates can be used to fabricate specialized products by various methods (Amass et al., 1998; Sudesh et al., 2000; and others). PHA properties vary depending on the structure of the lateral groups in the polymer chain and the distance between ester groups in a molecule. The linear structure of PHA molecules makes them thermoplastic. Furthermore, these polymers also have antioxidant and optical properties as well as piezoelectricity. PHAs are highly biocompatible and can be biodegraded in biological media. The combination of properties of PHAs makes them promising materials for various applications. This class of polymers can be used to produce materials with different physical and mechanical properties – from hard thermoplastics to construction elastomers.

One of the most important macroscopic parameters, characterizing polymer properties is molecular weight, which determines the processability of the material. PHA molecular weight is a variable parameter, depending on a number of factors, including the source of carbon nutrition for bacteria, the length of cultivation, and the method of polymer recovery. The molecular weights of PHAs differ considerably; for instance, the weight average molecular weight may vary from several hundred to several million Da.

Thermal properties of P(3HB) and its ability to crystallize in the native state are its most important parameters because they determine the processability of the polymer. PHAs, like many other polymers, have a heat distortion temperature somewhat lower, than the thermal degradation temperature. Thus, polymers cannot exist in the gaseous state, and the main type of phase equilibrium in them is a condensed state – crystalline, glassy, viscoelastic, and liquid. The ability of PHAs to crystallize is determined by the inner properties of its chains and is characterized by crystallization temperature, T_c. In a number of polymers, including PHAs, crystallization develops only partly for various reasons, and most of the polymers are semi-crystalline materials. The degree of crystallinity of PHAs with different structure can vary widely, between 10–20 and 70–80%, and this parameter can be controlled by changing the chemical composition of the polymers, produced under different conditions of cultivation of PHA-producing bacterial strains and different carbon nutrition conditions (Volova, Shishatskaya, 2011; Volova, Shishatskaya, Sinskey, 2013; Laucock et al., 2013).

P(3HB) is a homopolymer of D(-)-3-β-hydroxybutyric acid, an isotactic polyester with regular ($C_4H_6O_2$) units. The melting temperature of P(3HB) varies between 160 and 185°C, and the T_m proper is 176–182°C. The thermal decomposition temperature of P(3HB) lies within the range between 275 and 280°C. After reheating, the melting temperature of P(3HB) decreases, while its crystallization temperature remains unchanged. The pronounced difference between the melting point and the temperature for the onset of degradation is an essential processing property of the polymer, enabling fabrication of films, filaments, hollow constructs, etc. by conventional methods of polymer processing - solution casting, extrusion, and injection molding. The degree of crystallinity of different P(3HB) samples is only slightly influenced by the conditions of polymer production, ranging between 70 and 80% (Madison and Huisman, 1999; Volova et al., 2000; Laucock et al., 2013). A disadvantage of P(3HB) is that it cannot be strain-crystallized, and, thus, it is very difficult to process. The resulting products show low impact strength and hardness and are prone to ageing during the long-term storage.

The physicochemical properties of PHA copolymers are more diverse, and, thus, they show greater promise. However, production of PHA copolymers is a very complicated technological task, and it cannot be achieved without fundamental knowledge of the structural-functional organization of the PHA cellular cycle and the relationship between the physicochemical properties of these polymers and their chemical composition.

The T_m and T_d of PHA copolymers are lower, than those of P(3HB). The melting temperature of 3-hydroxybutyrate/3-hydroxyvalerate copolymers is lower, than the melting peak of homogeneous P3HB, and this difference increases with an increase in the 3HV molar fraction. The melting and thermal decomposition temperatures of the copolymers, consisting of 3-hydroxyhexanoate and 4-hydroxybutyrate monomer units, are also lower, than those of P(3HB). The low crystallization temperature of the homogeneous P(3HB) pose an obstacle to melt processing of this polymer. A possible way to increase the crystallization temperature of PHA, is to synthesize 3HB copolymers, tailored with 3HV and other monomers. The decrease in the melting temperatures and thermal decomposition temperatures of PHA copolymers does not reduce the difference between these parameters. Thus, different types of PHA copolymers retain their significant property – thermoplasticity.

The degrees of crystallinity of P(3HB/3HV)s are lower, than that of P(3HB). The incorporation of 3HV monomers into the 3HB chain decreases the degree of crystallinity of P(3HB/3HV) copolymers. P(3HB/3HV) copolymers exhibit isodimorphism due to co-crystallization of the 3HB and 3HV units. Incorporation of 3HV into the 3HB polymer chain considerably influences the kinetics of polymer crystallization, including the rate of the process and the size of the spherulites. The degree of crystallinity of these copolymers is linearly related to the molar fraction of 3HV only in the specimens containing up to 25-35 mol.% 3HV. Specimens with higher 3HV molar fractions (over 35–40 mol.%) showed the degree of crystallinity of about 50%. This is similar to the C_x of the copolymers containing lower 3HV molar fractions. This may be ascribed to a change in the crystal lattice that occurs when the 3HB to 3HV ratio is changed. At less than 35–40 mol.% 3HV, 3HV units can crystallize in the 3HB lattice and at greater than 40 mol.% 3HV, 3HB units can crystallize in the 3HV lattice. In specimens with 3HV as the major fraction, 3HB and 3HV units co-crystallize in one lattice, and this does not seem to influence the degree of crystallinity of P(3HB/3HV), in spite of an increase in the 3HV molar fraction.

Similar changes in C_x are observed in 3-hydroxybutyrate/3-hydroxyhexanoate P(3HB/3HHx) copolymers. Incorporation of 3HHx, similarly to 3HV in P(3HB/3HV), reduces the difference between the percentages of the amorphous and crystalline phases. As the 3HHx molar fraction is increased from 2.5% to 40–60%, the degree of crystallinity of the copolymer steadily decreases to 20–40%. Another PHA type – 3-hydroxybutyrate/4-hydroxybutyrate P(3HB/4HB) copolymers are highly elastic polymers, with elongation at break, reaching 1000%, which is two orders of magnitude higher than the corresponding parameter of P(3HB). The incorporation of 4HB influences considerably (to a greater extent than the incorporation of 3HV or 3HHx the ratio of crystalline to amorphous phase in the copolymer, significantly decreasing its crystallinity. P(3HB/4HB) copolymers with crystallinity degrees decreased to 10–12% have been described by some authors (Laucock et al., 2013; Volova et al., 2013; 2014 a,b).

Table 1. Companies engaged in scaling-up laboratory processes and establishing PHA production facilities (adapted from Chen, 2009; Ienczak et al., 2013; Kaur and Roy, 2015)

Company	Types of PHA	Production scale (tons/year)	Application
«ICI» (U.K.)	P(3HB/3HV)	300	Packaging
«Chemie Linz» (Austria)	P(3HB)	20–100	Packaging, drug delivery
«Biomers» (Germany)	P(3HB)	Unknown	Packaging, drug delivery
«BASF» (Germany)	P(3HB), P(3HB/3HV)	Pilot scale	Blending with Ecoflex
«Metabolix» (U.S.)	Several PHAs	Industrial scale	Packaging
«Tepha» (U.S.)	Several PHAs	Several hundred kg	Medical applications
«ADM» (U.S.) (with Metabolix)	Several PHAs	50 000	Feedstock
«P&G» (U.S.)	Several PHAs	Contract manufacture	Packaging
«Monsanto» (U.S.)	P(3HB), P(3HB/3HV)	Industrial production of PHAs	Feedstock
«Meredian» (U.S.)	Several PHAs	10 000	Feedstock
«Mitsubishi» (Japan	P(3HB)	10	Packaging
«Biocycles» (Brasil)	P(3HB)	100	Feedstock
«Bio-On» (Italy)	PHA	10 000	Feedstock
«Zhejiang Tian An» (China)	P(3HB/3HV)	2 000	Feedstock
«Yikeman, Shandon» (China)	PHA	3 000	Feedstock
«Shantou Lianyl Biotech» (China)	Several PHAs	Pilot scale	Packaging and medical applications
«Tianjing Green Bio-Science» (China)	P(3HB/4HB)	10 000	Feedstock and packaging
«Bioplast» (Russia)	P(3HB), P(3HB/4HB), P(3HB/3HV)	Pilot scale	Feedstock, experimental devices

Many companies have been engaged in commercialization of PHA production technologies. Since the 1980s, they have been producing PHAs on a pilot scale or industrially (Table 1). The best-known companies and corporations that have been engaged in PHA activities are: Monsanto Co., Metabolix Inc., Procter & Gamble, Berlin Packaging Corp., Bioscience Ltd., BioVentures Alberta Inc., and Merk, which produce polymers with the trademarks Biopol®, Biopol™, TephaFLEX™, DegraPol/btc®, Nodax ™, etc.

As mentioned previously, polyhydroxyalkanoates have physicochemical properties, similar to those of some synthetic polymers, such as polypropylene, which are produced in large quantities and cannot be degraded in the environment. At the present time, the use of PHAs is limited by their rather high cost, but the range of their applications is wide. The growing environmental concern on the one hand, and the possibility of reducing the cost of biopolymers by increasing the production efficiency, on the other, make polyhydroxyalkanoates promising materials of the 21st century.

There are two possible ways to increase production and broaden applications of PHAs. One way is to develop large-scale PHA production, i.e., to increase PHA outputs and reduce their cost by manufacturing inexpensive items such as packaging materials, everyday articles, films and pots for agriculture, etc. Researchers in the U.S., Japan, Europe, India, Malaysia are conducting extensive studies of PHAs for a variety of applications. They are mostly used to manufacture packaging items and garbage containers, food and cosmetic containers, and agricultural items (Plastics from Bacteria, 2010). These are extruded vials, jars, bottles, containers, and boxes for shampoos, lotions, etc. PHAs were initially used to make everyday articles such as shampoo bottles and packaging materials by Wella AG in Germany (Weiner, 1997). Short-chain-length PHAs are used to fabricate packaging films, shopping bags, containers and paper coatings, everyday use items, like as housings for TV sets and computers, toys, sports equipment, disposable dishes, hygiene products, and many others, by Biomers and Metabolix, and several other companies (Clarinval and Halleux, 2005; Noda, 2005).

Another way in industry of PHAs is to establish small-scale facilities for the production of high-cost specialized items. This type of biopolymers is demonstrate the greatest potential in medicine and pharmaceutics. The mild immune response to the PHA implants and the sufficient duration of PHA degradation in biological media make these polymers attractive candidates for use as drug carriers in controlled-release drug delivery systems, implants and grafts for tissue and organ regeneration, materials for tissue engineering and designing of bioartificial organs (Volova et al., 2003; Volova, Shishatskaya, 2011; Pouton, 2001; Williams, Martin, 1999; Sudesh, 2004; Sudesh et al., 2000; 2007; Volova, 2004; Volova, Shishatskaya, Sinskey, 2013; Polyhydroxyalkanoates (PHAs): Biosynthesis, Industrial Production, and Applications in Medicine, 2014; Luef et al., 2015).

Press releases of such well-known companies, as Tepha Inc., Metabolix, Procter & Gamble, and Monsanto suggest growing interest in PHAs and intensive research aimed at production, modification, and investigation of PHAs for cardiovascular surgery, dentistry, orthopedics, and pharmacology. Although PHAs are attracting more and more attention, there are rather few results of biomedical studies reported in the literature, as can be inferred from the analysis of biomedical studies of novel biomaterials, including PHAs, that are available in the major databases. Many aspects of PHA biotechnology and material science remain unclear. Among them are production of high-purity PHAs and processes, used to fabricate various PHA-based special biomedical items. Kinetics and mechanisms of PHA *in vivo* biodegradation need to be better understood. More studies should be performed to gain insight into mechanisms of *in vivo* interaction of PHA devices with cells and tissues and their medical and technical parameters in living organisms. The Food and Drug Administration (FDA) in the U.S. has approved the use of several products, manufactured by Tepha Inc., in clinical trials. These are suture material, mesh grafts, and films for uroplastic surgery.

Analysis of available literature suggests, that PHAs have been extensively studied as materials for cardiovascular surgery. These polymers are proposed as candidates for fabricating of vascular grafts and coatings for synthetic grafts (Marois et al., 1999 a, b; 2000). Perhaps the most remarkable results with PHA polymers have been obtained in the development of cell-seeded tissue-engineered heart valves. Stock et al. (2000) successfully replaced the polyglycolide-polylactide valves in animals with poly-3-hydroxyoctanoate (P3HO) pulmonary conduits. Porous scaffolds prepared from elastic poly-3-hydroxyoctanoate were used to fabricate heart valves (Sodian et al., 1999; 2000). For 8 days, the cells proliferated and filled the pores; they also synthesized collagen and generated connective tissue between the outer and inner surfaces of the scaffold. Constructs of porous P(3HO/3HHx) were seeded with cells of vascular tissue and evaluated under pulsatile flow *in vitro* (Sodian et al., 1999).

One of the most advanced applications of PHA polymers in cardiovascular products has been the development of a regenerative PHA patch that can be used to close the pericardium after heart surgery, without formation of adhesions between the heart and sternum (Malm et al., 1992; 1994; Martin, Williams, 2003). Researchers of the Department of Thoracic and Cardiovascular Surgery at the University Hospital in Uppsala, Sweden, examined P(3HB) patches used as pericardial substitutes (Duvernoy et al., 1995). The patch was gradually degraded and replaced by native tissues strong enough to prevent the development of postoperative adhesions between the patch and the cardiac surface.

There are very few data on using PHAs to enhance biocompatibility of vascular stents. Unverdorben et al. (2002) tried to use poly-3-hydroxybutyrate stents in experiments on rabbits, but the experiment was not quite successful. Tephas' researchers together with their German colleagues (Institute of Biomedical Engineering, Rostock) have tested polymer stents prepared from poly(tetrafluoroethane) and a blend of polylactide/poly-3-hydroxybutyrate (Grabow et al., 2007), comparing them with metallic stents. For the stents, to withstand the pressure in vessels, they were rather bulky. This caused adverse response of the vessel wall, exhibited as neointima growth and stronger inflammatory reaction, than that, caused by metallic stents.

PHA solutions can be used to prepare fibers. In one of the first studies of PHA fibers, Miller and Williams proved, that P(3HB/3HV) monofilaments are not biodegraded *in vitro* and *in vivo* (Miller, Williams, 1987). Tepha (U.S.) has developed suture material based on P(3HB/4HB). The filaments are melt-spun in a single-screw extruder by passing the material through 4 zones of the extruder, with temperatures 140, 190, 200, and 205°C, and multistage orientation (Martin et al., 2000). The extrusion process and subsequent orientation yield filaments with tensile strength over 126 MPa, which retain their properties for long periods of time. Having conducted all necessary tests, Tepha received the permission of FDA and marketed mono- and poly-filament fibers, meshes, and films under the trademark of TephaFLEX®.

PHAs are attractive materials for use in surgical reconstruction of bone tissues also. There are data on preparation of mechanically strong PHA/HA composites, proving that incorporation of HA into a PHA enhances polymer strength.

In recent years, much research effort has been devoted to the use of PHAs as matrices for drug delivery and as scaffolds for cell cultures intended to fabricate grafts for tissue engineering applications. In Russia, biomedical studies of polyhydroxyalkanoates and experimental prototypes of PHA products were initiated by the researchers of the Institute of Biophysics SB RAS and the Siberian Federal University, united in Research-and-Education Center "Yenisei". In cooperation with the Institute of Transplant Surgery and Artificial Organs (currently the V.I. Shumakov Federal Research of Transplant Surgery and Artificial Organs Center), the research team studied films of poly-3-hydroxybutyrate and P(3HB/3HV) copolymers and proved, that they did not produce any cytotoxic effect when contacting directly with the cultured cells and when implanted as sutures *in vivo*; high-purity specimens were suitable for contact with blood. Since then, the research team has considerably widened the scope of studies by synthesizing of PHAs with different chemical compositions and by designing and studying experimental films, barrier membranes, granules, filling materials, electrospunned ultrafine fibers, solid and porous 3D implants for bone defect repair, tubular biliary stents, mesh implants, modified by PHA-coating, microparticles for drug delivery, etc. In cooperation with the V.F. Voino-Yasenetsky Krasnoyarsk Federal Medical University, the research team has conducted pioneering clinical trials. Results have been covered by several Russian patents, reported in papers published in peer-reviewed Russian and international journals, summarized in books and reviews (Shishatsky, Shishatskaya, 2010; Volova, Shishatskaya, 2011; Volova, 2004; Volova, Shishatskaya, Sinskey, 2013).

2. Potentials of Polyhydroxyalkanoates as Spinning Materials for Cell Scaffolds in Tissue Engineering

Tissue engineering is intended to construct, outside the organism, living functional components that can be used to regenerate damaged tissues and/or organs. The task of tissue engineering is to provide constructions that would restore, maintain, or improve the function of damaged organs and tissues. Materials used in tissue engineering, TE, must have definite properties and make the tissue-engineered constructs (grafts) similar to living tissues. These constructs must be able to 1) regenerate themselves; 2) provide blood supply and 3) change their structure and properties in response to the effects of outer factors, including mechanical stress. The lifetime of implants is limited, and, thus, their main function is not only to replace the damaged tissue, but also to facilitate its regeneration (Hench, Jones, 2005). The approach to produce bioactive implants and bio-artificial organs is consists of following steps: 1) fabrication of TE-scaffolds for culturing the patient's autologous cells or cells, obtained from the cell bank; 2) culturing of cells and *in vitro* tissue formation; and 3) implantation of the resulting bioconstructs to the recipient organism. To induce tissue generation at the implantation site, initial cell concentration must be very high (10^7–10^8 cells). As introduction of cell suspension is insufficiently effective, so appropriate carrier materials for the delivery of cells are need to be found. The most important step in the use of pre-cultured cells is the transplantation of these cells to the defect body site. The success of this step depends on the proportion of cells that reach the defect site, their adhesion to the carrier, and their functional activity. One of the most difficult problems is the choice of an appropriate carriers to sertain type of cell, because cells need to stay attached to the carrier for a certain period of time.

The most widely-used scaffolds for today are membranes, films, and meshes. The flat surface of films is an appropriate substrate for the *in vitro* cell cultures. These systems are simple to prepare and to use.

Surface properties and porosity of TE-scaffolds are important for cell attachment and proliferation. Among promising approaches of the preparing of ultrafine fibers, membranes, and micro- and nano-particles, as models of cell scaffolds, are nanotechnological methods, such as nano- and microencapsulation and electrospinning. Depending on the polymer molecular weight, its solution density, and fabrication conditions, the resulting fibers may be of different diameters, and non-woven may have structures. Thus, construction of scaffolds for tissue engineering has received great attention lately, and perfect scaffolds may be designed in the nearest future.

There are several approaches for the application of cell technologies to tissue repair. One of them is to introduce cell suspension of the required phenotype and definite concentration, grown *in vitro,* into the damaged tissues, or into the bloodstream. Another, which is more complex technologically, approach, is to grow cells *in vitro*, on scaffold, and then to implant the resulting bioengineered construct (or the new tissue) to the recipient organism. Successful implementation of this approach much depends on the properties of cell scaffolds selected (Wang, 2003; Hench, Jones, 2005).

The main advantage of PHAs is that they can contain monomer units with different carbon chain lengths. PHA copolymers are more promising materials, as their properties can vary within a fairly broad range, depending upon the proportions of different monomer units contained in them (Sudesh et al., 2000; Volova, 2004; Laucock et al., 2013).

The structure and functional properties of cell scaffolds and other biomedical polymer devices are considerably influenced by the basic properties of the material they have been made of. Studies of PHAs as a materials for cell scaffolds mainly address to two types of PHA – homogenous P3HB and copolymers of 3-hydroxybutyrate and 3-hydroxyvalerate. The available literature data regarding other PHA types are scant and contradictory.

A number of processing parameters, such as an applied voltage, polymer solution feeding rate, solution density, working distance, capillary diameter, etc., can greatly influence fiber formation and structure of mats. In order to be able to tailor the properties of the resulting products, one needs to determine the processing parameters for each particular type of polymer material (Volova et al., 2006a; Goncharov et al., 2012; Volova et al., 2014 b). A number of studies described electrospinning of nonwoven PHA membranes and reported their structure, physical, mechanical, and biological properties, as related to electrospinning parameters and polymer composition. Ultrafine fibers in our research were electrospun from PHA solutions, using a Nanon 01A automatic set-up (MECC Inc., Japan). In our work we used polymers, synthesized in the Institute of Biophysics SB RAS. *Ralstonia eutropha* B5786 and B8562 and *Cupriavidus eutrophus* B10646, hydrogen-oxidizing bacterial strains, were used as PHA producers. The strains were grown under different conditions of carbon nutrition, which had been developed previously, and this enabled production of PHAs with different chemical compositions. Chloroform solutions with polymer concentrations, varied from 1 to 10 wt %, were prepared from all types of PHAs. Solution was poured into a plastic syringe, with 13 mm inside diameter, the syringe was fixed horizontally in the set-up, the solution feeding rate was varied from 4 to 8 ml/h, the applied voltage was from 15 to 30 kV, and the working distance was from 11 to 15 cm. Randomly oriented or aligned ultrafine fibers were collected on a flat steel plate or a rotating drum (at 1000 rpm), respectively; both collectors were covered with aluminum foil, to collect ultrafine fibers more effectively.

The effect of the density of polymer solutions to fiber properties was studied using the homopolymer of 3-hydroxybutyric acid, in order to avoid the influence of the chemical composition of the PHA on the electrospinning process and properties of the products. P(3HB) chloroform solutions with polymer concentration varied from 1 to 10 wt. % were used. The process parameters were as follows: needle diameter – 1 mm, applied voltage – 30 kV, solution feeding rate – 5 ml/h, and working distance – 15 cm, a flat steel collection plate. Polymer concentration directly influences the quality of electrospun fibers. Polymer solutions of the density under 2 wt. % could not yield high-quality fibers, due to their low viscosity (below 100 cP). These solutions yielded a few very thin ultrafine fibers and fine spray, which consisted of microdrops rather uniformly distributed on the collector. As P(3HB) concentrations increased, the solution viscosities increased too (from 60 to 800 cP), because the entanglement of polymer molecular chains prevented the breakup of the electrically driven jet and allowed the electrostatic stresses to further elongate the jet.

Stable electrospinning of ultrafine fibers in the Nanon 01A set-up was attained from P(3HB) solutions with polymer concentrations between 2 and 8 wt. % (solution viscosity 200–800 cP). Polymer concentration significantly influenced the diameter of the ultrafine fibers. Within the study range of polymer concentrations, the diameter of the ultrafine fibers was linearly related to the solution density. The viscosity of the solutions with polymer concentrations above 8 wt.% was too high (about 1000 cP) to allow successful formation of ultrafine fibers. Figure 1 shows SEM images of electrospun P(3HB) ultrafine fibers prepared from the polymer/chloroform solutions with different polymer concentrations. Most of the fibers were cylindrical and smooth; their surface was virtually defect-free; there were spaces between the fibers. As polymer concentration of the solution was increased, the range of fiber diameters became wider (between 1 μm and 3 μm). As the fiber diameter increased, spaces between fibers in the fibrous mat widened from about 2 to about 10 μm and the thickness of the mats increased too (from 10 to 75 μm). P(3HB) concentrations of the solution ranging between 2 and 8 wt.% yielded good-quality fibers. However, some of the fibers produced by electrospinning from solutions with P(3HB) concentration of 8 wt.% fused together at several points (Figure 1d), probably because of the presence of residual solvent in larger-diameter fibers.

Polymer solution concentration varied the diameter of ultrafine fibers, which were between 0.45 and 3.14 μm (Figure 1a). Within the study range of polymer concentration, the diameter of the fibers was linearly related to the solution density. As the fiber diameter increased, spaces between fibers in the mats increased from about 2 to about 10 μm, and the thickness of the mats increased also, from 0.010 to 0.075 μm.

The diameter of the fibers significantly influenced physical/mechanical properties of nonwoven membranes, comprised of them (Table 2). As fiber diameter increased from 0.45 to 3.14 μm, the membranes became more elastic, which was expressed as a considerable increase in elongation to break (from 4.5 to 10.6%), but less mechanically strong, with tensile strength, decreasing from 23.16 to 6.65 MPa and Young's modulus from 1.16 to 0.3 GPa. Young's modulus of the specimens electrospun from P(3HB) (0.3–1.16 GPa) was comparable to those of polyethylene (0.2 GPa) and polypropylene (1.5–2.0 GPa) (Table 2). The mechanical properties of the nonwoven membranes were similar to the mechanical properties of human tendons (Young's modulus 0.06 GPa) and skin (Young's modulus 15-150 MPa, tension stress 5–30 MPa) (Ying et al., 2008). Thus, we got a promising material for applications in engineering of soft tissues. The effect of the polymer solution feeding rate on the properties of the fibers was studied by varying this parameter between 2 and 8 ml/h. At the solution feeding rate below 2 ml/h, the jet was unstable; when the solution feeding rate reached 8 ml/h, polymer junctions were sufficiently formed.

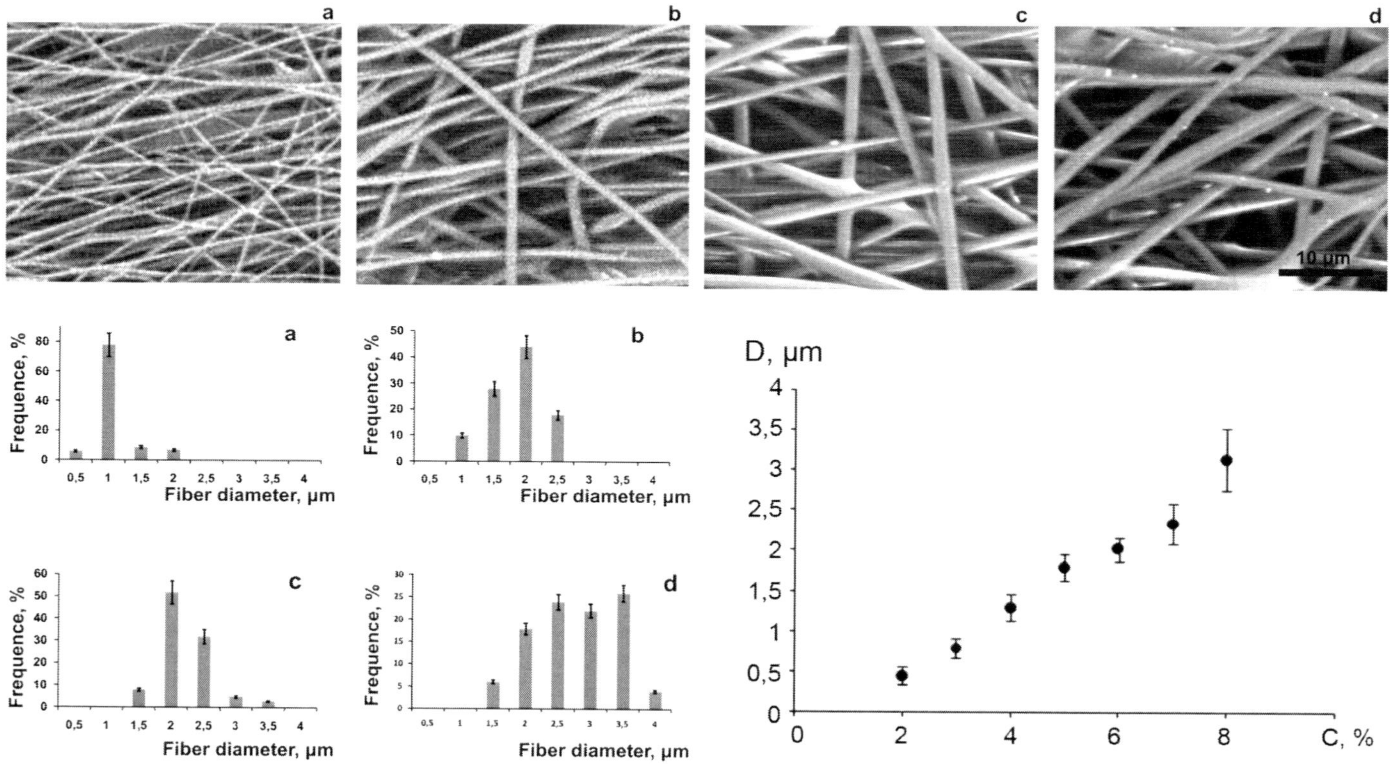

Figure 1. SEM images of nonwoven membranes (A) and diameter of ultrafine fibers (B) prepared by electrospinning from P(3HB) solutions of different concentrations (2, 4, 6, and 8 wt.%) (Goncharov et al., 2012).

Effects of changing of applied voltages from 15 to 30 kV on fiber morphology and diameter are shown in Figure 2. Other electrospinning parameters were maintained constant: needle diameter 1 mm, concentration of polymer solution 5 wt.%, solution feeding rate 5 ml/h, working distance 15 cm. Good fiber morphology was achieved at the voltage ranging between 15 and 30 kV. Within this voltage range, the average fiber diameter changed from 1.25 to 2.5 мm. At voltages below 10–12 kV, no fiber formation occurred, whatever the polymer concentration used.

Table 2. The effect of the density of P(3HB) chloroform solution on physical-mechanical properties of ultrafine fibers (Goncharov et al., 2012)

Polymer concentrations, % (w/w)	Thickness of membranes, μm	Fiber diameter, μm	Young's modulus E, MPa	Tensile strength σ, MPa	Elongation to break ε, %
2	0.010	0.45 ± 0.10	1160.22 ± 60.61	23.16 ± 0.74	4.5 ± 1.8
3	0.023	0.79 ± 0.12	709.21 ± 179.74	13.39 ± 1.48	5.78 ± 1.1
4	0.030	1.29 ± 0.16	623.41 ± 59.73	11.35 ± 0.60	6.9 ± 3.7
5	0.036	1.8 ± 0.17	540.85 ± 32.60	10.18 ± 0.33	9.9 ± 1.3
6	0.050	2.02 ± 0.15	421.05 ± 46.42	8.43 ± 0.48	10.3 ± 2.5
7	0.070	2.34 ± 0.24	344.82 ± 44.88	6.77 ± 0.83	10.5 ± 0.6
8	0.075	3.14 ± 0.38	329.18 ± 110.13	6.65 ± 2.37	10.6 ± 0.7

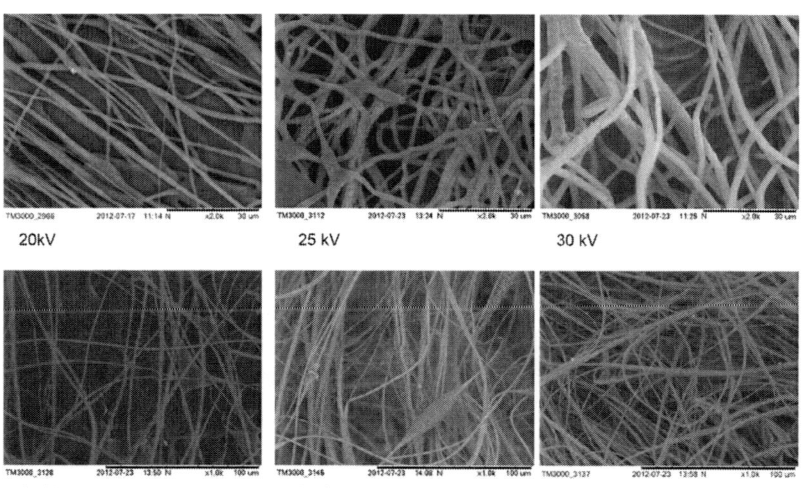

Figure 2. SEM images of nanofibers, electrospun from P(3HB) solutions under varied applied voltage (20–30 kV) and solution feeding rate (4–8 ml/h) (T. Volova's data).

Table 3. Surface properties of nonwoven membranes comprised of ultrafine fibers with different diameters electrospun from P(3HB) solutions (T. Volova's data)

Fiber diameter, μm	Water contact angle, θ °	Surface tension, γ, erg/cm^2	Interfacial free energy, γ_{SL}, erg/cm^2	Cohesive force, W_{SL}, erg/cm^2
0.45 ± 0.10	51.20 ± 1.06	68.54	2.54	118.42
0.79 ± 0.12	52.23 ± 0.70	68.88	2.73	117.39
1.29 ± 0.16	56.57 ± 1.50	70.27	3.67	112.91
1.8 ± 0.17	63.23 ± 0.75	72.25	5.50	105.59
2.02 ± 0.15	66.97 ± 1.23	73.30	6.74	101.28
2.34 ± 0.24	68.23 ± 0.31	73.64	7.20	99.80
3.14 ± 0.38	68.80 ± 0.26	73.79	7.42	99.13

Surface properties of nonwoven membranes comprised of ultrafine fibers of different diameters, electrospun from P(3HB) solutions of different concentrations, are listed in Table 3. Membranes, consisting of the smallest-diameter fibers (0.45–1.29 μm), had the lowest values of the water contact angle (51.20–56.57°).

The surface properties, such as surface tension (γ_S) and interfacial free energy (γ_{SL}), calculated using de Gennes equations, had the lowest values at the highest cohesive force (W_{SL}). As fiber diameter increased above 1.8 μm, the water contact angle increased. It was marked, that than the membranes became more porous, as fiber diameter increased. The finest, 0.45-μm diameter, fibers, showed the lowest porosity levels, about 43.5%. The porosity levels of the membranes, formed by the fibers of diameters between 0.79 and 3.14 μm, were similar to each other, but they were higher, than those of the mats, formed by the finest fibers (within the range of 62–65%).

Adhesive properties of the electrospun membranes comprised of ultrafine fibers of various diameters, were studied in the culture of NIH 3T3 mouse fibroblast cells (Figure 3). All membranes, regardless of the fiber diameter, showed good properties as cell scaffolds. DAPI staining did not show significant differences in the number of attached cells between the membranes consisting of the fibers prepared from 2 to 7% P(3HB) solutions and the control. On the membranes, prepared from the densest polymer solution and comprised by the fibers of the largest diameter, cell proliferation was considerably slower, than on other scaffolds; the membrane had defects in the form of junctions. One of the indications of the functionality of cell scaffolds is the ability of cells to synthesize an extracellular matrix proteins. SEM images of cells, obtained at Day 7 of the culture, showed formation of intercellular substance on all types of membranes, and the greatest deposits were observed on the membranes prepared from the 2–5% solutions, with fiber diameter between 0.45 and 1.8 μm, which was indicative of the high metabolic activity of fibroblasts. At Day 7, the greatest amounts of intercellular substance were observed on the membranes, consisting of the fibers between 0.45 and 1.8 μm in diameter. On the membranes, prepared from denser P(3HB) solutions (6–7%), which consisted of the fibers between 2.02 and 3.14 μm in diameter, proteins were aligned along the fibers, and the deposits were smaller. On the membranes, prepared from the densest polymer solutions, the number of cells was lower, almost by a factor of 2; no extracellular matrix proteins were detected.

Results of MTT assay of fibroblast cell viability are shown in Figure 4.

The fiber diameter and the thickness of the membrane, prepared from P(3HB) solutions of different concentrations (2–7%), did not significantly influence the physiological activity of fibroblasts. In 24 h after cell seeding, the number of cells on the membranes, prepared from the densest polymer solution, was comparable to the number of cells in the control on polystyrene. On other membranes, the number of cells was greater, than on polystyrene, almost by a factor of 2. The same results were observed in 3 days after seeding. Thus, all membranes, comprised of ultrafine fibers prepared from P(3HB) solutions, facilitated fibroblast cell proliferation. Membranes, consisting of the finer fibers, were better as a cell scaffolds, but they had poorer mechanical properties.

It is well-known, that the structure and properties of polymer products are determined both by the technique employed to fabricate them and by the properties of the material. Volova et al. (2014b) reported a study of the properties of membranes, prepared by electrospinning from four PHA types, which differed in their physicochemical properties, by using of different types of collectors.

Four types of PHAs were studied: a homopolymer of 3-hydroxybutyric acid [P(3HB)]; copolymers of 3-hydroxybutyric acid and 4-hydroxybutyric acid [P(3HB-*co*-4HB)]; copolymers of 3-hydroxybutyric acid and 3-hydroxyvaleric acid [P(3HB-*co*-3HV)]; and copolymers of 3-hydroxybutyric acid and 3-hydroxyhexanoic acid [P(3HB-*co*-3HHx)]. P(3HB-*co*-3HV) was extracted from bacterial biomass with chloroform and precipitated in hexane.

Ultrafine fibers were electrospun in the same conditions, as described earlier. We prepared ultrafine fibers using PHAs with different chemical structures. Two types of collectors were used: a flat plate, used for the formation of randomly oriented fibers, and a rotating drum (at 1000 rpm), for the formation of aligned fibers. High-quality randomly oriented ultrafine fibers were formed on the flat plate from solutions of all types of PHAs used (Figure 5A). Some of the aligned fibers (from solutions of P(3HB) and P(3HB-*co*-3HV) with 9.8 mol.% HV, which were collected on a rotating drum, had slight defects in the form of junctions (Figure 5B). In spite of that, fibrous mats, comprised of ultrafine fibers, electrospun from PHAs of different chemical compositions, were suitable for investigating of their surface structure and physical-mechanical properties.

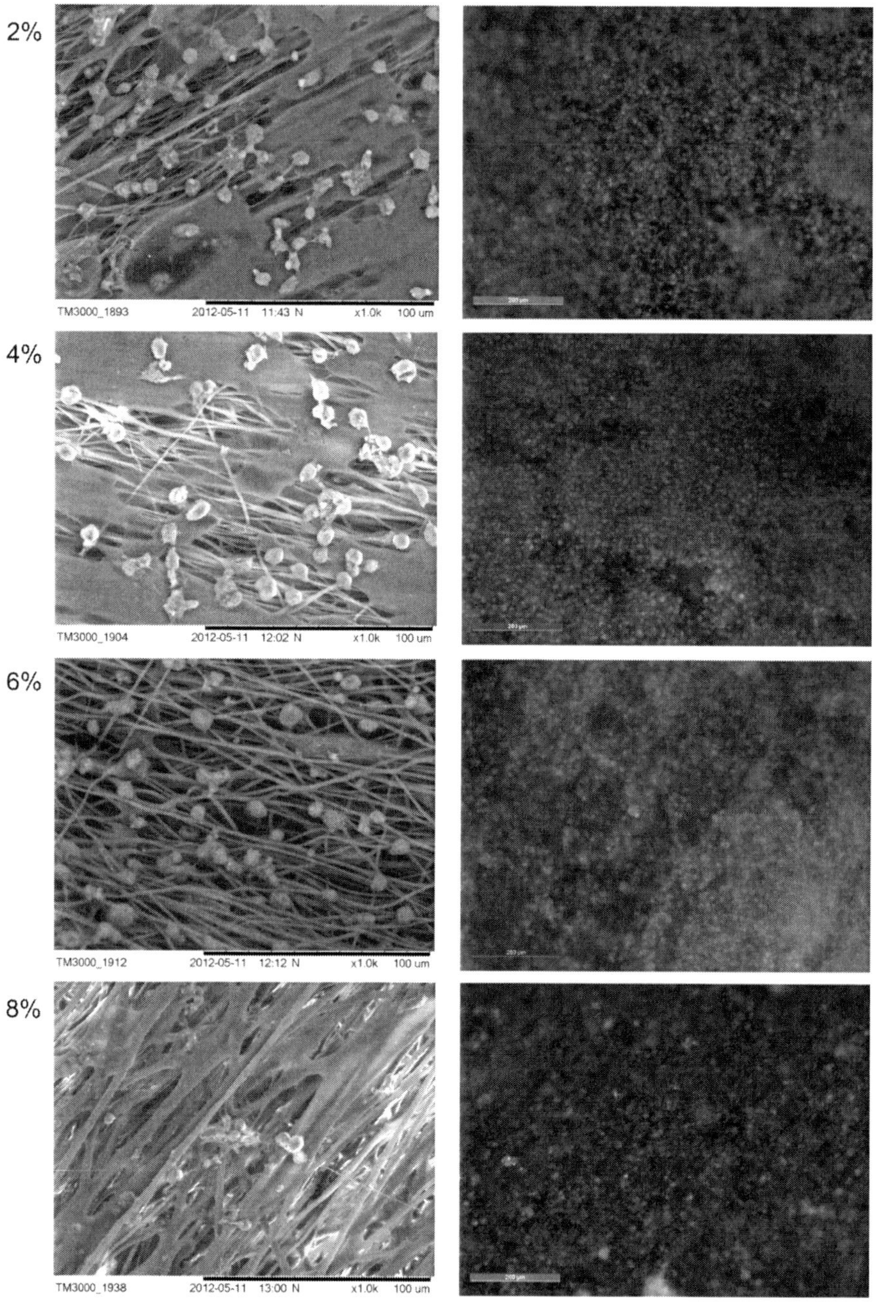

Figure 3. NIH 3T3 mouse fibroblast cells cultivated on membranes comprised of ultrafine fibers prepared from P(3HB) solutions of various concentrations; Day 7 of the culture: photographs to the left are SEM images, bar = 100 μm; photographs to the right are DAPI staining images, bar = 200 μm (Goncharov et al., 2012).

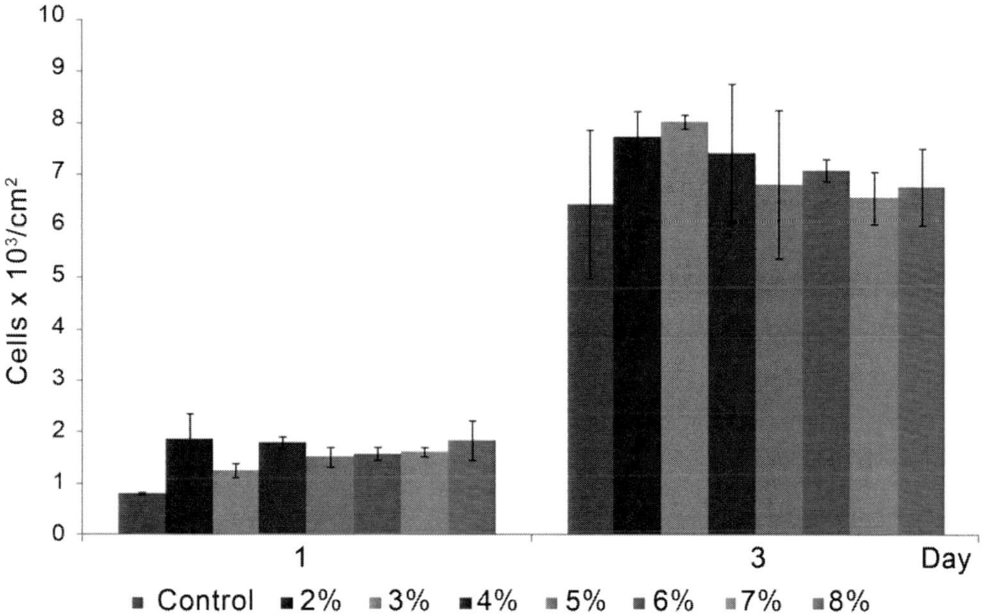

Figure 4. Viability of NIH 3T3 fibroblast cells on the membranes comprised of ultrafine fibers prepared by electrospinning from P(3HB) solutions of different concentrations (control is polystyrene) (Goncharov et al., 2012).

As Figure 5, the fibers were good quality but different in diameter. The average diameter of the fibers, prepared from P(3HB) was 2.9 μm, and the thickness of the membranes was 25 μm. Measurements of diameters of fibers prepared from copolymers with similar molar fractions of their second monomers showed that they had different average diameters and ranges of diameters, but the fibrous mats had similar thickness – about 20 μm. The average diameter of P(3HB)/10 mol.%-3HV fibers was 2.3 μm, while the average diameter of P(3HB-co-4HB) fibers was significantly smaller (1.7 μm). By contrast, the diameter of the fibers prepared from the solution of P(3HB-co-10 mol.%-3HHx) of the same concentration (5%) was twice larger (4.2 μm).

Surface properties of membranes, electrospun from PHAs of different chemical compositions, showing similar values of the water contact angle and properties of the membranes calculated based on the water contact angle (Table 4). Thus, polymer chemical composition did not influence surface properties of the membranes, comprised of electrospun ultrafine fibers. Likewise, no effect of the PHA chemical composition on the surface properties of nanofibrous membrane was revealed in the experiments with a rotating collector.

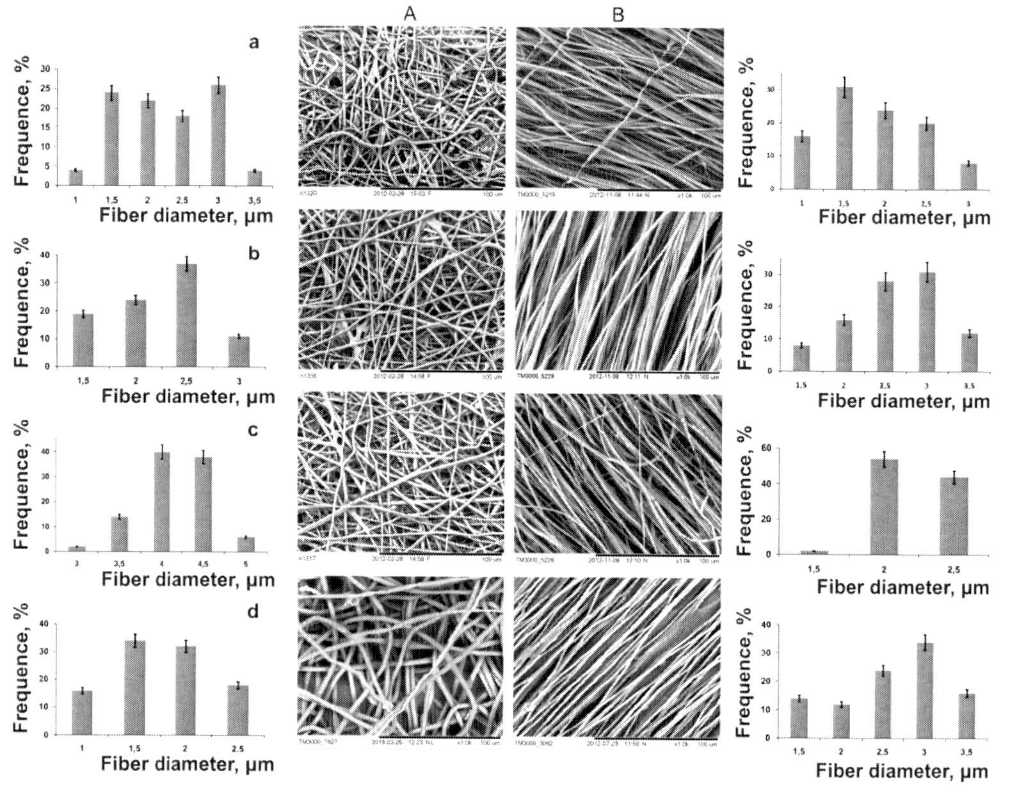

Figure 5. SEM images of randomly oriented (A) and aligned nanofibers (B)б produced by electrospinning from solutions of PHAs with different chemical compositions: a – P(3HB); b – P(3HB-*co*-3HV); c – P(3HB-*co*-4HV); d – P(3HB-*co*-3HHx) (T. Volova's data).

For randomly oriented fibers, no obvious relationship between their physical-mechanical properties and the molar fraction of the second monomer was observed. A more than 7-fold increase in the molar fraction of 3HV in P(3HB-co-3HV) (from 4.5 to 32.8%) caused a 1.6-fold increase in Young's modulus, but did not induce any change in tensile strength or elongation at break. However, a smaller (3-fold) increase in the molar fraction of 3HHx (from 4.9 to 13.6%) did not have any significant effect on Young's modulus, but reduced the tensile strength by half and caused a 3-fold decrease in elongation at break. A 7.5-fold increase in the molar fraction of 4HB in P(3HB-co-4HB) did not affect mechanical strength of the samples, but increased their elasticity considerably. The PHA samples with different chemical compositions had dissimilar degrees of crystallinity, which varied between 35 and 75%. These dissimilarities may be accounted for by differences in the micromolecular structure of polymer chains and crystallization processes of PHAs with different chemical compositions. Further work is required to establish this distinctly.

Table 4. Surface properties of nanofibrous membranes comprised of ultrafine fibers electrospun from solutions of PHAs with different chemical compositions (T. Volova's data)

Composition and type of PHA, mol.%	Water contact angle (θ, degrees)	Free surface energy (γ_S) (erg/cm^2)	Free interface energy (γ_{SL}) (erg/cm^2)	Cohesive force (W_{SL}) (erg/cm^2)
P(3HB)	64.33 ± 1.71	37.38	5.85	104.34
P(3HB-*co*-4HB) (90/10)	72.12 ± 0.55	31.19	8.69	95.30
P(3HB-*co*-4HB) (84/16)	73.23 ± 0.42	30.24	9.20	93.84
P(3HB-co-3HV (93/7)	83.51 ± 1.05	22.55	14.31	81.04
P(3HB-co-3HV) (91.2/9.8)	67.17 ± 1.12	35.20	6.76	101.25
P(3HB-co-3HV) (77.2/22.8)	72.63 ± 0.81	30.71	8.94	94.57
P(HB-co-3HHx) (95.7/4.3)	74.72 ± 1.35	29.07	9.86	92.01
P(HB-co-3HHx) (90/10)	69.85 ± 0.87	33.58	7.49	98.89

The tensile strength of the aligned mats was also higher, and this difference was more pronounced in copolymer-based specimens. The tensile strength of the aligned P(3HB-*co*-3HV) membranes was almost 4 times higher than that of the randomly oriented one. An even greater difference (nearly 6 times) was observed between aligned and randomly oriented P(3HB-*co*-4HB) membranes. On the other hand, fiber orientation had little, if any, influence to the elastic properties of P(3HB) and copolymer nanofibrous membranes. The chemical composition of the PHA did, however, influence the absolute values of elongation to break, which reached 16–22% for the mats from copolymers P(3HB-*co*-3HV) and P(3HB-*co*-4HB), but did not exceed 13–14% for P(3HB) membranes (either aligned or randomly oriented ones).

Aligned ultrafine fibers were prepared from PHAs of the same composition, as those, used in the previous study, and under the same electrospinning conditions, but with only a rotating drum, used as a collector. The average diameter of aligned fibers, prepared from P(3HB), was 2.1 μm. The diameter of copolymer aligned fibers, in contrast to randomly oriented ones, was similar to the diameter of P(3HB) fibers. The diameter of aligned P(3HB-co-3HV) fibers was similar to that of the corresponding randomly oriented fibers (about 2.5 μm); the average diameter of P(3HB-co-3HHx) fibers was 2.2 μm and that of P(3HB-co-4HB) fibers 2.7 μm. The diameter range of the aligned fibers was about 2 μm, and that was close to the diameter range of randomly oriented fibers

(Figure 6). The thickness of fibrous membranes comprised of aligned fibers was 25–30 μm, i.e., comparable to the thickness of randomly oriented scaffolds.

First, electrospun aligned membranes differed from randomly oriented ones in that they had much higher mechanical strength. Second, the effects of the second monomers of the copolymers, used to prepare the fibers on the properties of the aligned fibrous mats, were different from their effects on the properties of the randomly oriented membranes. The aligned fibrous mats, prepared from copolymers, containing 3HV and 3HHx, had similar values of tensile strength and Young's modulus, and they were not significantly lower, than those of P(3HB) fibers, but their elasticity values differed by a factor of two. In P(3HB-co-10 mol.%-4HB fibers, both parameters, characterizing mechanical strength, were lower than in P(3HB) ones, but this difference was not as significant as in randomly oriented fibers, while elasticity was more than 4 times higher.

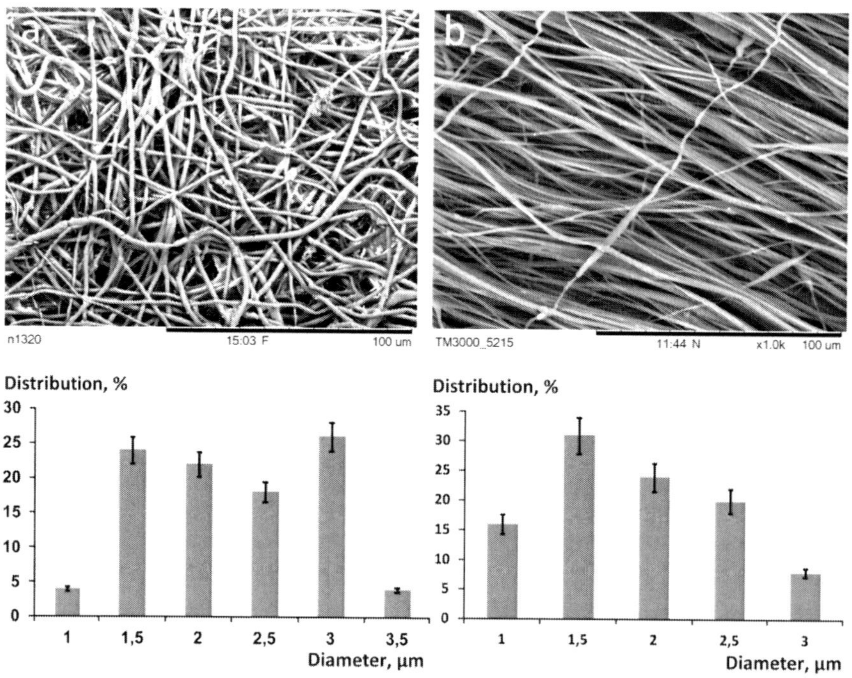

Figure 6. SEM images (a) and size distribution of diameters (b) of oriented and aligned ultrafine fibers produced by electrospinning from P(3HB) (Goncharov et al., 2014).

The most important difference between randomly and aligned oriented copolymer fibrous membranes was that in the latter, increased molar fractions of the second monomers had pronounced effect to the properties of mats. As the molar fraction of 3HV in P(3HB-co-3HV) was increased from 4.5% to 32.8%, Young's modulus consistently decreased from 824.04 ± 78.23 to 321.90 ± 27.33 MPa, while tensile strength remained practically unchanged, amounting to 14 MPa, and elongation at break increased from 10.11 ± 1.24% to 91.16 ± 7.32%. For P(3HB-co-4HB), the increase in the molar fraction of 4HB from 6.1% to 48.3% also caused a gradual and more pronounced decrease in Young's modulus, from 817.50 ± 76.81 to 4.12 ± 1.68 MPa, and an insignificant decrease in tensile strength, with elongation at break, rising from 13.10 ± 2.00 to 311.47 ± 45.37%. In the membranes, prepared from P(3HB-co-3HHx), the increase in the molar fraction of 3HHx from 4.9% to 13.6% did not cause any significant change in Young's modulus, but elongation at break gradually increased threefold.

The study revealed electrospinning parameters for the production of high-quality fibers from different types of PHA and determined, which parameters should be varied to tailor the properties of the products (fiber diameter, surface morphology, physical-mechanical properties). This study was the first to compare biological and physical-mechanical parameters of PHAs with different chemical compositions as dependent upon the fractions of monomers, constituting the polymers and fiber orientation.

Biological properties of fibrous membranes were studied in the culture of NIH 3T3 fibroblast cells. Considerable differences in cell culture parameters were revealed in experiments with membranes, prepared from PHAs with different chemical compositions. Figure 7 shows results of investigating of fibroblasts morphology in experiments with phalloidin staining, conjugated to FITC and DAPI, images showing the development of extracellular matrix. On randomly oriented fibers, cells were also arranged along the fibers; most cells were triangular or rectangular, with 3-4 appendages, used by cells to attach to the fibers (Figure 7A). Larger cells were observed on the randomly oriented membranes. On aligned membranes, cells, mostly spindle-shaped ones, were arranged along the fibers (Figure 7B).On the aligned P(3HB) membranes, the average cell size was 338.06 ± 45.19 μm^2, while on randomly oriented membranes it was 177.05 ± 45.20 μm^2. On randomly oriented membranes, prepared from PHA copolymers, the average cell sizes were also greater, than on copolymer aligned membranes: 381.73 ± 74.97 μm^2 on P(3HB-co-3HV), 398.77 ± 92.59 μm^2 on P(3HB-co-3HHx), and 429.93 ± 158 μm^2 on P(3HB-co-4HB) 387.38 ± 99.31 μm^2 on P(3HB-co-3HV), 370.82 ± 91.87 μm^2 on P(3HB-co-3HHx), and 274.79 ± 28.59 μm^2 on P3HB-co-4HB. However, significant differences ($P \leq 0.05$) were only obtained by comparing the results on aligned fibrous membranes, prepared from P(3HB) and from copolymer PHAs. The differences between randomly oriented membranes were insignificant.

At Day 7 after seeding, counts of viable cells, using MTT assay showed, that on randomly oriented fibrous membranes prepared from copolymers containing 3HV or 4HB as their second monomer the increase in the number of cells was about 1.4 times higher, than on P(3HB) membranes or on the membranes, prepared from the copolymer containing 3HHx (Figure 7). The number of cells on randomly oriented P(3HB), P(3HB-co-3HV), P(3HB-co-4HB), and P(3HB-co-3HHx) membranes reached $1.81 \pm 0.15 \cdot 10^5$, $2.33 \pm 0.17 \cdot 10^5$, $2.41 \pm 0.20 \cdot 10^5$, and $1.803 \pm 0.21 \cdot 10^5$ cells/cm^2, respectively. No statistically significant ($P \leq 0.05$) differences were found between P(3HB-co-3HV) and P(3HB-co-4HB) membranes. Also, fiber orientation had a significant effect on the growth and viability of fibroblast cells. It is apparent from Figure 7, that the number of viable fibroblasts on all aligned membranes was significantly lower ($1.14 \pm 0.19 \cdot 10^5$, $1.56 \pm 0.25 \cdot 10^5$, $1.83 \pm 0.31 \cdot 10^5$ and $1.16 \pm 0.12 \cdot 10^5$ cells/cm^2 at Day 7) than on randomly oriented fibrous membranes. The effect of the PHA chemical composition to the number of cells on aligned membranes was similar to that on randomly oriented ones; membranes, prepared from P(3HB-co-4HB) copolymers, provided the highest increase in cell numbers. On the reference scaffolds (polystyrene plates), the number of proliferating cells was lower too.

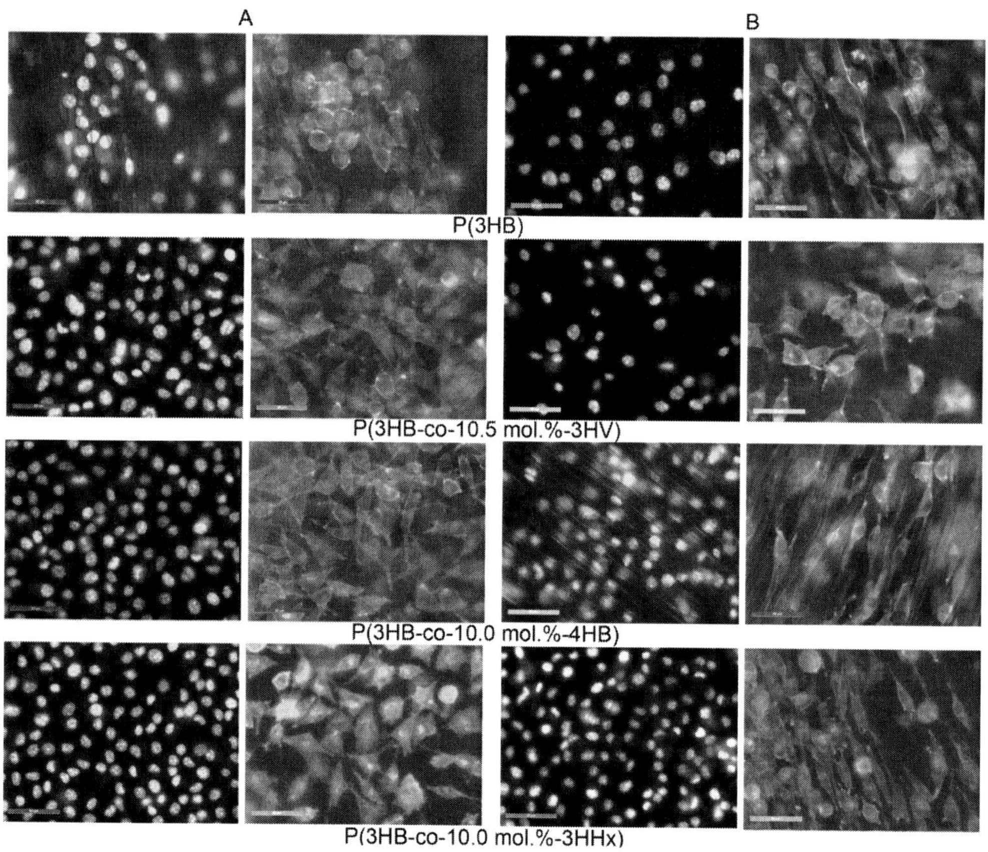

Figure 7. Light microscopy images of NIH 3T3 fibroblast cells, proliferating on randomly oriented fiber membranes (A), and on aligned oriented fiber membranes (B) prepared from P(3HB) and copolymers with different compositions and similar molar fractions of their second monomers (7 day): DAPI and FITC staining, bar = 50 μm (Nikolaeva's data).

Results of MTT assay suggest, that all types of fibrous membranes facilitate proliferation of fibroblast cells more effectively than the reference membranes and that randomly oriented membranes are more advantageous for growth and development of this kind of cells than aligned ones.

3. Potentials of Spinning Materials from PHA for the Repairing of Skin Defects

Reconstructive medicine needs novel materials for effective regeneration of skin, injured due to burns, traumas, and surgical interventions. There are hundreds of surgical and therapeutic devices for covering and healing skin defects and a great number of materials and drugs used to prepare these devices. Principles and methods of replacing the integrity of the skin are determined by such factors, as the depth and severity of the injury, the phase of the wound healing process, the wound location, the degree of microbial invasion, the patient's other diseases, and the drugs, taken by the patient. The basic principle of wound therapy is wound debridement and creation of the optimal conditions for wound healing. The ideal wound dressing must fulfill normal functions of healthy skin, which includes antimicrobial potential, promote moist wound environment, permit gaseous exchange, provide mechanical protection and be sufficiently elastic to fit the wound shape.

The fundamental studies underpinning cell biology, coupled with key clinical landmarks, led to invention of novel biomaterials, which paved their important roles in tissue-engineering of skin, which envisioned better understanding of skin biology (MacNeil, 2007). Studies also revealed three important factors in development of tissue-engineered materials, including the safety of the patient, clinical efficacy and convenience of usage. Perusal of scientific studies have reported considerable progress in development of tissue engineered skin for both, clinical and experimental medicine (MacNeil, 2007; 2008; Canto`n et al., 2010). The composition for the tissue engineered skin includes the culture of epidermal cells and biomaterials with cultured cells for replacing damaged epidermis or deeper skin layers. Initially, during development of tissue engineered skin, it is necessary to study the properties of the biomaterial, being used and determine its function in defect repair (Deshpande et al., 2013). Earlier suspensions of cell cultures – fibroblasts and keratinocytes - were used to treat skin wounds. However, administration of cell suspensions is not sufficiently effective for the skin defects repair. Later studies revealed, that the application of cells, pre-cultured on the scaffold, was more effective, than using of cell suspensions (Seland et al., 2011). Thus, in recent decade there has been tremendous interest towards using tissue-engineered constructs: scaffolds, carrying cells and drugs, and bioactive compounds (MacNeil, 2008; Metcalfe and Ferguson, 2007; Walker et al., 2010; 2012; Blais, 2013). Tissue-engineered skin has been successfully used to treat various diseases and skin defects such as vitiligo, melanoma, psoriasis, and blistering disorders (MacNeil, 2007).

Significant progress has been achieved since 25 years at creating tissue-engineered skin, yet there is a need for advancement, such as providing a barrier layer of renewable keratinocytes (the cells, that form the upper barrier layer of our skin), which is securely attached to the underlying dermis, is well vascularized and provides an elastic structural support for skin (MacNeil, 2008). Recent studies demonstrate the role of biomaterials used to create tissue-engineered skin. One of the major challenges is to choose an ideal material for constructing of grafts, which can be shaped as 2D and 3D constructs. Wound dressings, described in the literature, include tissue-engineered systems of keratinocytes or fibroblasts, seeded onto scaffolds of various materials, such as composites of polylactide/glycolide (Kim et al., 2005), polyethylene and silicon, collagen and glucosaminoglycan (Liu et al., 2008; Yang et al., 2000). These models can be used in clinical investigation of various skin diseases (MacNeil et al., 2011). The effective production and cultivation of keratinocytes in laboratory provided a basis for the clinical use (Sharma et al., 2014). Among the most promising cell scaffolds, nonwoven polymer membranes, sproduced by electrospinning, demonstrate better advantages, as they have similar structure to that of collagen fibers of living tissues (MacNeil, 2008; Canto`n et al., 2010, Sharma et al., 2014; Sill and von Recum, 2008; Rošic et al., 2013; Despande et al., 2013). Electrospinning can be used to produce 3D open porous structures and it is also possible to electrospin natural materials, such as collagen and chitosan or synthetic materials, such as poly-L-lactide (PLLA), polycaprolactone (PCL) and polyglycolic acid (PGA) (Ramalingman and Seeram, 2006). Scientific reviews highlight, that scaffolds of PHAs facilitate proliferation of various cells, including fibroblasts, osteoblasts, chondrocytes, neurons, and stem cells (Saad et al., 1997; Tezcaner et al., 2003; Liu et al., 2008; Lucchesi et al., 2008; Köse et al., 2005; Qu et al., 2005; Rentsch et al., 2010; Wang et al., 2010; You et al., 2011). Moreover, some data suggets, that fibroblasts and keratinocytes grow better on scaffolds of PHAs, than on other materials, including polylactides (Ji et al., 2008). Thus, there is a promising future for PHAs, as a materials for constructing of tissue-engineered grafts for healing of skin wounds.

In the present investigation, the main focus is to construct experimental wound dressings from degradable PHAs, intended for skin wound repair and evaluate their effectiveness in experiments on laboratory animals.

The nonwoven membranes, made from ultrafine fibers, were prepared by electrospinning from P(3HB/4HB) solutions, using a Nanon 01A automatic set-up (Figure 8). A chloroform solution with polymer concentration 6% was poured into a plastic syringe (13 mm inside diameter). The solution feeding rate was 8 ml/h, the applied voltage 25 kV, and the working distance was 15 cm. Randomly oriented ultrafine fibers were collected on a flat steel plate. The characterization of cell scaffolds results showed the presence of 3HB and 4HB monomer units, 90/10 mol. %.

The surface properties and physical/mechanical properties of the wound dressings obtained are given in Table 5. The nonwoven membranes had water contact angles at around 76.9°, with different diiodomethane contact angles at 43.5°. The elongation measurement at broken end indicated the elasticity of products with order of membranes, displaying higher parameters of mechanical strength including Young's modulus and tensile strength. The water vapor permeability of membranes P (3HB/4HB) was determined, and this parameter was higher by a factor of more than 20 in the electrospun membranes than in the solution cast films.

Table 5. Surface properties and physical/mechanical properties of experimental wound dressings prepared from P(3HB/4HB) (Shishatskaya et al., 2016)

Surface properties					
Samples	Water contact angle, o	Diiodo-methane contact angle, o	Surface free energy, эрг/sm2	Polar components mN/m)	Dispersive components mN/m)
Film	75,7 ± 2,7	55,1 ± 2,74	39,0 ± 0,76	7,6 ± 0,23	31,4 ± 0,54
Nonwoven membrane	76,9 ± 2,53	43,5 ± 1,41	43,2 ± 0,63	5,4 ± 0,27	37,8 ± 0,28
Physical/mechanical properties					
Samples	Thickness, μm	Young's modulus, E, MPa	Tensile strength σ, MPa	Elongation to break, %	Water vapor permeability, g/m^2/24 h
Film	24.0	1032.79 ± 5.64	17.48 ± 0.87	6.75 ± 3.37	432
Nonwoven membrane	25.0	1.59 ± 0.30	0.42 ± 0.08	72.98 ± 10.33	9312

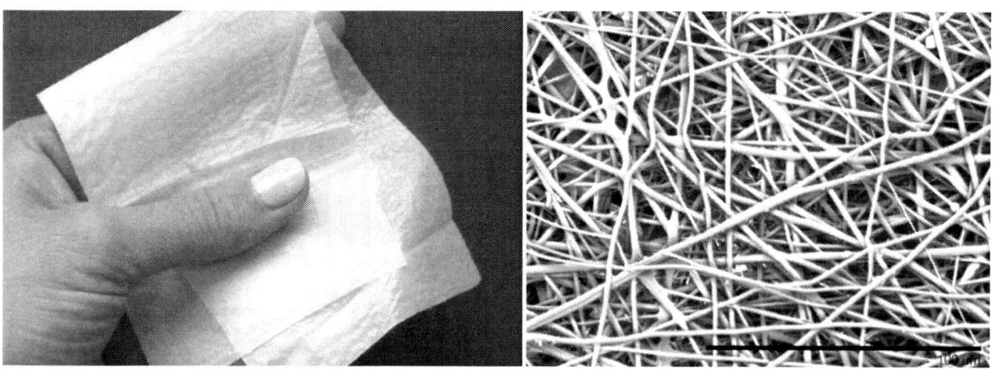

Figure 8. Photograph and SEM of nonwoven membranes (Shishatskaya et al., 2016).

The prepared membranes were seeded with mesenchymal stem sells cells, isolated from the adipose tissue of Wistar rats, which were fast euthanized by using an overdose of an anesthetic ether. The adipose tissue was isolated under aseptic conditions from abdominal and femoral regions, excised into small pieces to prepare a homogeneous mass and rinsed thrice with physiological saline buffered with phosphates, containing antibiotics. The cell suspension was transferred into 90-mm-diameter Petri dishes and placed into CO_2 incubator for 24 h. After the medium was replaced and unattached cells were removed. MSC differentiation into fibroblasts was induced by using the DMEM medium with 10% fetal bovine serum and a solution of antibiotics (100 units/ml of penicillin and 100 μg/ml of streptomycin). In DMEM medium these cells showed fibroblast-like morphology. After 3–4 passages, the cells were removed from Petri dishes with a trypsin solution and seeded in fresh dishes onto sterile PHA membranes at concentration of 10^5 cells per scaffold.

The nonwoven membranes, carrying fibroblast cells, were chosen for the constructing of hybrid tissue-engineered grafts. The electrospun membranes (scaffolds), used for constructing grafts, were composed of randomly oriented ultrafine fibers and during the electrospinning the fibers were collected on a flat plate.

The efficacy of nonwoven polymer membranes, prepared from P (3HB/4HB) copolymers, was studied on model skin defects in Wistar rats. Experiments were conducted in accordance with the Animal Welfare Act and the Guidelines for Ethical Treatment of Animals. The rats were given an inhalation anesthetic and a 2×2-cm section in the interscapular region of each rat was shaved and then excised (both epidermis and dermis, to its full thickness) under aseptic conditions and average wound area of 4.0–4.5 cm^2 was selected. The experiment was conducted with three sets of animals: two treatment groups, one with the grafts of nonwoven membranes and second with membranes, carrying epidermal cells, derived from adipose tissue. The third group served as control, whose wound was covered with sterile gauze. The dressings were fixed with 4 sutures and covered with sterile gauze. The state of the animals (motion activity, feeding behavior) was assessed daily throughout the experiment. The wounds were photographed and the area of the wound and the rate of healing were determined in order to monitor wound healing.

For histologic examination, skin samples were excised after the animals were euthanized, at Days 3, 7, and 14 of the experiment. The specimens were fixed in 10% neutral formalin and conventional histological techniques were used for the sampling. During investigation, evaluation of the inflammatory reaction and acanthosis (an indicator of increased proliferation of basal and spinous cells), counting of horn cysts (a marker of the lagging cell differentiation in the epidermis under the conditions of accelerated regeneration), quantification of sebaceous glands and hair follicles (a source of undifferentiated epithelial cells that can be involved in regeneration of the epidermis in the case of vast shallow wounds) were carried out.

To get an insight into the mechanism of the wound healing process, the gene expression studies were carried out, to detect the factors, that characterized the degree of inflammatory process, vascularization, and formation of the new connective tissue at the defect site. Real-time RT-PCR was performed in the region of quantification of gene expression for factors of rat angiogenesis (VEGF), inflammation (TNF-a), collagen type I (Col-1), as an indicator of connective tissue formation, keratin 10 (K10), and keratin 14 (K14), as indicators of the formation of the spinous and granulosa layers of the epidermis during regeneration, to determine the quantification level of transcription of genes, responsible for inflammation, vascularization, and connective tissue formation. Total RNA was isolated from the granulation tissue of the treatment and control groups by extraction with a guanidinium thiocyanate-phenol-chloroform mixture from the RNA-Extran reagent kit. Later, from RNA template by using reverse transcriptase, cDNA was synthesized with several types of oligonucleotide primers: with a mixture of random primers – hexa primers – and oligo-dT primer, following the procedure, recommended by the manufacturer (Sintol, Russia). Negative controls of reverse transcription reaction were prepared for all samples, to confirm the absence of DNA contamination in the initial RNA. Real-time PCR-amplification for quantification of cDNA fragments of rat VEGF, rat TNF-a, rat Col-1, rat K10, and rat K14 were performed by using a CFX-96 thermocycler, according to the manufacturer's protocol, using the color channel of HEX.

Throughout the postoperative observation period, all animals were healthy and active with normal eating behavior and moved on their own. After the treatment group animals awakened from anesthesia, they did not show any signs of pain.

Measurements of the wound area suggested, that in the treatment groups, the defects repaired faster. Photographs of the wounds taken during the experiment are shown in Figure 9. Histology of the skin samples excised at the wound regions showed usual tissue response to surgical intervention, characteristic of the healing process, including phases of post-traumatic inflammation, connective tissue formation, cicatrix formation and restructuring along with wound epithelialization.

Inflammation was observed in the wound region in all animals, but the hyperemia of the dermis vessels and cell infiltration of the dermis were pronounced to different extents, depending on the group. In the control group, large amounts of seropurulent exudate, containing leukocytes, were localized under the surface of necrotic masses. In the group with nonwoven P (3HB/4HB) membranes, seeded with epidermal cells, hyperemia of the vessels was less pronounced and there was no purulent exudate. That was a usual post-traumatic tissue response with moderate aseptic inflammation, which subsided rather quickly and was followed by tissue formation processes.

Measurements of the wound surface area showed significant changes in the group with membranes, seeded with epidermal cells. During the initial days, the wound decrease rate was the highest: 0.4–0.65 cm^2/d; at Day 3 the wound area was 3.6 cm^2 (81% of the initial wound area). Later at Day 5, the wound area constituted 62.7% of its initial area, similarly at Day 7 the wound area was found to be 57% and at Day 14 it was 9%. The group, consisting of PHA membranes showed lower healing rate of 0.3–0.4 cm^2/d. At Day 3, the wound are decreased by 9% (91% of the initial area) and at Day 7, the wound area constituted 78% of the initial area and at Day 14 it was found to be 9.1%. This result was comparable with the results, obtained from the group with membranes carrying cells. In the control group, during the first 24 h post-surgery, the healing rate was 0.16–0.23 cm^2/d (Figure 10).

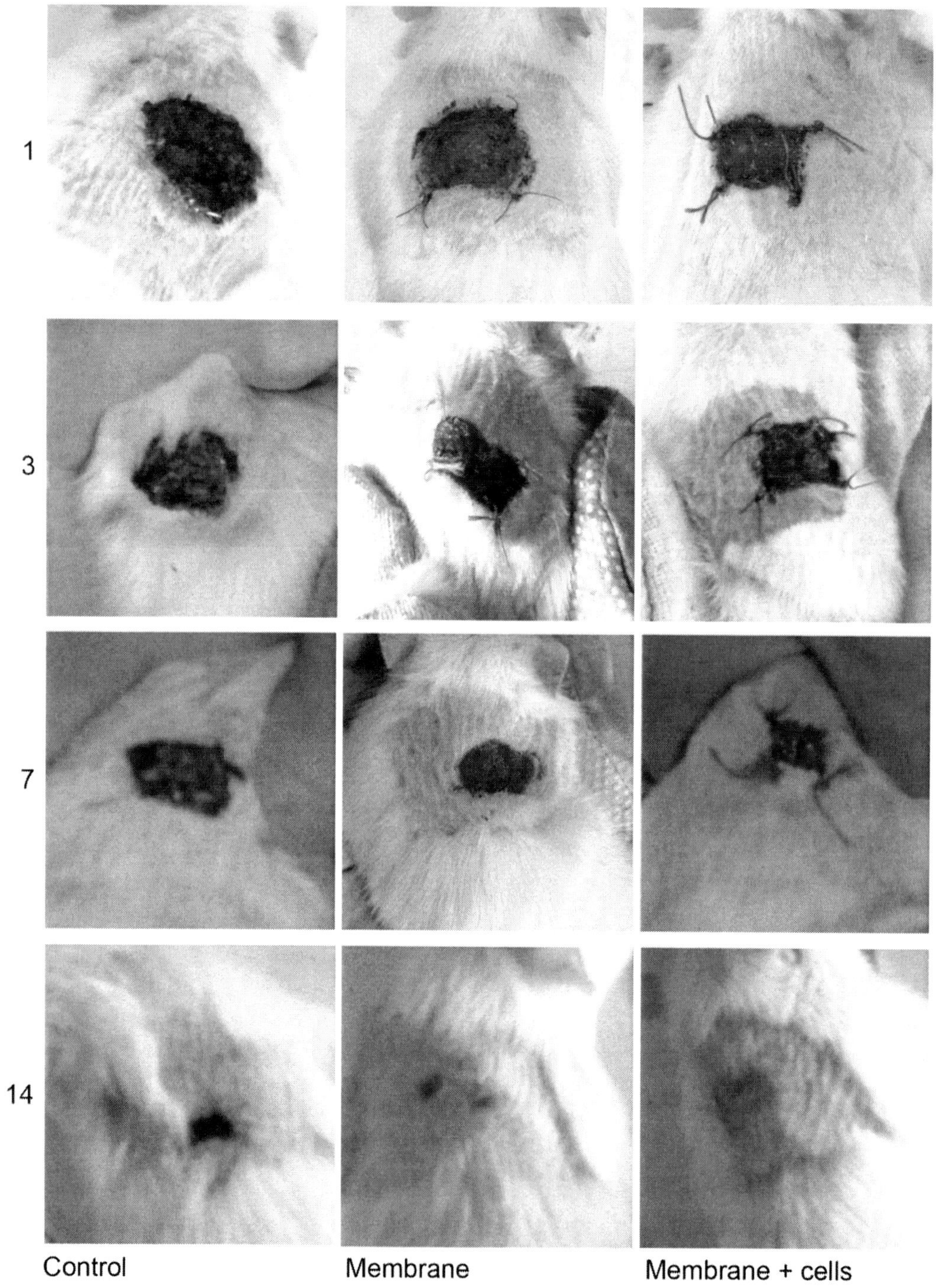

Figure 9. Photographs of skin wounds during healing (Shishatskaya et al., 2016).

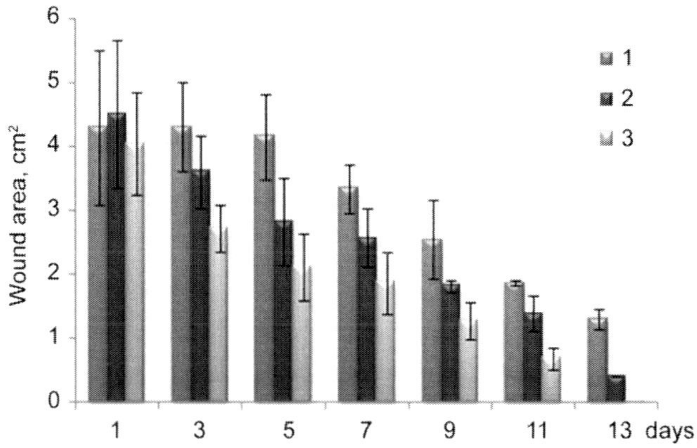

Figure 10. Dynamics of the decrease in the area of skin defects, created in laboratory rats, under the different types of wound dressings: 1 – control group; 2 – nonwoven membrane P(3HB/4HB); 3 – nonwoven membrane P(3HB/4HB), seeded with epidermal cells (Shishatskaya et al., 2016).

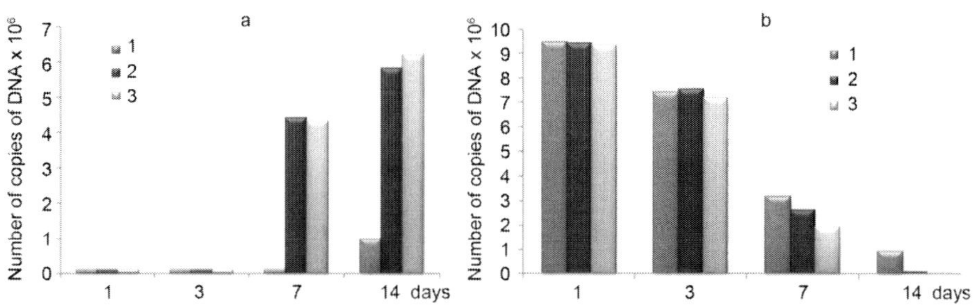

Figure 11. VEGF (a) and TNF-α (b) gene expression in laboratory rats under different types of wound dressings: 1 – control group; 2 – nonwoven membrane of P(3HB/4HB); 3 – nonwoven membrane of P(3HB/4HB), seeded with epidermal cells (Shishatskaya et al., 2016).

In the group with nonwoven membranes without cells, the average healing rate was lower: 0.45 cm^2/d. At Day 5, the area of the wound decreased to 62.7% in comparison with the initial wound area and at Day 7 it decreased to 57% and at Day 14 it was found to be 9.1%. In the control group, the wound healing rate was lower, in comparison with the treatment groups, which showed 0.16–0.23 cm^2/d and the area of the wound decreased by 4% by Day 5. At Day 7, a decrease in the wound area reached 23% and at Day 14 it was found to decrease by 30% of the initial wound area.

During the first 24 h, all animals developed edemas, which were more pronounced in the control group. The histological examination of the new tissue, collected from the defect site at Day 3, showed, that in the control group there was formation of connective tissue with very few collagen fibers and blood vessels. Vascularization was more pronounced under the experimental wound dressings, which was confirmed by the PCR of VEGF gene expression as an indicator of blood vessel formation (Figure 11a). The wounds covered with the polymer membrane dressings of P (3HB/4HB) displayed the density of newly formed collagen fibers which was higher than the control. Further, at

Day 7 the total cell counts in the dermis under the wound surface were slightly lower in the treated groups, which were studied under the microscope. It was also observed, that there was a clear shift towards fibroblast cells, suggesting faster reduction in the inflammatory process, which had developed at the defect site. The faster inflammation reduction in the treatment groups was confirmed in the PCR-based tests of TNF-α gene expression (inflammation factor) (Figure 11b). The results of planimetric measurements (Figure 10) and analysis of histological sections (Figure 12a), which suggested faster regeneration of the defects in the treatment groups, were confirmed by counting hair follicles, sebaceous glands, and horn cysts, as objective indicators of wound healing (Table 6).

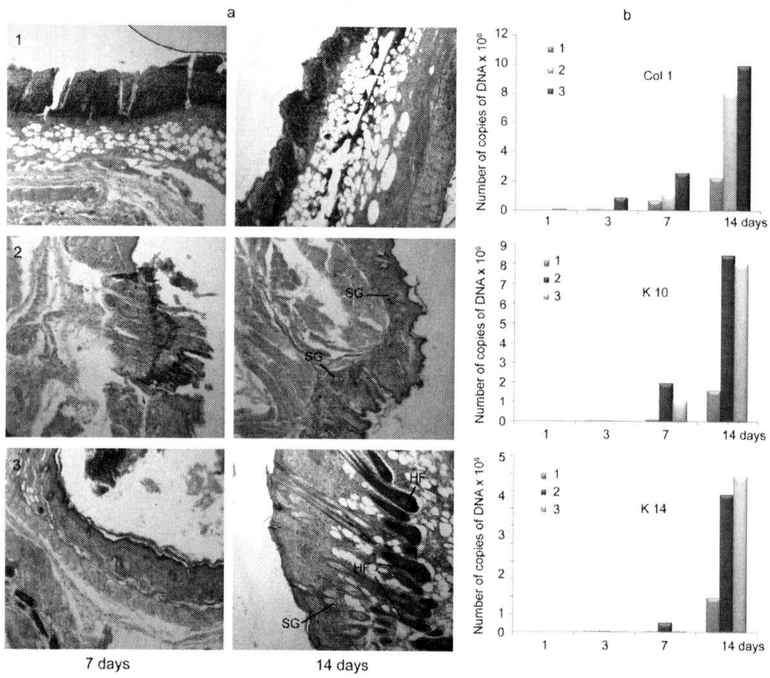

Figure 12. Histological sections from the skin defect sites. Wound healing (Day 7 post defect creation) under different wound dressings (a): 1 – control, 2 – nonwoven membrane of P(3HB/4HB); 3 – nonwoven membrane of P(3HB/4HB), seeded with epidermal cells. Notations: SG – sebaceous glands, HF – hair follicles. Hematoxylin and eosin staining, 100×. The number of Col-1, K10, and K14 cDNA copies during regeneration of skin defects in Wistar rats (b) (Shishatskaya et al., 2016).

Regeneration started earlier in the treatment groups, in which hair follicles and sebaceous glands were detected at Day 7, whereas only horn cysts, a marker of the lagging cell differentiation in the epidermis was detected in the control group. Counts of hair follicles, sebaceous glands, and horn cysts, as objective indicators of wound healing process, are listed in Table 6. Sebaceous glands and hair follicles are sources of undifferentiated epithelial cells (structurally the same as basal cells), which take part in skin regeneration.

The results of PCR-based assays of gene expression of collagen type I (Col-1), keratin 10 (K10) and keratin 14 (K14) showed, that new tissues developed were considerably better and wound healing rate was faster in the treated groups under experimental polymer membranes. The numbers of Col-1, K10, and K14 cDNA copies were higher, than those in the control by factors of 4.0–5.0, 3.5–4.0 and 4.0–4.5, respectively (Figure 12b).

Table 6. The history of regeneration of hair follicles and sebaceous glands in the wounds healing under different wound dressings (Shishatskaya et al., 2016)

Group	The numbers of hair bulbs, sebaceous glands, and horn cysts		
	Day 3	Day 7	Day 14
Control	–	5 horn cysts	7 hair bulbs 3 sebaceous glands 7 horn cysts
Treatment nonwoven membrane	–	4 hair bulbs 7 sebaceous glands	20 hair bulbs 16 sebaceous glands no horn cysts
Treatment nonwoven membrane +cells	–	6 hair bulbs 8 sebaceous glands	24 hair bulbs 17 sebaceous glands no horn cysts

The nonwoven polymer membranes and grafts, based on them, were investigated in experiments on laboratory animals with model skin defects. The experimental membranes fitted the wounds shape, protected them from external influences, and facilitated healing, promoting fast wound repair. Employing morphological, histological and molecular methods, we showed that nonwoven membranes, combined with cells, synthesizing growth factors, facilitated wound healing, neovascularization and regeneration, and enabled complete wound healing by Day 14 post surgery. The use of nonwoven membranes of degradable P(3HB/4HB) as atraumatic wound dressings can reduce the inflammation, enhance the angiogenic properties of the skin, and facilitate its healing.

4. Pilot Clinical Trials of Membranes, Comprised of Ultrafine PHA Fibers as Wound Dressings in the Treatment of Subcutaneous Septic Wounds

To enhance the therapeutic efficacy of wound dressings, they may be loaded with various drugs. In recent years, new processes of physical and chemical modification of wound dressings have been developed. Drugs can be immobilized on the surface of the dressings, enabling their slow release and prolonged therapeutic effect. To treat purulent wounds, the dressings are loaded with antiseptics, and the dressings themselves are fabricated from nonwoven polyvinyl alcohol fibers, activated with sodium dichloroisocyanurate or hydrogen peroxide, hydrogels, etc. A disadvantage of many wound dressings is that they stick to the wound surface. The adhesion of the dressing to the wound surface may be caused by various reasons, the most frequent of which is "gluing" of the dressing to the wound surface. The "glue" is the exudate, which dries and forms an eschar. As the hydrophilicity of the polymer material constituting the dressing is increased, it adheres to the wound surface more firmly. During the granulation phase, the adhesion of the wound dressing is associated with the growth of the granulation tissue into the pores of the dressing material.

A special group of wound dressings comprises the dressings, containing drugs, including antibacterial ones. They prevent the wound from being infected. These are such dressings as Iskom, DDB, and DDBM, which are fabricated from polyethylene film, spray-coated with a mixture of equal proportions of antibiotics (cephalexin, streptomycin, erythromycin, terramycin, tetracycline, vibramycin, synthomycin, neomycin, kanamycin, nystatin, daktarin, canesten, and rivanol) (5%) and talcum (95%). However, such dressings are impermeable to vapor and air, causing exudate accumulation on the wound. The DDBM film, a modification of the DDB film, has small drainage holes. Porous film Foliderm (Folium, St. Petersburg) is fabricated from hydrophobic material, which is permeable to gases and impermeable to bacteria. Films Aseplen, Foliderm, and DDBM can be used as wound dressings in the first phase of wound healing. Most of the films, however, are used as wound dressings in phases 2 and 3, as they protect the wounds without preventing tissue regeneration. Atraumatic absorptive wound dressings can be designed by using hydrophobic non-adhesive polymer materials, which may be loaded with antibacterial drugs.

Researchers carried out pilot clinical trials of the effectiveness of using of nonwoven membranes, comprised of ultrafine PHA fibers, which were prepared by electrospinning. A preliminary study was conducted to investigate antimicrobial properties of PHA-based wound dressings, loaded with ceftriaxone (5, 10, and 15% of the polymer weight). The antimicrobial effect of the dressings was evaluated by the diffusion method, by measuring the areas, where microbial culture growth was inhibited. Tests were performed with two cultures of Gram-negative bacteria, *Ps.aureginosa* and *E.coli*, potential pathogens to humans, which are recommended for evaluation of antibacterial activity of nonwoven and textile materials. Disks of 5 mm in diameter were cut out of the electrospun nonwoven membrane and placed on the agar medium with the bacterial cells seeded on it. The cultures were incubated at 37°C for 24 h, and then the inhibition area was measured. Paper disks loaded with ceftriaxone (Bio RAD) to the same concentrations were used as control. Nonwoven disks with no antibiotic were also tested, showing no inhibition regions. All membranes inhibited the growth of the both microbial cultures. The inhibition regions were very distinct, and their areas were easily determined. Changes in concentrations of the antibiotic in the membranes did not significantly influence the degree of inhibition, and the area of the inhibition regions on the membranes was comparable to that on the paper disks. Thus, dissolution of the drug in chloroform and the subsequent electrospinning did not decrease its efficacy. Of the two species, *E.coli* and *Ps.aureginosa*, *E.coli* was more sensitive to ceftriaxone.

The membranes, loaded with ceftriaxone, were used in the clinical trial. The purpose of the trial was to evaluate the efficacy of the wound dressing of degradable P(3HB/4HB), loaded with the antibacterial drug, ceftriaxone, in the treatment of purulent skin wounds. The trial was conducted with 22 patients, including 9 patients with acute purulent infections of soft tissues (abscesses, phlegmons, phlegmonous-necrotic erysipelas, trophic ulcers caused by venous disorders and diabetes mellitus), who were treated by using the proposed polymer dressings. The reference group consisted of the patients with the same diseases, who were treated by using wound dressing Voskopran (Russia). The groups were similar in respect of age, gender ratio, the type of purulent diseases of soft tissues, and the area of the wounds. The methods used in the trial were clinical evaluation of the wound healing, wound planimetry, pH measurement, laser Doppler flowmetry, and statistical processing. The patients were observed for between 14 and 45 days. When the patients with purulent diseases of soft tissues were admitted to the clinic, they underwent both the general physical examination and evaluation of the wound processes. The appearance of the wound, the presence or absence of skin hyperemia and infiltration of the wound edges, the time of the beginning of granulation and the type of the granulations, the start and development of epithelialization were evaluated during initial examination. All patients with purulent skin diseases (abscesses, phlegmons, phlegmonous-necrotic erysipelas) received immediate surgical treatment of the wounds in the operating room (lancing of abscesses and removal of as much necrotic tissue as possible, debridement of the wound, and drainage). All wounds were superficial, with the area no more than 1% of the body surface area, and the depth no more than 15 mm. After the wounds were debrided, they were covered with the dressings in accordance with the design of the trial. Subsequently, the medically indicated treatment included infusion, antibacterial, anti-inflammatory, and symptomatic therapies.

Topical medication was scheduled based on the wound healing phase, according to V.I. Struchkov's classification, accepted in Russia (Struchkov, 1975). In the first two days, the dressing was periodically removed, the wounds were cleansed with a 3% hydrogen peroxide solution, purulent-necrotic masses were removed mechanically, and the dressing was applied again (either Voskopran or an ultrafine PHA membranes). The treatment in the inflammation phase included the use of a 0.02% plivasept solution. During the regeneration phase, bandaging was performed once every 2–3 days, and before the wound was covered with the dressing, solcoseryl and methyluracil ointments were applied to it. After the granulation tissue was formed, the defect healed by secondary intention.

By using the ceftriaxone membranes of P(3HB/4HB) as a wound dressing, the researchers managed to optimize the wound healing process, speed up the development of the mature granulation tissue in the wound by 3 and 3–15 days, and increase the frequency of the epithelialization time by 28.7% as compared with the process where Voskopran wound dressing was used. In the group of patients with Voskopran, the body temperature reliably decreased at Day 7 post surgery, reaching normal values at Day 12–17. When the patients were admitted to the clinic, their laboratory data showed high levels of endogenous intoxication. In Group 1, the leukocyte counts reached $18.5 \pm 2.7\times10^9$/L; by Day 12, this parameter declined to $8.4 \pm 0.48 \times 10^9$/L ($p < 0.05$), reaching normal levels, $5.9 \pm 0.5 \times 10^9$/L ($p < 0.05$), by Day 17. During the first 24 h after wound debridement, the overall blood toxicity was reduced and the leukocyte counts decreased, but the differences were non-significant. In the first 24 h of the treatment, the leukocyte index of intoxication reached 5.42 ± 1.2 units, at Day 5, it was 4.17 ± 0.43 units ($p < 0.05$), at Day 10, it was lower by a factor of two, decreasing to normal values only at Day 17 – 1.52 ± 0.34 units ($p < 0.05$). In Group 2, with the experimental nanomatrices, the body temperature of the patient decreased at Day 3 after wound (trophic ulcer) debridement. At Day 6–7, the temperature was no more than 37°C. The leukocyte counts in the blood of the Group 2 patients were $16.1 \pm 1.2 \times 10^9$/L ($p < 0.05$) at Day 3, reaching normal levels – $7.8 \pm 1.2 \times 10^9$/L ($p < 0.05$) – at Day 10.

Clinical evaluation of the wound healing process was based on such parameters, lo7 as the time of disappearance of the edema, formation of the first granulations, filling of the wound by mature granulation tissue, the start of epithelialization, and complete epithelialization. The outcomes of the treatment showed that in Group 1, the transition from phase 1 to phase 2 of the healing process took a long time: in 6 patients (46.1%), epithelialization was not complete after 45 days. The rates of wound healing in the treatment group patients suggested good and adequate outcomes. At Day 45, complete wound epithelialization was observed in 8 patients (88.8%)

Thus, nonwoven membranes, comprised of ultrafine fibers, prepared by electrospinning and loaded with ceftriaxone, enables rapid epithelialization of purulent wounds when used as a wound dressing. When the dressing is removed, cell debris and bacteria are removed too. During the regeneration phase, ultrafine PHA membranes serves as a scaffold for the new tissue on the skin and soft tissue defects. The formation of the uniform and sufficiently vascularized tissue is a prerequisite for quicker wound healing and can serve as a basis for the subsequent skin grafting and spontaneous re-epithelialization of superficial wounds. The wound dressing, tested in this clinical trial, performs important physiological functions of natural skin, provides a barrier against secondary infection, reduces fluid loss, and, at the same time, does not keep the air out.

The wound dressing, tested in this clinical trial, performs important physiological functions of natural skin, provides a barrier against secondary infection, reduces fluid loss, and, at the same time, does not keep the air out.

CONCLUSION

This chapter is devoted to natural biodegradable materials – polyhydroxyalkanoates (PHAs), which have many attractive properties for biomedical applications. This is a new class of biodegradable and biocompatible polyesters, whose physicochemical properties can vary greatly depending on the PHA composition. PHAs have considerable advantages over polylactides. In addition to poly-3-hydroxybutyrate, there are many promising PHA copolymers, which, depending on their monomeric composition, have different basic properties (degree of crystallinity, melting point, ductility, mechanical strength, biodegradation rate, etc.).

In this study, electrospinning was used to prepare fibers from PHAs with different chemical compositions: P(3HB) and copolymers: P(3HB-*co*-4HB), P(3HB-*co*-3HV), and P(3HB-*co*-3HHx). The main process parameters that influence fiber diameter and properties (polymer concentration, solution feeding rate, working distance, and applied voltage) have been investigated and their effects evaluated. Mechanical strength of aligned fibers prepared from different PHAs is higher than that of randomly oriented ones; no significant effect of fiber orientation on surface properties has been found. The study revealed electrospinning parameters for the production of high-quality fibers and determined which parameters should be varied to tailor the properties of the products. This study is the first to compare biological and physical-mechanical parameters of PHAs with different chemical compositions as dependent upon the fractions of monomers constituting the polymers and fiber orientation. None of the nanofibrous membranes electrospun from PHAs had any adverse effects on attachment, growth, and viability of NIH 3T3 mouse fibroblast cells, and all of them were found to be suitable for tissue engineering applications.

Grafts – elastic nonwoven membranes carrying fibroblast cells derived from adipose tissue multipotent mesenchymal stem cells – were constructed and investigated. The effectiveness of nonwoven membranes of P(3HB/4HB) carrying the culture of allogenic fibroblasts was evaluated by using them as dressings of model skin defects in Wistar rats. Morphological, histological, and molecular studies showed that the presence of fibroblasts on the wound dressing facilitated wound healing, vascularization, and regeneration due to the effect of growth factors synthesized by the cells. Moreover, the cells created a layer of extracellular matrix proteins on the surface of the membranes, which additionally promoted migration of epidermal cells from the tissues surrounding the wound. The wounds under the P(3HB/4HB) membrane carrying cells healed 1.4

times faster than the wounds under the cell-free membrane and 3.5 times faster than the wounds healing under the eschar (control). In the "membrane+cells" group, complete healing was achieved at Day 14. The use of nonwoven membranes of degradable P(3HB/4HB) as atraumatic wound dressings can reduce the inflammation, enhance the angiogenic properties of the skin, and facilitate its healing.

Thus, nonwoven membrane comprised of ultrafine fibers prepared by electrospinning and loaded with ceftriaxone enables rapid epithelialization of purulent wounds when used as a wound dressing. When the dressing is removed, cell debris and bacteria are removed too. During the regeneration phase, ultrafine PHA nonwoven membrane serves as a scaffold for the new tissue on the skin and soft tissue defects. The formation of the uniform and sufficiently vascularized tissue is a prerequisite for quicker wound healing and can serve as a basis for the subsequent skin grafting and spontaneous re-epithelialization of superficial wounds. The wound dressing tested in this clinical trial performs important physiological functions of natural skin, provides a barrier against secondary infection, reduces fluid loss, and, at the same time, does not keep the air out.

Acknowledgments

The reported study was funded by RFBR and Government of Krasnoyarsk Territory according to the research project № 16-43-242024.

References

Amass, W; Amass, A; Tighe, B. A Review of Biodegradale Polymers: Uses, Current Developments in the Synthesis and Characterization of Biodegradable Polyesters, Blends of Biodegradable Polymers and Recent Advances in Biodegradation Studies. *Polymer International,* 1998, 47, 89–144.

Blais, M; Parenteau-Bareil, R; Cadau, S; Berthod, F. Concise review: tissue-engineered skin and nerve regeneration in burn treatment. *STEM CELLS Translational Medicine,* 2013, 2, 545–51.

Canto`n, I; Cole, DM; Kemp, EH; Watson, PF; Chunthapong, J; Ryan, AJ; MacNeil, S; Haycock, JW. Development of a 3D Human In Vitro Skin Co-Culture Model for Detecting Irritants in Real-Time. *Biotechnology and Bioengineering,* 2010, 106, 794–803.

Chen, GQ. A microbial polyhydroxyalkanoates (PHA) based bio- and materials industry. *Chemical Society Reviews,* 2009, 38, 2434–2446.

Chen, JY; Song, G; Chen, GQ. A lower specificity of PhaC2 synthase from *Pseudomonas stutzeri* catalyses the production of copolyesters consisting of short-chain-length and medium-chain-length 3-hydroxyalkanoates. *Antonie Van Leeuwenhoek,* 2006, 89, 157–167.

Clarinval, AM; Halleux, J. Classification of biodegradable polymers. In: Smith R, editor. *Biodegradable Polymers for Industrial Applications.* Woodhead Publishing. Cambridge; 2005; 3–31.

Deshpande, P; Ramachandran, C; Sangwan, VS; MacNeil, S. Cultivation of Limbal Epithelial Cells on Electrospun Poly(lactide-*co*-glycolide) Scaffolds for Delivery to the Cornea. In: Wright B, ConnonCJ editors. *Corneal Regenerative Medicine, Methods and Protocols.* New York: Humana Press; 2013; 179–185.

Duvernoy, O; Malm, T; Ramström, J; Bowald, S. A biodegradable patch used as a pericardial substitute after cardiac surgery: 6- and 24-month evaluation with CT. *Thoracic and Cardiovascular Surgeon,* 1995, 43, 271–274.

Goncharov, DB; Nikolaeva, ED; Sukovatyi, AG; Shabanov, AV; Shishatskaya, EI; Markelova, NM. Characterizaytion of ultrafine fibers prepared by electrospinning from poly-3-hydroxybutyrate. *Journal of Siberian Federal University. Biology,* 2012, 5 (4), 417–426 (in Russian).

Goncharov, DB; Sukovatyi, AG. Effect of Orientation on Properties of Ultrafine Fibers Produced by Electrostatic Molding from Poly-3-Hydroxybutyrate. *Journal of Siberian Federal University. Biology,* 2014, 7 (2), 186-194 (in Russian)

Grabow, N; Bünger, CM; Schultze, C; Schmohl, K; Martin, DP; Williams, SF; Sternberg, K; Schmitz, KP. A biodegradable slotted tube stent based on poly(L–lactide) and poly(4–hydroxybutyrate) for rapid balloon–expansion. *Annals of Biomedical Engineering,* 2007, 35, 2031–2038.

Hench, L; Jones, J. Biomaterials, artificial organs and tissue engineering. Woodhead Publishing Limited. Cambridge, England, 2005.

Ienczak, JL; Schmidell, W; de Aragao, GMF. High-cell-density culture strategies for polyhydroxyalkanoate production: review. *Journal of Industrial Microbiology and Biotechnology,* 2013, 40, 275–286.

Ji, Y; Li, XT; Chen, GQ. Interactions between a poly(3-hydroxybutyrate-co-3-hydroxyvalerate-co-3-hydroxyhexanoate) terpolyester and human keratinocytes. *Biomaterials,* 2008, 29, 3807–3814.

Kaur, G; Roy, I. Strategies for Large-scale Production of Polyhydroxyalkanoates. *Chemical and Biochemical Engineering Quarterly,* 2015, 29, 157–172.

Kim, SS; Gwak, SJ; Choi, CY; Kim, BS. Skin regeneration using keratinocytes and dermal fibroblasts cultured on biodegradable microspherical polymer scaffolds. *Journal of Biomedical Materials Research Part B: Applied Biomaterials,* 2005, 75, 369–377.

Köse, GT; Kokusuz, F; Özkul, A; Soysal, Y; Ozdemir, T; Yildiz, C; Hasirci, V. Tissue engineered cartilage on collagen and PHBV matrices. *Biomaterials,* 2005, 26, 5187–5197.

Laycock, B; Halley, P; Pratt, S; Werker, A; Lant, P. The chemomechanical properties of microbial polyhydroxyalkanoate. *Progress in Polymer Science,* 2013, 38, 536–583.

Lenz, RW; Marchessault, RH. Bacterial polyesters: biosynthesis, biodegradable plastics and biotechnology. *Biomacromolecules,* 2005, 6, 1–7.

Liu, P; Deng, Z; Han, S; Liu, T; Wen, N; Lu, W; Geng X, Huang S, Jin Y. Tissue-Engineered Skin Containing Mesenchymal Stem Cells Improves Burn Wounds. *Artificial Organs,* 2008, 32, 925–931.

Liu, P; Deng, Z; Han, S; Liu, T; Wen, N; Lu, W; Geng, X; Huang, S; Jin, Y. Tissue-Engineered Skin Containing Mesenchymal Stem Cells Improves Burn Wounds. *Artificial Organs,* 2008, 32, 925–931.

Lucchesi, C; Ferreira, BMP; Duek, EAR; Santos, Jr, AR; Joazeiro, PP.Increased response of Vero cells to PHBV matrices treated by plasma. *Journal of Materials Science: Materials in Medicine,* 2008, 19, 635–643.

Luef, KP; Stelzer, F; Wiesbrock, F. Poly(hydroxyl alkanoate)s in Medical Application. *Chemical and Biochemical Engineering Quarterly,* 2015, 29, 287–2912.

Luengo, JM; García, B; Sandoval, A. Bioplastics from microorganisms. *Current Opinion in Biotechnology,* 2003, 6, 251–260.

Luizier, WD. Materials derived from biomass/biodegradable materials. *Proceedings of the National Academy of Sciences of the United States of America,* 1992, 89, 839–842.

MacNeil, S. Biomaterials for tissue engineering of skin. *Materials Today,* 2008, 11, 26–35.

MacNeil, S. Progress and opportunities for tissue-engineered skin. *Nature,* 2007, 445, 874–80.

MacNeil, S; Shepherd, J; Smith, L. Production of Tissue-Engineered Skin and Oral Mucosa for Clinical and Experimental Use. In: Haycock JW, editor. *3D Cell Culture, Methods and Protocols.* New York: Humana Press; 2011; 129-153.

Madison, LL; Huisman, GW. Metabolic engineering of poly(3-hydroxyalkanoates): From DNA to plastic. Microbiol. *Microbiology and Molecular Biology Reviews,* 1999, 63, 21–53.

Malm, T; Bowald, S; Bylock, A; Busch, C; Saldeen, T. Enlargement of the right ventricular outflow tract and the pulmonary artery with a new biodegradazzble patch in transannular position. *European Surgical Research,* 1994, 26, 298–308.

Malm, T; Bowald, S; Karacagil, S; Bylock, A; Busch, C. A new biodegradable patch for closure of atrial septal defect. *Scandinavian Journal of Thoracic and Cardiovascular Surgery,* 1992, 26, 9–14.

Marois, Y; Zhang, Z; Vert, M; Beaulieu, L; Lenz, RW; Guidoin, R. *In vivo* biocompatibility and degradation studies of polyhydroxyoctanoate in the rat: A new sealant for the polyester arterial prosthesis. *Tissue Engineering,* 1999a, 5, 369–386.

Marois, Y; Zhang, Z; Vert, M; Deng, X; Lenz, RW; Guidoin, R. Bacterial polyesters for biomedical applications: *In vitro* and *in vivo* assessment of sterilization, degradation rate and biocompatibility of poly(*β*–hydroxyoctanoate (PHO). In: Agrawal CM, Parr JE, Lan ST, editors. *Synthesis Bioabsorbable Polymers for implants.* Scrawal: ASTM; 2000; 12–38.

Marois, Y; Zhang, Z; Vert, M; Deng, X; Lenz, RW; Guidoin, R. Effect of sterilization on the physical and structural characteristics of polyhydroxyoctanoate (PHO). *Journal of Biomaterials Science. Polymer Edition,* 1999b, 10, 469–482.

Martin, D; Williams, S. Medical application of polyhydroxybutyrate: a strong flexible absorbable biomaterial. *Biochemical Engineering Journal,* 2003, 16, 97–105.

Martin, DP; Peoples, OP, Williams, SF. Nutritional and therapeutic uses of 3-hydroxyalkanoate oligomers. PCT Patent Application No. WO 00/04895, 2000.

Metcalfe, AD; Ferguson, MWJ. Tissue engineering of replacement skin: the crossroads of biomaterials, wound healing, embryonic development, stem cells and regeneration. *Journal of the Royal Society Interface,* 2007, 4, 413–437.

Miller, ND; Williams, DF. On the biodegradation of poly-β-hydroxybutyrate (PHB) homopolymer and poly-*β*-hydroxybutyrate-hydroxyvalerate copolymers. *Biomaterials,* 1987, 8, 129–137.

Noda, I; Green, Ph; Satkowski, M; Schechtman, LA. Preparation and properties of novel class of polyhydroxyalkanoate copolymers. *Biomacromoleculas,* 2005, 6, 580–586.

Olivera, ER; Carnicero, D; García, B; Miñambres, B; Moreno, MA; Cañedo, L; Dirusso, CC; Naharro, G; Luengo, JM. Two different pathways are involved in the β-oxidation of n-alkanoic and n-phenylalkanoic acids in Pseudomonas putida U: genetic studies and biotechnological applications. *Molecular Microbiology,* 2001b, 39, 863–874.

Olivera, ER; Carnicero, D; Jodrá, R; Miñambres, B; García, B; Abraham, GA; Gallardo, A; Román, JS; García, JL; Naharro, G; Luengo, JM. Genetically engineered *Pseudomonas:* a factory of new bioplastics with broad applications. *Environmental Microbiology,* 2001a, 3, 612–618.

Plastic from Bacteria. Natural Functions Applications. In: Chen GQ, editor. Berlin: Springer-Verlag; 2010.

Polyhydroxyalkanoates (PHA): Biosynthesis, Industrial Production and Applications in Medicine. In: Wu LP, editor. NY USA: Nova Science Pub Inc; 2014.

Pouton, CW. Polymeric materials for advanced drug delivery. *Advanced Drug Delivery Reviews,* 2001, 53, 1–3.

Qu, XH; Wu, Q; Liang, J; Qu, X; Wang, SG; Chen, GQ. Enhanced vascular-related cellular affinity on surface modified copolyesters of 3-hydroxybutyrate and 3-hydroxyhexanoate (PHBHHx). *Biomaterials,* 2005, 26, 6991–7001.

Ramalingman, M; Seeram, R. Nano-featured scaffolds for tissue engineering: a review of spinning methodologies. *Tissue Engineering,* 2006, 12, 437–4470.

Rentsch, C; Rentsch, B; Breier, A; Hofmann, A; Manthey, S; Scharnweber, D; Biewener, A; Zwipp, H. Evaluation of the osteogenic potential and vascularization of 3D poly(3)hydroxybutyrate scaffolds subcutaneously implanted in nude rats. *Journal of Biomedical Materials Research. Part A,* 2010, 92, 185–195.

Rošic, R; Kocbek, P; Pelipenko, J; Kristl, J; Baumgartner, S. Nanofibers and their biomedical use. *Acta Pharmaceutica,* 2013, 63, 295–304.

Saad, B; Hirt, TD; Welti, M; Uhlschmid, GK, NeuenschwanderP,Suter UW. Development of degradable polyesterurethanes for medical applications: in vitro and in vivo evaluations. *Journal of Biomedical Materials Research,* 1997;36;65–74.

Seland, H; Gusafson, CJ; Johnson, H; Junker, JPE; Kratz, G. Transplantation of acellular dermis and keratinocytes cultured on porous biodegradable microcarriers into full-thickness skin injuries on athymic rats. *Burns,* 2011, 37, 99–108.

Sharma, K; Bullock, A; Ralston, D; MacNeil, S. Development of a one-step approach for the reconstruction of full thickness skin defects using minced split thickness skin grafts and biodegradable synthetic scaffolds as a dermal substitute. *Burns,* 2014, 40, 957–965.

Shishatskaya, EI; Nikolaeva, ED; Vinogradova, ON; Volova, TG. Experimental wound dressings of degradable PHA for skin defect repair. *Journal of Material Science: Materials in Medicine,* 2016, 27, 1–16.

Shishatsky, ON; Shishatskaya, EI. Analysis of the market for materials and devices for medical applications. Krasnoyarsk: Krasnoyarskii Pisatel; 2010 (in Russian).

Shtilman, MI. Polymers intended for biomedical applications. Moscow: Akademkniga Publishers; 2006 (in Russian).

Sill, TJ, von Recum, HA. Electrospinning: Applications in drug delivery and tissue engineering. *Biomaterials,* 2008, 29, 1989–2006.

Sodian, R; Hoerstrup, SP; Sperling, JS; Daebritz, SH; Martin, DP; Schoen, FJ; Vacanti, JP; Mayer, JE Jr. Tissue engineering of heart valves: *in vitro* experiences. *The Annals of thoracic surgery,* 2000, 70, 140–144.

Sodian, R; Sperling, JS; Martin, DP; Stock, U; Mayer, JE Jr; Vacanti, JP. Tissue engineering of a trileaflet heart valve. Early *in vivo* experiences with a combined polymer. *Tissue Engineering,* 1999, 5, 489–493.

Stock, U; Nagashima, M; Khalil, PN; Nollert, GD; Herden, T; Sperling, JS; Moran, A; Lien, J; Martin DP; Schoen, FJ; Vacanti, JP; Mayer, JE Jr. Tissue-engineered valved conduits in the pulmonary circulation. *The Journal of thoracic and cardiovascular surgery,* 2000, 119, 732 –7 40.

Struchkov, VI; Grigoryan, AV; Gostishchev, VK. Purulent wound. Moscow: Meditsina; 1975 (in Russian).

Sudesh, K. Microbial polyhydroxyalkanoates (PHAs): an emerging biomaterial for tissue engineering and therapeutic applications. *The Medical journal of Malaysia,* 2004, 59, 55–66.

Sudesh, K; Abe, H; Doi, Y. Synthesis, structure and properties of polyhydroxyalkanoates: biological polyesters. Progress in Polymer Science, 2000, 25, 1503–1555.

Sudesh, K; Loo, CY; Goh, LK; Iwata, T; Maeda, M. The oil-absorbing property of polyhydroxyalkanoate films and its practical application: a refreshing new outlook for an old degrading material. *Macromolecular Bioscience,* 2007, 7, 1199–1205.

Taylor, G. Electrically driven jets. *Proceedings of the Royal Society of London. Series A, Mathematical and Physical Sciences,* 1969, A313(1515), 453–475.

Tezcaner, A; Bugra, K; Hasirci, V. Retinal pigment epithelium cell culture on surface modified poly(hydroxybutyrate-cohydroxyvalerate) thin films. *Biomaterials,* 2003, 24, 4573–4583.

Tong, HW; Wang, M. Electrospinning of aligned biodegradable polymer fiber and composite fibers for tissue engineering applications. *Journal of nanoscience and nanotechnology,* 2007, 7, 3834–3841.

Tong, HW; Wang, M; Lu, WL. Electrospinning of Poly(Hydroxybuturate-co-hydroxyvalerate) Fibrous Membranes Consisting of Paralled-Aligned Fibers or Cross-Aligned Fibers: Characterization and Biological Evaluation. *Journal of Biomaterials Science. Polymer Edition,* 2012, 22, 2475–2497.

Unverdorben, M; Spielberger, A; Schywalsky, M; Labahn, D; Harting, S; Schneider, M; Lootz, D; Behrend, D; Schmitz, K; Degenhardt, R; Schaldach, M; Vallbracht, C. A Polyhydroxybutyrate Biodegradable Stent: Preliminary Experience in the Rabbit. *CardioVascular and Interventional Radiology,* 2002, 25, 127–132.

Volova, TG. Polyhydroxyalkanoates – Plastic Materials of the 21st Century: production, properties, application. NY, USA: Nova Science Pub Inc; 2004.

Volova, TG; Goncharov, DB; Sukovatyi, AG; Shabanov, AV; Nikolaeva, ED; Shishatskaya, EI. Electrospinning of polyhydroxyalkanoate fibrous scaffolds: effect on electrospinning parameters on structure and properties. *Journal of Biomaterials Science. Polymer Edition,* 2014b, 25, 370–393.

Volova, TG; Kiselev, EG; Vinogradova, ON; Nikolaeva, ED; Chistyakov, AA; Sukovatyi, AG; Shishatskaya, EI. A glucose-utilizing strain, *Cupriavidus eutrophus* B-10646: growth kinetics, characterization and synthesis of multicomponent PHAs. *PloS One,* 2014a, 9, 87551–87566.

Volova, TG; Sevastyanov, VI; Shishatskaya, EI. Polyhydroxyalkanoates – biodegradable polymers for medicine. In: Shumakov VI, editor. Novosibirsk: SB RAS Publishers, 2003 (in Russian).

Volova, TG; Shishatskaya, EI. Biodegradable polymers: synthesis, properties, applications. In: Sinskey AJ, editor. Krasnoyarsk: Krasnoyarskii Pisatel; 2011 (in Russian).

Volova, TG; Shishatskaya, EI. Results of biomedical studies of PHAs produced in the Institute of Biophysics SB RAS and Siberian Federal University. In: Wu LP, editor. *Polyhydroxyalkanoates (PHA): Biosynthesis, Industrial Production and Applications in Medicine.* NY, USA: Nova Scienses Pub Inc; 2014, 273–330.

Volova, TG; Shishatskaya, EI; Gordeev, SA. Characterization of ultrafine fibers electrospun from a thermoplastic polyester, poly(3-hydroxybutyrate-co-3-hydroxyvalerate). *Perspektivnyye materialy (Advanced materials),* 2006a, 3, 25–29 (in Russian).

Volova, TG; Shishatskaya, EI; Sinskey, AJ. Degradable Polymers: Production, Properties and Applications. NY, USA: Nova Science Pub Inc; 2013.

Volova, TG; Vasiliev, AD; Zeer, EP. Investigation of molecular structure of poly(3-hydroxybutyrate), a thermoplastic and degradable polymer. *Biofizika (Biophysics),* 2000, 45, 33–439 (in Russian).

Volova, TG; Voinov, NA; Muratov, VS; Bubnov, NV; Gurulev, KV; Kalacheva, GS; Gorbuova, NV; Plotnikov, VF; Zhila, NO; Shishatskaya, EI; Belyaeva, OG. Pilot production of degradable biopolymers. *Biotekhnologiya (Biotechnology),* 2006b, 6, 28–34 (in Russian).

Walker, MNM; Wright, KT; Fuller, HR; MacNeil, S; Johnson, WEB. Mesenchymal stem cell-conditioned medium accelerates skin wound healing: An *in vitro* study of fibroblast and keratinocyte scratch assays. *Experimental Cell Research,* 2010, 316, 1271–1281.

Walker, NG; Mistry, AR; Smith, LE; Eves, PC; Tsaknakis, G; Forster, S; Watt, SM; MacNeil, S. A Chemically Defined Carrier for the Delivery of Human Mesenchymal Stem/Stromal Cells to Skin Wounds. *Tissue Engineering. Part C, Methods,* 2012, 18, 143–155.

Wang, L; Wang, ZH; Shen, CY; You, ML; Xiao, JF; Chen, GQ. Differentiation of human bone marrow mesenchymal stem cells grown in terpolyesters of 3-hydroxyalkanoates scaffolds into nerve cells. *Biomaterials*, 2010, 31, 1691–1698.

Wang, M. Developing bioactive composite materials for tissue replacement. *Biomaterials,* 2003, 24, 2133–2151.

Wang, Y; Cao, R; Wang, PP; Jian, J; Jiang, XL; Yan, C; Lin, X; Wu, L; Chen, GQ; Wu, Q. The differential effects of aligned electrospun PHBHHx fibers on adipogenic and asteogenic potencial of MSCs through the regeneration of PPARг signaling. *Biomaterials,* 2012, 33, 485–493.

Weiner, RM. Biopolymers from marine prokaryotes. *Trends in Biotechnology,* 1997, 15, 390–394.

Williams, SF; Martin, DP; Horowitz, DM; Peoples, OP. PHA applications: addressing the price performance issue. I. Tissue engineering. *International Journal of Biological Macromolecules,* 1999, 25, 11–121.

Yang, EK; Seo, YK; Youn, HH; Lee, DH; Park, SN; Park, JK. Tissue Engineered Artificial Skin Composed of Dermis and Epidermis. *Artificial Organs,* 2000, 24, 7–17.

Ying, TH; Ishii, D; Mahara, A; Murakami, S; Yamaoka, T; Sudesh, K; Samian, R; Fujita, M; Maeda, M; Iwata, T. Scaffolds from electrospun polyhydroxyalkanoate copolimers: Fabrication, characterization, bioabsorbtion and tissue response. *Biomaterials,* 2008, 29, 1307–1317.

You, M; Peng, G; Li, J; Ma, P; Wang, Z; Shu, W; Peng, S; Chen, GQ. Chondrogenic differentiation of human bone marrow mesenchymal stem cells on polyhydroxyalkanoate (PHA) scaffolds coated with PHA granule binding protein PhaP fused with RGD peptide. *Biomaterials,* 2011, 32, 2305–2313.

Yu, BY; Chen, PY; Sun, YM; Lee, YT; Young, TH. Response of Human Mesenchymal Stem Cells (hMSC) to the Topographic Variation of Poly(3-Hydroxybutyrate-co-3-Hydroxyhexanoate) (PHBHHx) Films. *Journal of* Biomaterials Science. Polymer Edition, 2012, 23, 1–26.

Biographical Sketches

Tatiana Grigorievna Volova

Affiliation: Professor, Doctor of biological sciences in microbiology

Education: Krasnoyarsk State Pedagogical University

Business Address: Institute of Biophysics SB RAS, Akademgorodok, Krasnoyarsk 660036, Russia. +7(3912)2494428. volova45@mail.ru;

Research and Professional Experience:

Professor Volova is conducting research in the field of physico-chemical biology and biotechnology. She is well-known expert in the field of microbial physiology and biotechnology. Tatiana Volova has created and developed a new and original branch in chemoautotrophic biosynthesis, in which the two main directions of the XXI century technologies are conjugate – hydrogen energy and biotechnology. The obtained fundamental results had provided a significant outputs – were developed the unique biotechnical producing systems, based on hydrogen biosynthesis for single-cell protein, amino-acids, enzymes; under the guidance of Prof. Volova the pilot production facility of single cell protein, utilizing hydrogen, had been created and run into operation. The possibility of involvement of man-made sources of hydrogen into biotechnological processes as a substrate, including synthesis gas from brown coals and vegetable wastes, was demonstrated in the research of Prof. Volova. She had initiated and deployed in Russia the comprehensive research on microbial degradable bioplastics; results of this research are covering various aspects of biosynthesis, metabolism, physiological role, structure and properties of these biopolymers, polyhydroxyalcanoates (PHAs), and have made a scientific basis for their biomedical applications. and allowed to deploy the topping biomedical research. Professor TatianaVolova is the author of more than 300 scientific works, including 12 monographs, 16 inventions; series of textbooks for universities.

Professional Appointments: Head of Laboratory of Chemoautotrophic Biosynthesis at the Institute of Biophysics, Siberian Branch of the Russian Academy of Sciences; Head of Biotechnology Department at the Siberian Federal University. Russia. Sc. D. Professor.

Honors: State Award of Russian Federation - Second Class Medal of the Order "For Merit to the Fatherland"; diplomas and notes of thanks of President of Russian Federation, Presidium of Russian Academy of Science.

Publications from the Last 3 Years:

Volova, TG; Shishatskaya, EI. Results of biomedical studies of PHAs produced in Institute of Biophysics SB RAS and Siberian Federal University. In: Wu LP, editor. Polyhydroxyalkanoates (PHA): Biosynthesis, Industrial Production and Applications in Medicine. NY, USA: Nova Sciensеs Publ. Inc.; 2014; 331–349.

Volova, TG; Kiselev, EG; Vinogradova, ON; Nikolaeva, ED; Chistyakov, AA; Sukovatyi, AG; Shishatskaya, EI. A glucose-utilizing strain, Cupriavidus eutrophus B-10646: growth kinetics, characterization and synthesis of multicomponent PHAs. Plos One, 2014, 9, 1–15.

Volova, TG; Goncharov, DB; Sukovatyi, AG; Shabanov, AV; Nikolaeva, ED; Shishatskaya, EI. Electrospinning of polyhydroxyalkanoate fibrous scaffolds: effect on electrospinning parameters on structure and properties. Journal of Biomaterials Science. Polymer Edition, 2014b, 25, 370–393.

Shishatskaya, EI; Volova, TG; Goreva, AV; Nikolaeva, ED; Sinskey, AJ. An in vivo study of 2D PHA matrixes of different chemical compositions: tissue reactions and biodegradations. Materials Science and Technology, 2014, 30, 549–557.

Zhila, NO; Kalacheva, GS; Volova, TG. Fatty acid composition and polyhydroxyalkanoates production by Cupriavidus eutrophus B-10646 cells grown on different carbon sources. Process Biochemistry, 2015, 50, 69–78.

Volova, TG; Zhila, NO; Shishatskaya, EI. Synthesis of poly(3-hydroxybutyrate) by the autotrophic CO-oxidizing bacterium Seliberia carboxydohydrogena Z-1062. The Journal of Industrial Microbiology and Biotechnology, 2015, 42, 1377–1387.

Volova, TG; Tarasevich, AA; Golubev, AI; Boyandin, AN; Shumilova, AA; Nikolaeva, ED; Shishatskaya, EI. Laser processing of polymer constructs from poly(3-hydroxybutyrate). Journal of Biomaterials Science. Polymer Edition, 2015, 26, 1210–1228.

Shishatskaya, EI; Nikolaeva, ED; Vinogradova, ON; Volova, TG. Experimental wound dressings of degradable PHA for skin defect repair. Journal of Materials Science: Materials in Medicine, 2016, 27, 1–16.

Volova, TG; Zhila, NO; Kiselev, EG; Prudnikova, SV; Vinogradova, ON; Nikolaeva, ED; Shumilova, AA; Shershneva, AM; Shishatskaya, EI. Poly(3-hydroxybutyrate)/metribuzin formulations: characterization, controlled release properties, herbicidal activity, and effect on soil microorganisms. Environmental Science and Pollution Research, 2016. DOI 10.1007/s11356-016-7636-7.

Volova, TG; Prudnikova, SV; Vinogradova, ON; Syrvacheva, DA; Shishatskaya, EI. Microbial degradation of polyhydroxyalkanoates with different chemical compositions and their biodegradability. Microbial Ecology, 2016. DOI: 10.1007/s00248-016-0852-3.

Volova, TG; Prudnikova, SV; Zhila, NO; Vinogradova, ON; Shumilova, AA; Nikolaeva, ED; Kiselev, EG; Shishatskaya, EI. Efficacy of tebuconazole embedded in biodegradable poly-3-hydroxybutyrate to inhibit the development of Fusarium moniliforme in soil microecosystems. Pest Management Science, 2016. DOI 10.1002/ps.4367.

Volova, TG; Vinogradova, ON; Zhila, NO; Peterson, IV; Kiselev, EG; Vasiliev, AD; Sukovatiy, AG; Shishatskaya, EI. Properties of a novel quaterpolymer P(3HB/4HB/3HV/3HHx). Polymer, 2016, 101, 67–74.

Syromotina, DS; Surmenev, RA; Surmeneva, MA; Boyandin, AN; Epple, M; Ulbricht, M; Oehr, C; Volova, TG. Oxygen and ammonia plasma treatment of poly(3-hydroxybutyrate) films for controlled surface zeta potential and improved cell compatibility. Materials Letters, 2016, 163, 277–280.

Volova, TG; Zhila, NO; Kiselev, EG; Shishatskaya, EI. A study of synthesis and properties of poly-3-hydroxybutyrate/diethylene glycol copolymers. Biotechnology Progress, 2016, 32, 1017 – 1028.

Volova, TG; Zhila, NO; Vinogradova, ON; Nikolaeva, ED; Kiselev, EG; Shumilova, AA; Shershneva, AM; Shishatskaya, EI. Constructing herbicide metribuzin sustained-release formulations based on the natural polymer poly-3-hydroxybutyrate as a degradable matrix. Journal of Environmental Science and Health, Part B. 2016, 51, 113–125.

Syromotina, DS; Surmenev, RA; Surmeneva, MA; Boyandin, AN; Nikolaeva, D; Prymak, O; Epple, M; Ulbricht, M; Oehr, C; Volova, TG. Surface wettability and energy effects on the biological performance of poly-3-hydroxybutyrate films treated with RF plasma. Materials Science & Engineering C, 2016, 62, 450–457.

Volova, TG; Prudnikova, SV; Boyandin, AN. Biodegradable poly-3-hydroxybutyrate as a fertilizer carrier. Journal of the Science of Food and Agriculture, 2016, 96, 4183–4193.

Boyandin, AN; Zhila, NO; Kiselev, EG; Volova, TG. Constructing slow-release formulations of metribuzin based on degradable poly(3-hydroxybutyrate). Journal of Agricultural and Food Chemistry, 2016, 64, 5625–5632.

Volova, TG; Syrvacheva, DA; Zhila, NO; Sukovatiy, AG. Synthesis of P(3HB-co-3HHx) copolymers containing high molar fraction of 3-hydroxyhexanoate monomer by Cupriavidus eutrophus B10646. Journal of chemical technology and biotechnology, 2016, 91, 416–425.

Volova, TG; Zhila N., Vinogradova, ON; Shumilova, AA; Prudnikova, SV; Shishatskaya, EI. Characterization of biodegradable poly-3-hydroxybutyrate films and pellets loaded with the fungicide tebuconazole. Environmental Science and Pollution Research. 2016. V.23. P.5243-5254.

Shumilova, AA; Myltygashev, MP; Kirichenko, AK; Nikolaeva, ED; Volova, TG; Shishatskaya, EI. Porous 3D implants of degradable poly-3-hydroxybutyrate used to enhance regeneration of rat cranial defect. Journal of Biomedical Materials Research: Part A, 2017, 105, 566–577.

Volova, TG; Vinogradova, ON; Zhila, NO; Kiselev, EG; Peterson, IV; Vasil'ev, AD; Shishatskaya, EI. Physicochemical Properties of Multicomponent Polyhydroxyalkanoates: Novel Aspects. Polymer Science, Series A, 2017, 59, 98–106.

Ekaterina Igorevna Shishatskaya

Affiliation: Professor, Doctor of biological sciences in biotechnology

Education: Krasnoyarsk State Medical University named after Professor V.F. Voino-Yasenetsky

Business Address: Akademgorodok, Krasnoyarsk 660036,
Russia. +7(3912)2494428. shishatskaya@inbox.ru.

Research and Professional Experience:

Ekaterina I. Shishatskaya is supervises the direction of biomedical research of new materials. Field of research experience of Dr. Shishatskaya – an investigation of interaction mechanisms between biomaterials and biological objects, and development of high-tech biomedical devices. This actual science direction is oriented to the development of new reconstructive biomedical technologies, includes cell biology and tissue engineering. Biodegradable polymers of carbon acids – polyhydroxyalkanoates, PHAs – are new class of materials for medicine, are under active investigation in a world; Dr. Shishatskaya is Russian leader in comprehensive medical and biological studies of this class of polymers. Completed pioneer study of developed polymer compounds and products of them have shown fool compliance with the requirements for materials and devices for medicine, and proved suitability of PHAs for reconstruction of defects in soft and hard tissues, in a forms of film coatings, an independent implants, surgical sutures and matrixes for various cell types; also, PHAs have big potential as a carriers in modern drug delivering systems. Professional activity of Dr. Shishatskaya also is aimed to the implementation of the obtained results into practice, and contains communication with clinical centers and topping specialists in regenerative medicine. Dr. Shishatskaya is author of about 150 research works, including 5 monographs and 8 patents. She is the winner of the President of Russian Federation for youth in the field of science and innovations; has State Prize of Krasnoyarsk Region in the area of high education and science and is a laureate of L'Oréal-UNESCO for young women in science.

Professional Appointments: Institute of Biophysics, Leading Researcher of Laboratory of Chemoautotrophic Biosynthesis; Siberian Branch of the Russian Academy of Sciences; the Siberian Federal University. Head of Department of Medical Biology.

Honors: A laureate of the Prize of President of Russian Federation for young people in the area of science and innovetions; a laureate of the State Prize of Krasnoyarskiy kray; a prize-winner of awards of eminent scientists of Siberian Branch of RAS; a laureate of the Russian National Prize «Future of suture materials», the Prize of Academician Lavrentiev, the Prize of the Association "Siberian Agreement"; a laureat of the L'Oréal-UNESCO Award for Women in Science.

Publications from the Last 3 Years:

Volova, TG; Shishatskaya, EI. Results of biomedical studies of PHAs produced in Institute of Biophysics SB RAS and Siberian Federal University. In: Wu LP, editor. Polyhydroxyalkanoates (PHA): Biosynthesis, Industrial Production and Applications in Medicine. NY, USA: Nova Scienses Publ. Inc.; 2014; 331–349.

Shishatskaya, EI; Kamendov, IV; Starosvetsky, SI; Vinnik, YS; Markelova, NN; Shageev, AA; Khorzhevsky, VA; Peryanova, OV; Shumilova, AA. An in vivo study of osteoplastic properties of resorbable poly-3-hydroxybutyrate in models of segmental osteotomy and chronic osteomyelitis. Artificial Cells, Nanomedicine and Biotechnology, 2014, 42, 344–355.

Volova, TG; Kiselev, EG; Vinogradova, ON; Nikolaeva, ED; Chistyakov, AA; Sukovatyi, AG; Shishatskaya, EI. A glucose-utilizing strain, Cupriavidus eutrophus B-10646: growth kinetics, characterization and synthesis of multicomponent PHAs. Plos One, 2014, 9, 1–15.

Volova, TG; Goncharov, DB; Sukovatyi, AG; Shabanov, AV; Nikolaeva, ED; Shishatskaya, EI. Electrospinning of polyhydroxyalkanoate fibrous scaffolds: effect on electrospinning parameters on structure and properties. Journal of Biomaterials Science. Polymer Edition, 2014b, 25, 370–393.

Shishatskaya, EI; Volova, TG; Goreva, AV; Nikolaeva, ED; Sinskey, AJ. An in vivo study of 2D PHA matrixes of different chemical compositions: tissue reactions and biodegradations. Materials Science and Technology, 2014, 30, 549–557.

Eke, G; Kuzmina, AM; Goreva, AV; Shishatskaya, EI; Hasirci, N; Hasirci, V. In vitro and transdermal penetration of PHBV micro/nanoparticles. Journal of Materials Science: Materials in Medicine, 2014, 25, 1471–1481.

Volova, TG; Zhila, NO; Shishatskaya, EI. Synthesis of poly(3-hydroxybutyrate) by the autotrophic CO-oxidizing bacterium Seliberia carboxydohydrogena Z-1062. The Journal of Industrial Microbiology and Biotechnology, 2015, 42, 1377–1387.

Volova, TG; Tarasevich, AA; Golubev, AI; Boyandin, AN; Shumilova, AA; Nikolaeva, ED; Shishatskaya, EI. Laser processing of polymer constructs from poly(3-hydroxybutyrate). Journal of Biomaterials Science. Polymer Edition, 2015, 26, 1210–1228.

Shishatskaya, EI; Nikolaeva, ED; Vinogradova, ON; Volova, TG. Experimental wound dressings of degradable PHA for skin defect repair. Journal of Materials Science: Materials in Medicine, 2016, 27, 1–16.

Volova, TG; Zhila, NO; Kiselev, EG; Prudnikova, SV; Vinogradova, ON; Nikolaeva, ED; Shumilova, AA; Shershneva, AM; Shishatskaya, EI. Poly(3-hydroxybutyrate)/metribuzin formulations: characterization, controlled release properties, herbicidal activity, and effect on soil microorganisms. Environmental Science and Pollution Research, 2016. DOI 10.1007/s11356-016-7636-7.

Volova, TG; Prudnikova, SV; Vinogradova, ON; Syrvacheva, DA; Shishatskaya, EI. Microbial degradation of polyhydroxyalkanoates with different chemical compositions and their biodegradability. Microbial Ecology, 2016. DOI: 10.1007/s00248-016-0852-3.

Volova, TG; Prudnikova, SV; Zhila, NO; Vinogradova, ON; Shumilova, AA; Nikolaeva, ED; Kiselev, EG; Shishatskaya, EI. Efficacy of tebuconazole embedded in biodegradable poly-3-hydroxybutyrate to inhibit the development of Fusarium moniliforme in soil microecosystems. Pest Management Science, 2016. DOI 10.1002/ps.4367.

Volova, TG; Vinogradova, ON; Zhila, NO; Peterson, IV; Kiselev, EG; Vasiliev, AD; Sukovatiy, AG; Shishatskaya, EI. Properties of a novel quaterpolymer P(3HB/4HB/3HV/3HHx). Polymer, 2016, 101, 67–74.

Volova, TG; Zhila, NO; Kiselev, EG; Shishatskaya, EI. A study of synthesis and properties of poly-3-hydroxybutyrate/diethylene glycol copolymers. Biotechnology Progress, 2016, 32, 1017–1028.

Volova, TG; Zhila, NO; Vinogradova, ON; Nikolaeva, ED; Kiselev, EG; Shumilova, AA; Shershneva, AM; Shishatskaya, EI. Constructing herbicide metribuzin sustained-release formulations based on the natural polymer poly-3-hydroxybutyrate as a degradable matrix. Journal of Environmental Science and Health, Part B. 2016, 51, 113–125.

Volova, TG; Zhila N., Vinogradova, ON; Shumilova, AA; Prudnikova, SV; Shishatskaya, EI. Characterization of biodegradable poly-3-hydroxybutyrate films and pellets loaded with the fungicide tebuconazole. Environmental Science and Pollution Research. 2016. V.23. P.5243-5254.

Piperigkou, Z; Karamanou, K; Engin, AB; Gialeli, C; Docea, AO; Vynios, D; Pavao, M;. Golokhvast, K; Shtilman, M; Argiris, A; Shishatskaya, E; Tsatsakis, A. Emerging aspects of nanotoxicology in health and disease: from agriculture and food sector to cancer therapeutics. Food and Chemical Toxicology, 2016, 91, 42–57.

Shishatskaya, EI; Nikitovic, D; Shabanov, A; Tzanakakis, GN; Tsatsakis, AM; Menzianova, NG. Short-term culture of monocytes as an in vitro evaluation system for bionanomaterials designated for medical use. Food and Chemical Toxicology, 2016, 96, 302–308.

Shumilova, AA; Myltygashev, MP; Kirichenko, AK; Nikolaeva, ED; Volova, TG; Shishatskaya, EI. Porous 3D implants of degradable poly-3-hydroxybutyrate used to enhance regeneration of rat cranial defect. Journal of Biomedical Materials Research: Part A, 2017, 105, 566–577.

Volova, TG; Vinogradova, ON; Zhila, NO; Kiselev, EG; Peterson, IV; Vasil'ev, AD; Shishatskaya, EI. Physicochemical Properties of Multicomponent Polyhydroxyalkanoates: Novel Aspects. Polymer Science, Series A, 2017, 59, 98–106.

Elena Dmitrievna Nikolaeva

Affiliation: PhD of biological sciences in biotechnology, researcher

Education: Siberian Federal University

Business Address: Institute of Biophysics SB RAS, Akademgorodok, Krasnoyarsk 660036, Russia. +7(391) 2905491, nikolaeva-lena@mail.ru

Research and Professional Experience:
Elena D. Nikolayeva is a member of staff of Laboratory of Chemoautotrophic Biosynthesis and Laboratory of Biotechnology of New Biomaterials in Siberian Federal University. Area of scientific interests is cell biology and tissue engineering. Nikolaeva is researching the biocompatibility of new types of biopolymers, design of bioartificial skin, and investigation of interaction between cells and biopolymeric substrates.

Professional Appointments: Institute of Biophysics, Researcher of Laboratory of Chemoautotrophic Biosynthesis.

Publications from the Last 3 Years:

Volova, TG; Kiselev, EG; Vinogradova, ON; Nikolaeva, ED; Chistyakov, AA; Sukovatyi, AG; Shishatskaya, EI. A glucose-utilizing strain, *Cupriavidus eutrophus* B-10646: growth kinetics, characterization and synthesis of multicomponent PHAs. *Plos One,* 2014, 9, 1–15.

Volova, TG; Goncharov, DB; Sukovatyi, AG; Shabanov, AV; Nikolaeva, ED; Shishatskaya, EI. Electrospinning of polyhydroxyalkanoate fibrous scaffolds: effect on electrospinning parameters on structure and properties. *Journal of Biomaterials Science. Polymer Edition,* 2014b, 25, 370–393.

Shishatskaya, EI; Volova, TG; Goreva, AV; Nikolaeva, ED; Sinskey, AJ. An *in vivo* study of 2D PHA matrixes of different chemical compositions: tissue reactions and biodegradations. *Materials Science and Technology,* 2014, 30, 549–557.

Volova, TG; Tarasevich, AA; Golubev, AI; Boyandin, AN; Shumilova, AA; Nikolaeva, ED; Shishatskaya, EI. Laser processing of polymer constructs from poly(3-hydroxybutyrate). *Journal of Biomaterials Science. Polymer Edition,* 2015, 26, 1210–1228.

Shishatskaya, EI; Nikolaeva, ED; Vinogradova, ON; Volova, TG. Experimental wound dressings of degradable PHA for skin defect repair. *Journal of Materials Science: Materials in Medicine,* 2016, 27, 1–16.

Volova, TG; Zhila, NO; Kiselev, EG; Prudnikova, SV; Vinogradova, ON; Nikolaeva, ED; Shumilova, AA; Shershneva, AM; Shishatskaya, EI. Poly(3-hydroxybutyrate)/metribuzin formulations: characterization, controlled release properties, herbicidal activity, and effect on soil microorganisms. *Environmental Science and Pollution Research,* 2016. DOI 10.1007/s11356-016-7636-7.

Volova, TG; Prudnikova, SV; Zhila, NO; Vinogradova, ON; Shumilova, AA; Nikolaeva, ED; Kiselev, EG; Shishatskaya, EI. Efficacy of tebuconazole embedded in biodegradable poly-3-hydroxybutyrate to inhibit the development of Fusarium moniliforme in soil microecosystems. *Pest Management Science,* 2016. DOI 10.1002/ps.4367.

Volova, TG; Zhila, NO; Vinogradova, ON; Nikolaeva, ED; Kiselev, EG; Shumilova, AA; Shershneva, AM; Shishatskaya, EI. Constructing herbicide metribuzin sustained-release formulations based on the natural polymer poly-3-hydroxybutyrate as a degradable matrix. *Journal of Environmental Science and Health, Part B.* 2016, 51, 113–125.

Syromotina, DS; Surmenev, RA; Surmeneva, MA; Boyandin, AN; Nikolaeva, D; Prymak, O; Epple, M; Ulbricht, M; Oehr, C; Volova, TG. Surface wettability and energy effects on the biological performance of poly-3-hydroxybutyrate films treated with RF plasma. *Materials Science & Engineering C,* 2016, 62, 450–457.

Shumilova, AA; Myltygashev, MP; Kirichenko, AK; Nikolaeva, ED; Volova, TG; Shishatskaya, EI. Porous 3D implants of degradable poly-3-hydroxybutyrate used to enhance regeneration of rat cranial defect. *Journal of Biomedical Materials Research: Part A,* 2017, 105, 566–577.

Borovkova, NV; Evseeva, AK; Makarova, MS; Goroncharovskaya, IV; Vinogradova, ON; Nikolaeva, ED; Goncharov, DB. Study of Biocompatible Films and Nonwoven Membranes Made of Copolymer of 3-hydroxybutyric Acid and 4-hydroxybutyric Acid *in vitro. Journal of Siberian Federal University. Biology,* 2016, 9, 43–52.

Dmitrii Boricovich Goncharov

Affiliation: Researcher

Education: Siberian Federal University. Post-graduate student in Biotechnology.

Business Address: Akademgorodok, Krasnoyarsk 660036,
Russia. +7(3912)2494428. e.mail: dima281088@mail.ru

Research and Professional Experience:

D.Goncharov is a specialist in the area of electrostatic polymer formation. He has investigated conditions of electrostatic polymer formation from solutions of polyhydroxyalkanoates of different chemical composition and has fine-tuned a technology of obtaining good-quality non-woven nanomembranes. He has demonstrated high biocompatibility of electrospun polymeric goods and their suitability for cell technologies in cell tissue and animal experiments. He has prepared and submitted for defense his thesis “Biosynthesis of polyhydroxyalkanoates: the effect of the chemical composition on polymer properties and characteristics of non-woven electrospun materials”

Professional Appointments: Researcher of Laboratory of Chemoautotrophic Biosynthesis; Siberian Branch of the Russian Academy of Sciences

Honors: Diplomas of the winner of young scientist competitions of different Russian and International scientific forums

Publications from the Last 3 Years:

Volova, TG; Goncharov, DB; Sukovatyi, AG; Shabanov, AV; Nikolaeva, ED; Shishatskaya, EI. Electrospinning of polyhydroxyalkanoate fibrous scaffolds: effect on electrospinning parameters on structure and properties. *Journal of Biomaterials Science. Polymer Edition,* 2014b, 25, 370–393.

Borovkova, NV; Evseeva, AK; Makarova, MS; Goroncharovskaya, IV; Vinogradova, ON; Nikolaeva, ED; Goncharov, DB. Study of Biocompatible Films and Nonwoven Membranes Made of Copolymer of 3-hydroxybutyric Acid and 4-hydroxybutyric Acid *in vitro. Journal of Siberian Federal University. Biology,* 2016, 9, 43–52.

Borovkova, NV; Evseeva, AK; Andreeva, YV; Goncharov, DB; Shishatskaya, EI. Wound Dressings Made of Biodegradable Natural Polymers Polyhydroxyalkanoates (PHAs): Production and Properties. *Journal of Siberian Federal University. Biology,* 2016, 9, 88–97.

Goncharov, DB; Sukovatyi, AG. Rheology of Polyhydroxyalkanoate Solutions. *Journal of Siberian Federal University. Biology,* 2016, 9, 190–197.

Goncharov, DB; Sukovatyi, AG. Properties of Fibrous Scaffolds from Poly(3-Hydroxybutyrate), Polylactide, Polyglycolide and Poly(Lactide-Glycolide) with Various Methods of Electrostatic Forming. *Journal of Siberian Federal University. Biology,* 2016, 9, 212–222.

In: Electrospinning and Electroplating
Editor: Toby Jacobs
ISBN: 978-1-53612-363-0

Chapter 2

The Use of Water-Soluble Polymers in Electro-Spinning and Their Application Fields

Renato Carajelescov Nonato and Sílvia Vaz Guerra Nista
School of Chemical Engineering, State University of Campinas,
Campinas, SP, Brazil

Abstract

With the increasing dominance of the electrospinning process, the diversity of materials that have already been tested in this area increases, so an interesting group of polymers is highlighted due to its solubility in water. A great advantage in the use of these polymers is that they have low indices of toxicity and biocompatible features, what give to them a wide range of applications. Among the water-soluble polymers most commonly used in electrospinning, we can mention PVA, PVP, PEG, PEO, collagen, chitosan, alginate among others, with applications in industry, commerce, medical and food. A highly exploited application of water-soluble polymer nanofibers is in the field of medicine, including tissue engineering, drug delivery vehicles, cell growth, curatives, etc. A new area that has been highlighted is the use of these polymers as sacrificial polymers, helping in the production of ceramic nanofibers. Ceramic nanofibers have been gaining attention because of their good mechanical properties, thermal and corrosion resistance. They have been studied as agents for the release of drugs in the health area, but also as components for photoelectrodes, such as sensors, catalysts, filtering agents, among others.

This chapter aims to give an insight into the use of this interesting class of polymers in electrospinning as well as to explore the wide range of possible applications.

Keywords: water-soluble polymers, electrospinning, ceramic nanofibers

Introduction

The dominance of the electrospinning process is increasing, and an interesting group of polymers gains prominence due to its solubility in water. Water-soluble polymers have a great advantage in their use due to the low toxicity rates and biocompatible characteristics, making them present a wide range of applications.

Water-soluble polymers have a wide range of applications currently in various fields, including food and pharmaceutical industries, paint, textiles, paper, construction, adhesives, coatings and water treatment (Halake et al., 2014). Traditional uses include additives to thickeners and antifoams, binders, electrolytic solvents, lubricants, stabilizers, dispersants, surfactants, laxatives, and excipients. These polymers are substances which dissolve, disperse or swelling in water and thus modify the physical properties of aqueous systems in form of gelling, thickening or emulsification/stabilization. The polymer chains contain hydrophilic groups which may be nonionic, anionic, cationic or amphoteric (Kadajji et al., 2011).

Electrospinning is an incredibly simple and versatile technique for the preparation of nanostructured materials with a wide range of compositions for various applications. The process is based on one electrode connected to a high voltage source, which is fixed in the capillary tube containing the polymer solution, while the other electrode is fixed to a metal collector, usually a copper or aluminum plate. The capillary and the collector are usually kept at a short distance from each other, and during the tests, the polymer solution is pressed by the syringe plunger, until it reaches the tip of the needle. The drop formed at the needle tip is initially pendant due to the surface tension, with a nonzero net charge due to the action of the electric field. Electrical charges on the surface of the counter electrode cause a force directly opposite to the surface tension. Increasing the electric field to a critical value, electrostatic forces overcome the surface tension, resulting in a hollow cone of fluid, which is ejected, known as the Taylor cone. From the time when the solution is transferred from the syringe until the time it is collected, the solvent evaporates and the dry fibers are deposited, 1 usually in the form of a nonwoven blanket. Alternatively, one could obtain these electrospun fibers aligned, with various degrees of order and direction, by using a dynamic collector (Nista et al., 2012).

When organic solvents are used in the electrospinning process, residual solvent is found in the nanofiber membranes, because of this there are several drawbacks regarding the use of these in some applications. In the electrospinning process, the evaporation of organic solvents would result in air pollution with solvent residues, and when nanofiber membranes are used as scaffolds for cell growth, they may present problems including decreased cell binding, proliferation, growth, and so on. Thus, electrospun nanofibers from water-soluble polymers should be considered as potential options in biomaterial, application in tissue engineering and development of eco-friendly materials (Sun et al., 2010).

The hydrophilic functional groups, such as ether, alcohol, amide and pyrrolidone, are biocompatible and non-toxic. While linear polymers dissolve readily in water, crosslinked polymers form insoluble hydrogels. The use of water-soluble polymer in electrospinning is very promising due to the non-toxicity. However, the number of water-soluble polymers is limited and furthermore, the electrospun materials produced will dissolve in a future application in contact with water. The water stability of water-soluble polymers electrospun, when necessary, is accomplished by various cross-linking methods (Khorshidi et al., 2016). The use of hydrogen bonding or copolymerization is often an excellent strategy for increasing their insolubility in the final material (Halake et al., 2014).

These polymers are divided into two categories: natural and synthetic. Among the available water-soluble synthetic polymers are polyethylene glycol, polyvinyl alcohol, polyacrylamide, polyvinylpyrrolidone and poly (N-isopropyl acrylamide) and naturals we can mention alginate, chitosan, collagen and others (Halake et al., 2014).

The recent nanotechnology developments in environmental engineering, biomedical engineering, and information technology, these polymers with biocompatible and environmentally properties have received increased attention (Halake et al., 2014). These new applications cover a wide range in the medical field such as transporters in drug delivery, scaffolds in tissue engineering, medical devices implantation and artificial organs, prostheses, ophthalmology, dentistry, bone repair, but also as components for photoelectrodes such as sensors, catalysts, filtering agents, environmental applications such as heavy metal removers, among others (Halake et al., 2014).

In tissue engineering these materials have received great attention from the scientific community because, when properly designed, they are able to replace and allow the growth and regeneration of the body tissues, permanently, without toxic effects and with inflammatory processes, and when present, are discrete and tolerable. Electrospinning has been shown to be a powerful tool for manufacturing scaffolds for tissue engineering as it is simple, inexpensive, versatile and capable of forming structures that serve as a substitute for the native extracellular matrix (ECM) and plays a crucial role in tissue regeneration by providing support cells during the formation of natural ECM (Khorshidi et al., 2016).

There is increasing interest in bioabsorbable polymeric materials, such as most water-soluble materials, which undergo hydrolysis and enzymatic degradation processes when in contact with organic tissues and fluids. The degradation process results in the release of microparticles which are absorbed by the body and can be incorporated into the tissues or further metabolized and eliminated via excretion. The possibility of the material being eliminated after having fulfilled its function makes these materials extremely attractive.

The membranes of nanofibers produced by electrospinning from water-soluble polymers have also attracted special attention in the food industry because of their potential as vehicles for controlled release. An area of great interest to both academia and industries is the use of these polymers in the encapsulation of bioactive compounds and probiotic bacteria within prebiotic substances to protect or even enhance their survival while passing through the upper gastrointestinal tract (Ghorani et al., 2015). Electrospinning is shown as a promising technique as a new vehicle for the delivery of supplemental food compounds because the process can work with an aqueous solution at room temperature and without coagulation chemistry (Ghorani et al., 2015).

Electrospinning is also a remarkably simple method for generating nanofibers of polymers. When combined with conventional sol-gel processing, it provides a versatile technique for producing ceramic nanofibers with either a solid, porous, or hollow structure. The production of ceramic nanofibers by electrospinning depends fundamentally on the use of water-soluble polymers as precursors with high affinity to the ceramic materials and the salts. There is no doubt that electrospinning has become one of the most favored techniques also for the manufacture of ceramic nanofibers in a cost-effective and controllable way. Electrospun ceramic nanofibers exhibit a number of unique features and properties, such as morphology, extraordinary length, large surface area and porous structure.

Electrospun ceramic nanofibers are promising for applications in areas where high porosities and surface areas are desired, for example as components for structural reinforcement and thermal insulation, active detection units, catalysis supports, electrodes in energy converters or Storage devices including batteries, dye-sensitized solar cells, supercapacitors and actuators, in various applications in tissue engineering, electronic devices, optoelectronic devices, photocatalysis, sensors, electrochemical energy storage devices, photographic sensors, semiconductors, photo-sensor devices High performance, due to its unique polycrystalline nature and rough surfaces (Wu et al., 2012; Li et al., 2006). In non-conventional applications we can mention, for example, possible models to synthesize new types of nanostructures, functional coatings to control the wettability of surfaces, nanoscale channels in micro and nanofluids (Li et al., 2006).

As already mentioned, the large surface area presented by nanofibers produced by electrospinning also provides unique characteristics for application as membranes for purification and separation, which aid in the selective capture of contaminants or functional portions. Nanosized ceramic material for membrane applications is an emerging field and little information is available in the literature. Electrospun ceramic materials using as precursors water-soluble polymers are also being indicated for use as membranes for liquid/liquid or gas/liquid separation and for chemical reactions as catalysts (Ramaseshan et al., 2007).

Significant progress has been made in the electrospinning process of water-soluble polymers over the past few years and the resulting nanostructures have been exploited for a wide range of applications. There are still many challenges to be overcome in this process and a number of key issues remain open. So far, only a relatively small number of water-soluble polymers have been tested for the production of nanofibers by electrospinning, with very limited understanding of the electrospinning process for these polymers. Extensive research and development in all areas are needed to increase the understanding and feasibility of these eco-friendly polymers, which will certainly contribute to the development of new ecologically sustainable materials.

Poly(Vinyl Alcohol) (PVA)

Polyvinyl alcohol (PVA) is a synthetic polymer used since the early 1930s in a wide range of industrial, commercial, medical and food applications including resins, lacquers, surgical threads and food-contact applications. The physical characteristics of PVA are dependent on its method of preparation from the hydrolysis, or partial hydrolysis, of polyvinyl acetate. PVA is generally classified into two groups, partially hydrolyzed and fully hydrolyzed (Demerlis and Schoneker, 2003).

PVA is approved for use in several medical applications including transdermal patches, the preparation of jellies that dry rapidly when applied to the skin and in immediate and sustained release tablet formulations. Cross-linked poly(vinyl alcohol) are also used for controlled release of oral drugs. Ophthalmic solutions, such as synthetic tears, may also contain PVA because it provides good dispersion and coating properties (Wade and Weller, 1994).

The minimum PVA concentration that allowed the electrospinning was measured by Koski et al. (2004), the authors found that it was possible to spin PVA as long as $[\eta].c > 5$, where $[\eta]$ was the intrinsic viscosity and c was the concentration. As some applications needs water resistance and PVA is a water soluble polymers, some treatments could be done. Yao et al. (2003) observed that electrospun PVA fibers could be stabilized in water by simple soak in methanol. Shalumon et al. (2009) achieved the stabilization by cross linking with glutaraldehyde.

A common feature of PVA fibers is their low mechanical strength and integrity, which have triggered alternatives such as post-treatment (Jeun et al., 2009), cross-linking (Ding et al., 2002) and blending (Ding et al., 2004; Huang et al., 2009). Peresin et al. (2010) studied the addition of cellulose nanocrystals (CN) in PVA electrospun nanofibers. The nanofibers diameters obtained vary from 182 nm to 295 nm. The addition of CN leads to an increase in thermomechanical properties, but this increase is influenced by the hydrolysis degree of the PVA used.

PVA nanofibers has a potential application in wound dressing for skin regeneration. Zhou et al. (2008) studied membranes of PVA with carboxyethyl chitosan (CECS/PVA), observing that the ratio of CECS and PVA strongly influence the diameter and the presence of beams in the electrospun membrane. The membranes demonstrated to be stable in water after a cross-linked process and in vitro cytotoxicity tests with mouse connective tissue, fibroblast-like cells (L929), indicated no cytotoxic effect of the membranes.

Tarun and Gobi (2012), studied nanocomposites of calcium alginate and PVA using electrospinning. Chemical structures of natural polymers and their derivatives (chitosan, dextran, N-O-carboxymethyl chitosan, hydroxyethyl starch and (1,3), (1,6)-b-glucan) were blended with PVA hydrogel to form wound dressing materials. The authors demonstrated that the nanofiber with the maximum calcium alginate content showed the maximum water vapor transmission rate, which indicate that this composite maintain the local moist which could accelerate wound healing. In vivo tests made on rats showed that, apparently, new epithelium was formed without any harmful reaction when the wound is covered with PVA/calcium alginate nanofibers.

Li et al. (2013) showed that nanofibers of PVA/chitosan/Ag nanoparticle have inhibited the growth of *E. Coli* and *S. Aureus* bacteria due to Ag nanoparticles. In a similar way, Shalumon et al. (2011) incorporate Zinc Oxide nanoparticles into PVA/Sodium alginate nanofibers. Results showed that the incorporation of low Zinc Oxide nanoparticle is less toxic and good L929 cells spread than those with higher concentration of Zinc Oxide. Moreover, the final material showed good antibacterial activity against *E. Coli* and *S. Aureus* due to the presence of Zinc Oxide nanoparticles. The results should potential in scaffolds or wound dressing applications.

Sundaramurthi et al. (2012) produced chitosan/PVA (C-PVA) nanofibers for application in scaffolds. *In vivo* studies revealed that C-PVA nanofibers along with R-Spondin 1 are promising dermal substitute which could accelerate the wound healing and skin regeneration.

Ignatova et al. 2007 evaluate the crosslinking method of PVA/Q-chitosan mats using photocrosslinking electrospinning in the growth of Gram-positive and Gram-negative bacteria. The results suggested that the PVA/Q-chitosan mats efficient inhibited the growth of both Gram-positive and Gram-negative bacteria. The results showed the potencial application for scaffolds and wound dressing materials.

Shalumon et al. (2009) studied carboxymethyl chitin (CMC) and PVA nanofibrous for scaffolds, observing that the ratio of CMC and PVA strongly influence in the final morphology of the nanofibers. Mineralization studies showed the capacity of the material forming calcium phosphate by alternate soaking technique. Human mesenchymal stem cells were capable to adhere and proliferate on the membranes, showing that the material may be suitable for tissue engineering applications.

The use of PVA nanofibers as a protein delivery system were studied by Zeng et al. (2005), the authors loaded PVA nanofibers with proteins (FITC-BSA or luciferase), observing that the release of FITC-BSA is fast under physiological conditions but can be retarded by additional polymer coatings on the nanofiber. Even very solvent resistant polymers such as poly(p-xylene) (PPX) allow the release of FITC-BSA.

PVA nanofibers shows applications in drug release systems too. Taepaiboon et al. (2006) studied PVA nanofibers with different drugs (Sodium Salicylate, Diclofenac Sodium, Naproxen and Indomethacin), observing that the PVA in nanofiber form had a higher release then PVA made by casting and the total amount of the drugs released decreased with increasing molecular weight of the drugs.

Jannesari et al. (2011) studied composites of poly(vinyl alcohol)/poly (vinyl acetate) nanofibers, loaded with ciprofloxacin HCL, for drug release. The addition of the drug reduced the nanofibers diameter, which the authors attribute to the reduce in solution viscosity. The amount of drug loaded in nanofibers affect the initial drug release and the release behavior. The authors still observed that in pure PVA nanofibers the release rate was much faster than in pure poly(vinyl acetate) nanofibers, 3 days for almost 100% drug release for PVA against 10 days for a 30% of the drug released for poly(vinyl acetate). The composite with PVA/poly(vinyl acetate) (50:50 by weight) showed an intermediate drug release (in 3 days it released 70% however in 10 days the amount increased to just 80%), however, the addition of poly(vinyl acetate) made nanofibers more flexible and increase the degree of swelling, showing that this material could have applications in the fields of wound dressing.

Azarbayjani et al. (2010) developed a drug delivery system for levothyroxine using nanofibrous membranes made by electrospinning of blends of PVA and poly-N-isopropylacrylamide (PNIPAM). These membranes showed a reduction in deposition of adipose tissue on the skin. The release of levothyroxine showed to be a function of PNIPAM concentration, which could be explaining by the high water solubility of PNIPAM which dissolved almost instantly leading to a rapid release of levothyroxine. In vitro skin permeation tests showed that blending of PVA and PNIPAM increased the skin retention of levothyroxine when compared with pure PNIPAM.

Gold nanoparticles poly(vinyl alcohol) (Au NPs-PVA) were made and tested for applications in biosensors by Wang et al. (2012). The authors made nanofibrous films of PVA using 3-mercaptopropyltrimethoxysilane in electrospun membranes to produce the porosity, which triggered successful homogeneous decoration of Au NPs through gold-sulfur bonding interactions. The Au NPs-PVA nanofibrous mats were embedded with horseradish peroxidase by electrostatic interactions and used as biosensor for H_2O_2 detection. The detection limit were 0.5 μM at a signal-to-noise ratio of 3.

Tang et al. (2009) studied ultrafiltration UV-cured poly(vinyl alcohol) nanofibrous membranes. A membrane based on UV-cured PVA barrier layer and chemically cross-linked PVA nanofibrous scaffold were made. The coating of the barrier layer were made using the UV-reactive PVA with a rapid UV curing process. The thickness of the UV-cured barrier could be controlled by the concentration of UV-PVA added. The UV-PVA membranes showed a capacity to maintain a high flux, high rejection rate and good fouling resistance in a system with oil/water emulsion.

Another field of application of PVA as a sacrifice polymer in the manufacture of ceramic nanofibers made by electrospinning. PVA were used to made CeO_2 (Yang et al., 2005), Fe_2O_3 (Zheng et al., 2009), SnO_2 (Yang et al., 2008; Zhang et al., 2008), ZnO (Nonato et al., 2016; Nonato et al., 2017), Cr_2O_3/Al_2O_3 (Yang et al., 2007), NiO/ZnO (Shao et al., 2004). In these cases, PVA carried a precursor for the ceramic material and is removed lately with a process like calcination. In some cases the calcination still convert the precursor in the material of interest (Nonato et al., 2016).

Poly(Vinyl Pyrrolidone) (PVP)

PVP is a bulky, non-toxic (Jadhav et al., 2013), non-ionic (Lu et al., 2011) polymer with C=O, C–N and CH_2 functional groups (Ziaei-Azad and Semagina, 2014) that is widely used. The PVP molecule contains a strongly hydrophilic component (the pyrrolidone moiety) and a considerable hydrophobic group (the alkyl group). Water and many non-aqueous liquids are excellent solvents for PVP, as a result of the highly polar amide group within the pyrrolidone ring and apolar methylene and methine groups in the ring and along its backbone (Graf et al., 2006).

Hwang and Sunghoon (2011) prepared PVP nanofibers by electrospinning with nanosilver particles (NSPs). In their research, three kinds of nanosilver particles were prepared using the seed mediate growth method and added to electrospinning solutions. The electrospun PVP/NSPs nanocomposites were photocross-linked to improve their water stability. The antibacterial efficacy of the PVP/NSPs nanocomposites was assessed against three types of bacteria: *S. aureus, Klebsiella pneumoniae* and *E. coli*. The photocross-linked PVP/NSPs nanocomposites had high water stability and significant antibacterial efficacy against all three types of bacteria, showing the potential of these materials for antimicrobial applications.

Ignatova et al. (2007), studied nanofibers containing poly(vinyl pyrrolidone)–iodine complex (PVP–iodine) obtained by electrospinning with potential application in wound dressings. Different approaches were used to obtain the nanofibers: (1) a one-step method based on electrospinning of PVP–iodine or poly(ethylene oxide)/PVP–iodine solutions and (2) a three-step method based on electrospinning of PVP or poly(ethylene oxide)/PVP mixed solutions followed by photo-mediated crosslinking of the obtained nanofibers and subsequent complexation with iodine. The diameters of the nanofibers vary from 150nm to 470nm and it depends on the composition and on the applied field strength. Higher applied field strength resulted in greater fiber diameter and in size distribution broadening. Photo-mediated crosslinking in the presence of 4,4′–diazidostilbene–2,2′–dissulfonic acid disodium salt successfully stabilized the electrospun PVP and PEO/PVP nanofibers against water and water vapor.

Ignatova et al. (2007), prepared nanofibers by electrospinning of quaternized chitosan (QCh) and poly(vinyl pyrrolidone). The average fiber diameter significantly decreases from 2.8 to 1.5 μm on increasing the polyelectrolyte content. In order to stabilize QCh/PVP electrospun fibers to water and water vapor, the fibers have been crosslinked by incorporation of photo-crosslinking additives into QCh/PVP spinning solutions and subsequent UV irradiation for 10 hours of the electrospun fibers. Photo-crosslinked QCh-containing electrospun mats show high antibacterial activity against the *S. aureus* and *E. Coli*. The results show a possibility of application in biomedical area such as wound dressing applications.

Li et al. (2012) studied poly(vinyl pyrrolidone)/poly(L-lactide-co-ε-caprolactone) (PVP/PLCL) produced by coaxial electrospinning. Electrospun PLCL and chitosan membranes were also prepared by traditional electrospinning as controls. The electrospun PVP/PLCL membranes showed the largest water absorption (501.3%) due to introduction of the PVP component and the fiber structure. The PVP/PLCL membranes possessed higher tensile strength and elongation-at-break, and lower Young's modulus than those of PLCL and chitosan membranes in both dry and wet states. Studies on cell adhesion showed that PVP/PLCL membranes could mimic the structure of natural extracellular matrices and positively promote cell–cell and cell–matrix interactions because of hydrophilicity/hydrophobicity balance.

PVP can be used as a stabilizing and shape-directing agent in the polyol synthesis of metallic nanoparticles. Examples of these nanoparticles include plasmonic elements (Ag, Au, Cu) (Sun and Xia, 2002; Wang et al., 2006; Dreaden et al., 2012), catalytic elements (Pd, Pt) (Shen et al., 2009; Ye et al., 2012; Wang et al., 2013), magnetic elements (Co, Ni) (Zhang et al., 2008; Zhou et al., 2011) and bimetallic compositions (Au–M, Pt–M) (Zhang et al., 2012; Singh et al., 2013).

Jiang et al. (2012) studied PVP/zein nanofibers for biphasic drug release profiles with ketoprofen as the model drug. In vitro dissolution tests showed that the nanofibers could provide an immediate release of 42.3% of the contained ketoprofen, followed by a sustained release over 10 h of the remaining drug, the study showed a simple and useful approach to systematically design and fabricate nanostructures using electrospinning for providing biphasic drug release profiles.

PVP is one of the most popular polymers employed as a sacrificial polymer for electrospinning of ceramic nanofibers. It happens due to its high solubility in ethanol or water and its good compatibility with many metal alkoxides and salts, including titanium isopropoxide and zirconium acetylacetonate (Dai et al., 2010). PVP were used to made Al_2O_3 (Azad, 2006), TiO_2 (Li and Xia, 2003), ZnS (Lin et al., 2009), ZnO/SnO_2 (Song et al., 2009), ZrO_2/SnO_2 (Wang et al., 2009), $NiFe_2O_4$ (Li et al., 2003). The solvents used in these researches can vary from water (Min et al., 2007), ethanol (Azad, 2006), isopropanol (Li et al., 2003) and DMF (Song et al., 2009).

POLY(ETHYLENE GLYCOL) (PEG)

PEG is a linear branched, neutral polyether, available in a variety of polymeric weights and soluble in water and most inorganic solvents. It is focus of interest in the biotechnical and biomedical fields. PEG is usually effective at excluding other polymers from it presence when in an aqueous environment, which includes protein rejection, formation of two-phase systems with other polymers, non-immunogenicity and non-antigenicity. PEG is nontoxic and does not harm active proteins or cells even interacting with cell membranes. When attached to other molecules it has little effect on their chemistry but controls their solubility and increases their size (Harris, 1992). PEG can be used as phase transfer catalysis for a variety of organic reactions. PEG provide a lower cost, nontoxic phase transfer catalyst relative to crown ethers (Totten and Clinton, 2008).

Chen et al. (2013) prepared by electrospinning polyethylene glycol/poly (dl-lactide) (PEG/PLA) blends with various PEG/PLA mass ratios. The better results on morphology appeared when the mass ratio of PEG/ PLA varies from 100/100 to 200/100, and the average fiber diameter increases with increasing PEG content. The composite fibers have available heat storage capacity with maximum melting enthalpy of 74.7 J/g (PEG/PLA 200/100), and the degradation temperatures of the fibers are higher than 320°C. The composite fibers show form stable characteristic, balanced phase change behaviors and good heat storage/release properties after thermal treatment. The prepared phase change composite fibers have potential applications in smart textiles, medicine cares and electric devices for thermal energy storage and temperature regulation.

Chen et al. (2011) studied PEG/cellulose acetate (PEG/CA) blends by electrospinning with potential application in thermal energy storage and temperature regulations. The results show that the latent heats of the phase change fibers increase with the increasing of PEG content in the fibers, and the PEG/CA fibers with high enthalpies have a good capability to regulate their interior temperature as the ambient temperature alters.

PEG can be used as a sacrificial polymer too. Skotak et al. (2011) prepared Gelatin-based nanofibrous scaffolds with and without micrometer-sized PEG fibers, using PEG fibers as sacrificial templates. Upon fabrication of the scaffolds via electrospinning, the gelatin fibers were crosslinked with glutaraldehyde, and the PEG templates were removed using tert-butanol. Fibroblasts were seeded onto both types of the gelatin-based nanofibrous surfaces and cultured. Cell penetration up to a depth of 250 and 90 μm was noted in gelatin scaffolds prepared with sacrificial templates. The results show that the scaffold preparation protocol allowed the structural integrity to be maintained even with high template content (95%) and could be extended toward other classes of electrospun polymer matrices for tissue engineering.

Zong et al. (2005) studied poly(lactide) and poly(glycolide) (as PEG) based scaffolds for heart tissue constructs. Electrospinning was used to fabricate the scaffolds. In vitro studies confirmed a dose–response effect of the poly(glycolide) concentration on the degradation rate and the pH value changes. Structural analysis by confocal microscopy indicated that cardiomyocytes had a preference for relatively hydrophobic surfaces. Cardiomyocytes on the scaffolds show a superior response on poly(lactide) when compared with poly(lactide) with poly(glycolide). The final conclusion is the scaffolds can be applied as cardiac tissue constructs.

Nguyen and Park (2011) studied blends of polyvinylidene fluoride and polyethylene glycol (PVDF/PEG) made by electrospinning. Addition of fumed silica to electrospun fibers helped prevent the leakage of molten PEG during the solid-liquid phase change and improve the mechanical strength of PVDF/PEG mats. The PVDF/PEG mats showed high thermal stability confirmed by differential scanning calorimetry. The fumed silica had large energy storage capacity, which allows applications in energy storage and in the manufacture of thermoregulating textiles.

Cui et al. (2009) evaluate the application of electrospun scaffolds of poly(dl-lactide)/(poly(ethylene glycol) (PDLLA/PEG) for tissue engineering. The surface hydrophilicity was improved, and the degradation patterns of PDLLA/PEG mats changed from surface erosion to bulk degradation with the increase in PEG contents. Human dermal fibroblasts integrated well with the surrounding fibers containing 20% and 30% PEG, which provided significantly better environment for biological activities than pure PDLLA mats. It indicated that electrospun mats containing 30% PEG exhibited the most balanced properties, including moderately hydrophilic surface, minimal dimensional changes, adaptable bulk biodegradation pattern and enhancement of cell penetration and growth within fibrous mats.

Fu et al. (2012) studied scaffolds of electrospun poly(ε-caprolactone)/poly(ethylene glycol)/poly(ε-caprolactone) and 30 wt.% nano-hydroxyapatite (n-HA). The study investigate *in vitro* and *in vivo* performance by means of hydrolytic degradation, muscle pouch implantation and repair the calvarial defects in New Zealand white rabbits. The results show that the degradable scaffold held good biocompatibility, which suggested that the composite scaffold had better activity of guided bone regeneration than that of self-healing.

Poly(Ethylene Oxide) – PEO

Poly(ethylene oxide) (PEO) is a crystalline, thermoplastic, water-soluble polymer with the general formula $(OCH_2CH_2)_n$. Unlike most polymer systems, PEO is commercially available in a wide range of molecular weights. PEO is soluble in water and a wide number of organic solvents (Bailey and Koleske, 1976).

Zhang et al. (2009) studied PEO/chitosan electrospun nanofibers. The blending ratio of PEO and chitosan, molecular weight of chitosan and temperature of electrospinning looks like to be the key influence factors on the formation of the structures. Because of the chitosan outer layer and shell thickness being controllable, the core-shell structure nanofiber shows a potential application for the biomedical fields.

Jin et al. (2002) explored electrospinning for protein-based biomaterials to fabricate scaffolds and membranes from regenerated silkworm silk, *Bombyx mori*, solutions for high-performance filters and biomaterial scaffolds for vascular grafts or wound dressings. A variety of compositions of the silk/PEO aqueous blends were successfully electrospun. Fiber diameters were uniform and less than 800 nm. Traditional silk fibroin conformational transitions were induced with methanol treatment of the fibers, suggesting that native structural features of the silk were preserved in the electrospinning process. The results open new directions in the fabrication of silk-based biomaterial scaffolds for biomedical applications.

The antibacterial activity of electrospun chitosan/poly(ethylene oxide) (PEO/CS) fibers containing silver nanoparticles were evaluated by An et al. (2009). In the study the silver nanoparticles were distributed in PEO/CS ultrafine fibers with the size less than 5 nm. X-ray photoelectron spectroscopy suggested that the existence of Ag—O bond in the composite led to the tight combination between Ag and CS. Evaluation of antimicrobial activities of the electrospun PEO/CS membranes against *E. coli* showed that the silver nanoparticles in the ultrafine fibers significantly enhanced the inactivation of bacteria.

Antimicrobial activity of electrospun membranes of chitosan/poly (ethylene oxide) (CS/PEO) incorporated with poly(hexamethylene biguanide) hydrochloride (PHMB) were studied by Dilamian et al. (2013). In the study, the authors electrospun CS/PEO in the presence of PHMB. Results revealed that the incorporation of PHMB in chitosan/PEO solutions led to decrease in the zero-shear rate viscosity up to 20%. Moreover, increasing PHMB from 0.5 mM to 1 mM led to formation of thinner fibers with diameters ranging from 240 nm to 60 nm, respectively. Inhibition of the bacteria growth for both *E. Coli* and *S. Aureus* were achieved on the PHMB loaded nanofibers. Also, a burst release of PHMB from mats has been observed in the first hour. The results suggest a great potential in fabrication of biomaterials with incorporation of PHMB using electrospinning.

Kriegel et al. (2009) fabricated nanofibers of PEO and cationic chitosan by electrospinning. To broaden the processing window under which nanofibers are produced, surfactants of different charge were added at concentrations well above their critical micellar concentrations (cmc). Pure chitosan did not form fibers and was instead deposited as beads but the addition of PEO and surfactants induced spinnability. The spinnability of all the constituents may be of significant commercial importance since micelles could serve as carriers of lypophilic components such as pharmaceuticals, nutraceuticals, antimicrobials, flavors or fragrances thereby further enhancing the functionality of nanofibers.

Ma et al. (2012) studied nanofibers of sodium alginate/poly(ethylene oxide) (SA/PEO) prepared by electrospinning. An one-step cross-linking method through being immersed in $CaCl_2$ solution was investigated to improve the anti-water property of the electrospun nanofibers mats in order to facilitate their practical applications as tissue engineering scaffolds, and the changes of the structural of nanofibers before and after cross-linking was characterized. Indirect cytotoxicity assessment indicated that SA/PEO nanofibers membrane was nontoxic to the fibroblasts cells, and cell culture suggested that SA/PEO nanofibers tended to promote fibroblasts cells attachment and proliferation. The results indicate that the electrospun SA/PEO membrane could be used for tissue engineering scaffolds.

Brun et al. (2011) studied nanofibrous electrospun scaffolds of poly(ethylene oxide) and self-assembling peptides in aqueous solution. Biological assays confirmed greater adhesion of human osteoblasts to the electrospun matrices when they were enriched with b-hairpin or b-sheet peptides. This scaffold significantly promoted growth and differentiation of human osteoblasts. The work discuss the importance of topographical, morphological and biochemical aspects that must be optimized and integrated, together with mechanical properties, to decrease the difference between the extra cellular matrix and the extra cellular matrix mimetic materials. The results show a potential application for bone tissue engineering.

Honarbakhsh and Pourdeyhimi (2011) prepared electrospun scaffolds of Poly(lactic acid) (PLA) and poly(lactic acid)/(poly(ethylene oxide) (PLA/PEO), focusing in the development of a biodegradable, controlled, and potentially targeted drug delivery system. In the work, they produce a highly porous biodegradable fibrous structures suitable for biomedical applications and as a matrix for drug delivery, one made of electrospun PLA and the other structure has enhanced hydrophilicity compared to PLA matrix and is formed by blending PLA/PEO. The incorporation of PEO in the matrix introduces preferable sites for aqueous compounds to be attached to while retaining the overall structural integrity and porous morphology. It is hypothesized that the existence of alternative hydrophilic and hydrophobic segments in the structure may reduce post-implantation complications such as platelet adhesion.

CHITOSAN

Chitosan-based biomaterials are an emerging class with application in various biomedical fields. The high hydrophilicity of chitosan, due to a large number of hydroxyl and amino groups present in the polymer chain, allows its use as a biomaterial in the form of microparticles, gel, nanofibers and membrane in various applications. It is obtained by the deacetylation reaction of chitin in alkaline medium, derived from the exoskeleton of crustaceans, insects etc. Chitosan is a non-toxic natural polymer, improves healing and bone formation, has hemostatic properties, and exhibits excellent biocompatibility (Jayacumar et al., 2010).

Chitosan has excellent biological properties, such as biodegradability, biocompatibility, antibacterial activity and healing activity. Besides this, chitosan can reach hemostasis and promote normal tissue regeneration. For these reasons, chitosan was considered one of the most promising biomacromoleculcs for the development of scaffolds for tissue engineering and dressings for skin lesions (Zhou et al., 2008).

The concept of tissue engineering was born when several researchers realized that when cells are placed close enough to each other they form structures identical to those formed by these cells in a living body (Sell et al., 2010). This, apparently, can be obtained thanks to signs that living cells are able to exchange with neighbors. This technique may allow an overcoming of the problems encountered in the reconstruction of various tissues and organs and establish a new basis for regenerative medicine. Among natural and synthetic polymeric materials which have been discovered and are suitable for tissue engineering applications, particular attention has recently been given to chitosan derivatives in combination with various polysaccharides (Jagur-Grodzinsk, 2006).

Chitosan nanofibrous matrices have demonstrated enormous promises as scaffolds for tissue engineering and as skin substitutes for serious injuries. The advantages of a scaffold composed of ultrafine continuous fibers are high porosity, oxygen permeability, variable pore size distribution, high surface/volume ratio and, most importantly, the morphological similarity with the extracellular matrix (ECM) in the skin, which promote migration and proliferation of cell adhesion (Zhou et al., 2008).

The work of Nie et al. (2009) demonstrated the use of PLGA- chitosan nanofibers containing hydroxyapatite bone morphogenetic protein (BMP-2) encapsulated. BMP-2 is known to be able to induce bone healing, while hydroxyapatite may increase binding to bone cells. The presence of hydroxyapatite increased the release of BMP-2 due to its hydrophilicity in a hydrophobic matrix. The authors also implanted the PLGA scaffolds in mice and reported that the composite nanofiber of PLGA-hydroxyapatite with BMP-2 coated with chitosan can improve the healing of segmental bone defects, increasing the efficiency of transfer of BMP-2 to a higher level (Leung et al., 2011).

In the work of Huang et al. (2011), collagen-chitosan-poly (urethane) blends were electrospun for biocompatible scaffolds for application in tissue engineering. Pig arterial endothelial cells and Schwann cells were seeded in the scaffolds and showed increased proliferation in the oriented and randomly aligned nanofibers, suggesting that these scaffolds potentially allow for faster repair of blood vessels and regeneration of nerves.

Biopolymers, in general, have low mechanical strength, aiming to improve their physical properties several groups are working on the incorporation of reinforcement materials in these nanofibres. The work of Sambudi et al. (2015) incorporated $CaCO_3$ nanoparticles as a reinforcing agent increasing the mechanical properties of chitosan/polyvinyl alcohol (PVA) nanofibers. The loading concentration of $CaCO_3$ nanoparticles ranged from 1 to 5% by weight and the fiber diameter ranged from 71.5 ±

23.4 nm to 140.7 ± 15.1 nm. The tensile test on $CaCO_3$-reinforced nanofibers (4% m/m) revealed young's modulus nearly sixty times greater than that of fibers without $CaCO_3$. The biocompatibilities of the $CaCO_3$-loaded fibers were also tested in a simulated 14-day incubation of body fluid (FBS) to induce the formation of apatite minerals and in a 14-day cell proliferation assay with ATDC5 cells. It has been found that the material provides the most suitable environment for cell growth compared to the unbranched material. Based on the results obtained, this group concluded that the $CaCO_3$-reinforced nanofibers have the potential to be a promising alternative for artificial cartilage since it presented exceptional mechanical resistance, biocompatibility and is suitable to develop chondrocyte cells. Also in this line, Koosha et al. (2015) prepared chitosan/polyvinyl alcohol nanofibers reinforced with montmorillonite nanoceramics (MMT) prepared by electrospinning technique. The incorporation of nanoceramics into the nanofibers increased the tensile strength and increased the glass transition of the membranes. Cytotoxicity was examined by MTT assay using the A-431 cell line and had no significant effect on cell viability.

Controlled drug release technology is an interdisciplinary challenge for pharmacists, chemical engineers, biomaterial engineers, and the medical community (Liechty et al., 2010). Development of polymers for controlled drug release has been booming since the 1960s. Since then, extensive progress has been made in the synthesis and fabrication of these sophisticated polymer systems.

Polymeric systems for controlled drug release have numerous advantages, compared to normal dosage forms (VERRECK et al., 2003). Several polymers have already been tested in controlled release systems, some because of their physical properties, and others because of their chemical properties. Chitosan has adequate properties in drug delivery systems and has been investigated as a drug delivery vehicle because it is able to reduce transepithelial electrical resistance, transiently opening a strong channel between epithelial cells (Elgadir et al., 2015). In addition to the aforementioned characteristics, chitosan exhibits favorable biological behavior, such as bio-adhesion, permeability, and interesting physicochemical characteristics, which make this biopolymer a unique material for the design of transmucosal release systems. (Lonso et al., 2003).

Chitosan is considered a good system of drug release in the oral cavity, because its antibacterial activity may be due to electrostatic interactions between amino groups and anionic groups on the cell walls of bacteria from residues of carboxylic acids and phospholipids. Abruzzo et al. (2012) developed and characterized chitosan/gelatin films as an innovative mucoadhesive system for oral delivery of propanolol hydrochloride. The presence of higher amounts of chitosan in the chitosan/gelatin films allowed the lower percentage of water uptake and a longer residence time in vivo in the oral cavity. Besides that, the presence of mannitol in the formulation allowed 80% permeation of the drug through the buccal mucosa in 5 h. Another interesting aspect of the chitosan/gelatin films was their compatibility with oral microflora in the absence of drug and their ability to determine inhibition of growth of pathogenic bacteria, but not for probiotic species, when loaded with the drug.

It has been reported in the literature that chitosan is degraded by the microflora that is available in the colon. Due to this property, chitosan can be considered a promising polymer matrix specific for drug release in the colon (Nunthanid et al., 2009). Ardeshirzadeh et al. (2015) prepared polyethylene oxide (PEO)/chitosan (CS)/graphene oxide (GO) nanofibrous membranes by electrospinning process. Doxorubicin hydrochloride, an anticancer drug, was successfully encapsulated in nanofibrous scaffolds for controlled release. Nanofibers with diameter of 85 nm were obtained, and the material had 98% drug loading and controlled DOX release. Cell viability of DOX-loaded nanofibers exhibited lower cytotoxicity compared to free DOX, suggesting that this system could be a promising candidate for controlled and targeted drug delivery for the treatment of lung cancer.

The incorporation of natural active principles also presents itself as a trend in the area of electrospun nanofibers. We can cite the work of Sarhan et al. (2015) that prepared nanofibers with a high concentration of honey. Honey has profound medicinal and nutritional properties, presents antimicrobial activity, debridement and deodorization, as well as anti-inflammatory activities, antioxidants and wound healing. In this study, polyvinyl alcohol/chitosan was electrospun with honey concentrations of 20% to 40%. The nanofibers showed pronounced antibacterial activity against Staphylococcus aureus and the material had no cytotoxicity effects on fibroblast culture. The group concluded that this material has potential as an effective dressing for wounds.

The electrospinning membranes of nanofibers are considered of great potential in the field of tissue regeneration since they can mimic the architecture of the extracellular matrix. The electrospinning process also provides operational flexibility for the incorporation of multiple components into nanofibers, such as metal nanoparticles and inorganic nanoparticles. Magnetic nanoparticles (NPs) are of enormous importance for their biomedical applications, such as magnetic resonance imaging, tissue repair, immunoassay, biological fluid detoxification, hyperthermia and drug delivery. Also, the electrospinning technique had been used successfully in the manufacture of magnetic fibrous scaffolds (Nicknejad et al., 2015). In the field of drug release, Fe_3O_4 nanoparticles are used because of their ability to be moved by external magnetic force and thus achieve, In addition, a magnetic nanoparticle, once exposed to an alternative magnetic field, could be used for controlled release of drug components incorporated within a polymer. Therefore, the incorporation of magnetic particles in electrospun nanofibers could offer improved efficacy of drug delivery (Nicknejad et al., 2015).

Wei et al. (2011), prepared magnetic nanofibers of chitosan for purposes of bone regeneration. The Nicknejad group (2015) developed a magnetic (PVA)/magnetic chitosan crosslinked membrane with Fe_3O_4 addition for use in load and release applications of proteins. Bovine serum albumin (BSA) was used as a model of protein drugs. The average diameter of the nanofibers produced was 45 nm and the Fe_3O_4 nanoparticles were uniformly dispersed. A slow and controlled release rate was obtained with a greater amount of BSA release of 60% after 30 h. Liu et al. (2015) prepared chitosan/PVA nanofibers with the incorporation of silver nanoparticles in order to obtain an antimicrobial material for biomedical applications. The silver ion release behavior at a concentration of 0.5 wt% in nanofiber, indicated that these nanofibers released silver continuously for 16 days, exhibiting antibacterial activity against *S. aureus* and *E. Coli*.

In addition to the biomedical area, chitosan has also been used extensively in many areas ranging from the food to the treatment of industrial effluents due to its affinity with metallic ions (kadajji et al., 2011). Chitosan, an alkaline deacetylated product of chitin, has been widely used in biosorption due to its low cost, hydrophilicity, nontoxicity and high levels of amino and hydroxyl functional groups, which have high activity as adsorption sites. The development of chitosan-based adsorbents for the removal of metal ions from aqueous solutions has become a hot topic in the water treatment field due to its excellent properties (min et al., 2015). Arsenic is an element commonly distributed in the natural environment, particularly in groundwater. Contamination of arsenic in water leads to a number of health problems. People who drink water contaminated with an arsenic concentration greater than 0.05 mg/L are likely to increase the risk of lung and bladder cancer and arsenic-associated skin lesions (Min et al., 2015). Min and co-workers (2015) prepared a membrane of chitosan nanofibers by electrospinning was an adsorbent for removal of arsenate in water. A SEM observation demonstrated that the material was highly porous and had a large specific surface area, favorable to adsorption the adsorption of arsenate was established in 30 minutes, indicating that the absorption of As (V) occurred very fast. Experiments of the adsorption isotherm showed a maximum adsorption capacity of 30.8 mg/g. The study suggested that an electrophilic nanofiber membrane based on eco-friendly polymers could be applied as a promising adsorbent for arsenic and other immersed organic pollutants due to its fast adsorption kinetics, high adsorption capacity and easy separation of water.

ALGINATE

Sodium alginate is extracted mainly from 3 algae species, namely Macrocystis pyrifera, Laminaria Hyperborea and Ascophyllum nodosum. Chemically it is an anionic biopolymer, composed of linear chains of β-D-manuronic acid (unit M) and α-L-guluronic acid (unit G) (Kleinubing et al., 2013). This polysaccharide is water-soluble, mucoadhesive, biocompatible used in drug delivery, wound dressing, and tissue engineering, and other areas (Bonino et al., 2011). Alginate crosslinking can be carried out in the presence of divalent cations, due to its ability to form gels with calcium by ionic bonds. When used in vivo, the ionically crosslinked alginate degrades when calcium ions are exchanged with other ions in the body, such as Na^+. Shorter degradation times may be more ideal for some tissue regeneration applications wishing to combine tissue formation with the degradation rate of the polymer (Bonino et al., 2011). Thus, low PM alginate composite nanofibers are attractive for in vivo biomedical applications where body degradation and clearance are desirable (Bonino et al., 2011). Studies on the preparation of mucoadhesive polymer systems prepared by electrospinning are still scarce in the scientific literature due to their complexity. Electrospinning of biopolymers with mucoadhesive properties has been a major challenge due to the limited solubility of these in most organic solvents, poor molecular flexibility (due to the difficulty of entanglement of the polymer chains caused by the rigid and prolonged conformation of the chain) and the ease of forming hydrogen bonds in the three-dimensional structure (its polycationic characteristic in aqueous solution, increases the surface tension of the solution, requiring very high electrical voltages to be electrospun). Alginate nanofiber membranes can be successfully fabricated by electrospinning, when the solutions was prepared with a second material, usually an auxiliary polymer, for example, PEO, which is also mucoadhesive, widely used to facilitate electrospinning by reducing conductivity of the polysaccharide solution and increase the interlacing of the chains.

Nanofibers of sodium alginate/poly (ethylene oxide) were prepared via electrospinning by the group of Ma (2012) in aqueous solution. The membranes formed were crosslinked by immersion in $CaCl_2$ solution, to improve the water solubility property and facilitate their practical applications as tissue engineering scaffolds. Indirect evaluation of cytotoxicity indicated that the SA/PEO nanofibrous membrane was non-toxic to fibroblast cells, and cell culture suggested that the nanofibers tended to promote the binding and proliferation of fibroblast cells.

In the study by Alborzi et al. (2010), the electrospinning process of sodium alginate, PEO and pectin fibers was investigated to be used as a vehicle for the stabilization of folic acid. Thus, electrospun fibers were obtained with different morphological transitions, depending on the mixture ratio of the alginate/pectin and PEO used, and the viscosity of the solution. Fang et al. (2011) also fabricated sodium alginate nanofibers by electrospinning from aqueous solutions. In this study, the electrospinning capacity was improved by the introduction of cations (Ca^{+2}) in the solutions.

In the work of Wei Lu et al. (2006), sodium alginate was also electrospun from an aqueous solution containing polyethylene oxide (PEO), whose smooth fibers had a diameter of around 250 nm. The water dissolution of the electrospun membranes was crosslinked, with a combination of aqueous calcium chloride and hexamethylene diisocyanate.

Chae et al., (2013) prepared membranes of hydroxyapatite/alginate nanofibers by electrospinning technique with the objective of imitating mineralized collagen fibers in the bone tissue. The growth of HAp nanocrystals was induced in the alginate nanofibers impregnated with PO_4^{-3} ions. This new process resulted in a uniform deposition of HAp nanocrystals on the nanofibers. The in vitro cell study showed that the rat calvarial osteoblasts were more stablely attached to the surface of the scaffolds with HAp than in the pure alginate scaffold, indicating a potential use of this material for the regeneration of bone tissue.

In the medical field, a serious shortage of good quality cornea donors presents itself as an international crisis in public health. Alternatives to donor tissue need to be urgently developed to meet the growing demand for corneal transplantation. The work of Tonsomboon et al., (2013) shows that the mechanical properties of corneal transplant with compatible hydrogels can be substantially increased with the reinforcement of electrospinning nanofiber. This work shows that mechanically reinforced transparent hydrogels can be simply manufactured from two cheap and readily available natural polymers: gelatin and alginate. Nano-random and aligned electrospun gelatin fibers were used to strengthen the hydrogels, increasing the mechanical properties of the alginate hydrogels in one order of magnitude. These new nanofibrous composites have great promise as scaffolds for engineering applications of corneal tissues due to their optical transparency.

In the drug release area, Sharma et al. (2013) have developed an oral formulation of an antidiabetic drug release provide a controlled and sustained release profile. A transmucosal membrane composed of electrospun poly (vinyl alcohol) (PVA) and sodium alginate (NaAlg) was developed, and the insulin was incorporated by active loading. In vivo studies were performed on male Wistar rats via the sublingual route. The in vitro activity provided a pattern of controlled release of the drug from the nanofiber membrane. A 99% encapsulation effect of the experimental formulation provides a sufficient indication that the composite nanofibers serve as an ideal carrier for sublingual insulin administration. Thus, the present investigation gives an impetus to work towards the administration of antidiabetic drugs (proteins and peptides) via the transmucosal route.

Following the use of bacterial filters, the work of Moon et al. (2012) produced nanofibers composed of poly (ethylene oxide) (PEO)/hydrated iron oxide (HIO)/sodium alginate (SA) with high tensile strength, with significant bacterial decontamination properties (removal of Vibrio vulnificus in 92.5%) and high absorption properties. These properties of bacterial decontamination and good mechanical properties enable various applications of this material as biomedical, absorbent material and in clinical, food, and environmental applications as well as protective clothing, composites, and other areas.

Also in this line, the work of Shalumon et al. (2011), membranes of sodium alginate (SA)/polyvinyl alcohol (PVA) nanofibers was prepared by electrospinning technique with addition of ZnO in different concentrations (0.5, 1, 2 and 5%). The objective was the preparation of an ideal biomaterial for wound dressing applications due to ZnO antibacterial activity. The study of antibacterial activity of the 1% ZnO membranes was examined with *S. Aureus* and *E. Coli* and verified that they show activity due to the presence of ZnO.

The membranes of electrospun alginate nanofibers also present a potential in the environmental area, in the removal of toxic waste in an aqueous medium. In recent years, the removal of heavy metals from aqueous solution has received considerable attention. Heavy metals are highly dangerous to humans, even at low levels of concentration. When they enter the human body, they cause various disorders and diseases. Exists various methods to remove the toxic waste but it is found that the adsorption method is more effective for the removal of heavy metals (Karthik et al., (2015).) Sodium alginate (SA) has received more attention as an adsorbent for the presence of carboxylate groups (COOH) in SA provides the ability to form a complex with the variety of multivalent ions. Karthik et al. (2015) prepared the sodium alginate-polyaniline (SAP) nanofibers for use as an adsorbent for the removal of Cr (VI) ions from an aqueous solution. Thermodynamic parameters indicated that the adsorption process was spontaneous endothermic and physiognomic in nature. The kinetic data are well expressed by the pseudo-second-order model and the results revealed that SAP nanofibers could be used as adsorbents for the removal of Cr(VI) ions from Cr(VI) contaminated water and could be reused for more than three consecutive cycles.

Alginate is also one of the most studied anionic polyelectrolytes in complexation with chitosan because the poly complex formed between these two polymers is still biodegradable, biocompatible and mechanically more resistant (Hamman et al., 2010).

Polyelectrolytes are macromolecules which play an important role in the transport of a relatively large number of charged functional groups, or which may become charged. They may have the function of polycations or polyanions, since the net charge of these macromolecules in solution depends on the functional groups, which may be positively or negatively charged, depending on the pH of the medium (Simsek-Ege et al., 2003).

Chitosan and alginate are well known, biocompatible, biodegradable and mucoadhesive polyelectrolytes, allowing several pharmaceutical and biomedical applications (Sarmento et al., 2007). They can be used as thickening agents in the food industry; Such as drug delivery systems, in pharmaceutical applications, and as biomaterials in cell culture and wound healing. These two polysaccharides can also be used together, forming a polyelectrolyte complex, widely used to encapsulate proteins, cells, and enzymes (Simsek-Ege et al., 2003).

The formation of the polyelectrolyte complex is facilitated by an electrostatic mechanism, where charge neutralization occurs through interactions such as hydrogen bonds, Coulomb forces and Van der Waals forces (Meng et al., 2010). Studies on the biodegradability of chitosan-alginate polyelectrolyte complexes showed that while chitosan alone was degraded by lysozymes, the effect of these enzymes on the polyelectrolyte complex was negligible. The complex showed high adsorption capacity of lysozyme, but enzymatic degradation was hampered by the strong interaction between chitosan and alginate polymer chains (Hamman et al., 2010).

A major advantage of the chitosan-alginate polyelectrolyte complex is its preparation that occurs in water, dispensing with the use of toxic organic solvents, in the preparation of coating membranes for controlled release systems. The membranes thus obtained are biodegradable and insoluble in water, with great potential for biomedical applications (Meng et al., 2010). In the field of nanotechnology, the formation of this polyelectrolyte has been widely explored in the production of several polysaccharide-based nanoparticles controlled drug delivery systems for application to various sites in the human body (Goycoolea et al., 2009). Its use may have promising applications in the dentistry area, such as the transmucosal administration of bioactive macromolecules, due to several interesting properties, such as mucoadhesion and bio-adhesiveness. This system has a high ability to associate and release therapeutic macromolecules in their bioactive form as well as improve the transport of bioactive compounds through well-organized epithelial barriers such as ocular, nasal, oral and intestinal (Goycoolea et al., 2009).

The work of Nista et al. (2015) explored the electrospinning of two mucoadhesive polymers, chitosan and alginate, to form coaxial nanofibers for applications as controlled drug administration. The formation of coaxial nanofibres was evidenced by the use of transmission electron microscopy (TEM). Other characterization techniques such as scanning electron microscopy (SEM), differential scanning calorimetry (DSC), thermogravimetric analysis (TGA), infrared spectroscopy (FTIR) and XRD (XRD) strongly suggest the formation of different molecular structures membranes obtained by the complexation of chitosan and alginate. The swelling rate and weight loss tests followed by SEM analyzes confirmed that the nanofiber structure of these membranes was maintained even after incubation for 24 h in water.

Only a few examples of the application of water soluble polymers nanofibers have been shown in this work. The number of researches has been growing every day, showing the great application of this polymers and the versatility of this materials.

REFERENCES

An, J; Zhang, H; Zhang, J; Zhao, Y; Yuan, X. (2009) Preparation and antibacterial activity of electrospun chitosan/poly(ethylene oxide) membranes containing silver nanoparticles. *Colloid and Polymer Science 287*, 1425-1434.

Abruzzo, A; Bigucci, F; Cerchiara, T; Cruciani, F; Vitali, B; Luppi, B. (2012) Muchoadesive Chitosan-Gelatin Film for Buccal Delivery of Propanol Hydrochloride. *Carbohydrate Polymers 87*, 581–588.

Alborzi, S; Lim, L; Kakuda, Y. (2010) Electrospinning of Sodium Alginate-Pectin Ultrafine Fibers. *Journal of Food Science 75*, 1, C100-C107.

Alonso, MJ; Sanchez A. (2003) The potential of chitosan in ocular drug delivery. *Journal of Pharmacy and Pharmacology 55*, 1451-1463.

Ardeshirzadeh, B; Anaraki, NA; Irani, M; Rad, LR; Shamshiri, S. (2015) Controlled release of doxorubicin from electrospun PEO/chitosan/graphene oxide nanocomposite nanofibrous scaffolds. *Materials Science and Engineering C 48*, 384–390.

Azad, A-M. (2006) Fabrication of transparent alumina (Al_2O_3) nanofibers by electrospinning. *Materials Science and Engineering: A 435-436*, 468-473.

Azarbayjani, AF; Venugopal, JR; Ramakrishna, S; Lim, PFC; Chan, YW; Chan, SY. (2010) Smart polymeric nanofibers for topical delivery of levothyroxine. *Journal of Pharmacy & Pharmaceutical Sciences 13*, 400-410.

Baile, FE; Koleske, J.V. Poly(ethylene oxide). Academic Press, USA, 1976.

Bonino, CA; Krebs, MD; Saquing, CD; Jeong, SI; Shearer, KL; Alsberg, E; Khan, SA. (2011) Electrospinning alginate-based nanofibers: From blends to crosslinked low molecular weight alginate-only systems. *Carbohydrate Polymers 85*, 111–119.

Brun, P; Ghezzo, F; Roso, M; Danesin, R; Palù, G; Bagno, A; Modesti, M; Catagliuolo, I; Dettin, M. (2011) Electrospun scaffolds of self-assembling peptides with poly(ethylene oxide) for bone tissue engineering. *Acta Biomaterialia 7*, 2526-2532.

Chae, T; Yang, H; Leung, V; Ko, F; Troczynski, T. (2013) Novel biomimetic hydroxyapatite/alginate nanocomposite fibrous scaffolds for bone tissue regeneration. *Journal of Materials Science: Materials in Medicine 24*, 1885-1894.

Chen, C; Liu, K; Wang, H; Liu, W; Zhang, H. (2013) Morphology and performances of electrospun polyethylene glycol/poly (dl-lactide) phase change ultrafine fibers for thermal energy storage. *Solar Energy Materials & Solar Cells 117*, 372-381.

Chen, C; Wang, L; Huang, Y. (2011) Electrospun phase change fibers based on polyethylene glycol/cellulose acetate blends. *Applied Energy 88*, 3133-3139.

Cui, W; Zhu, X; Yang, Y; Li, X; Jin, Y. (2009) Evaluation of electrospun fibrous scaffolds of poly(DL-lactide) and poly(ethylene glycol) for skin tissue engineering. *Materials Science and Engineering C 29*, 1869-1876.

Dai, Y; Liu, W; Formo, E; Sun, Y; Xia, Y. (2011) Ceramic nanofibers fabricated by electrospinning and their applications in catalysis, environmental science, and energy technology. *Polymers Advanced Technologies 22*, 326-338.

Demerlis, CC; Schoneker, DR. (2003) Review of the oral toxicity of polyvinyl alcohol (PVA). *Food and Chemical Toxicology 41*, 319-326.

Dilamian, M; Montazer, M; Masoumi, J. (2013) Antimicrobial electrospun membranes of chitosan/poly(ethylene oxide) incorporating poly(hexamethylene biguanide) hydrochloride. *Carbohydrate Polymers 94*, 364-371.

Ding, B; Kim, H-Y; Lee, S-C; Lee, D-R; Choi, K-J. (2002) Preparation and characterization of nanoscaled poly(vinyl alcohol) fibers via electrospinning. *Fibers Polymers 3*, 73-79.

Ding, B; Kimura, E; Sato, T; Fujita, S; Shiratori, S. (2004) Fabrication of blend biodegradable nanofibrous nonwoven mats via multi-jet electrospinning. *Polymer 45*, 1895-1902.

Dreaden, EC; Alkilany, AM; Huang, X; Murphy, CJ; El-Sayed, M. (2002) The golden age: Golden nanoparticles for biomedicine. *Chemical Society Reviews 41*, 2740.

Elgadir, MA; Uddin, MS; Ferdosh, S; Adam, A; Chowdhury, AJK; Sarker, MZI. (2015) Impact of chitosan composites and chitosan nanoparticle composites on various drug delivery systems: A review. *Journal of Food and Drug Analysis 23*, 619-629.

Fang, D; Liu, Y; Jiang, S; Nie, J; Ma, G. (2011) Effect of intermolecular interaction on electrospinning of sodium alginate. *Carbohydrate Polymers 85*, 276–279.

Fu, S; Ni, P; Wang, B; Chu, B; Peng, J; Zheng, L; Zhao, X; Luo, F; Wei, Y; Qian, Z. (2012) In vivo biocompatibility and osteogenesis of electrospun poly(ε-caprolactone) poly(ethyleneglycol) poly(ε-caprolactone)/nano-hydroxyapatite composite scaffold. *Biomaterials 33*, 8363-8371.

Ghorani, B; Tucker, N. (2015) Fundamentals of electrospinning as a novel delivery vehicle for bioactive compounds in food nanotechnology. *Food Hydrocolloids 51*, 227-240.

Goycoolea, FM; Lollo, G; Remunan-Lopez, C; Quaglia, F; Alonso, MJ. (2009) Chitosan-Alginate Blended Nanoparticles as Carriers for the Transmucosal Delivery of Macromolecules. *Biomacromolecules 10*, 1736–1743.

Halake, K; Birajdar, M; Kim, BS; Bae, H; Lee, C; Kim, YJ; Kim, S; Kim, HJ; Ahn, S; An, SY; Lee, J. (2014) Recent application developments of water-soluble synthetic polymers. *Journal of Industrial and Engineering Chemistry 20*, 3913–3918.

Hamman, J.H. (2010) Chitosan Based Polyelectrolyte Complexes as Potential Carrier Materials in Drug Delivery Systems. *Marine Drugs 8*, 1305-1322.

Harris, J.M. (Ed.). Poly(Ethylene Glycol) Chemistry: Biotechnical and Biomedical Applications, 1992.

Honarbakhsh, S; Pourdeyhimi, B. (2011) Scaffolds for drug delivery, part I: electrospun porous poly(lactic acid) and poly(lactic acid)/poly(ethylene oxide) hybrid scaffolds. *Journal of Materials Science 46*, 2874-2881.

Huang, C; Chen, R; Ke, Q; Morsi, Y; Zhang, K; Mo, X. (2011) Electrospun collagen-chitosan-TPU nanofibrous scaffolds for tissue engineered tubular grafts. *Colloids and Surfaces B: Biointerfaces 82*, 307–315.

Huang, CC; Lin, CK; Lu, CT; Lou, CW; Chao, CY; Lin, JH. (2009) Evaluation of the Electrospinning Manufacturing Process based on the Preparation of PVA Composite Fibres. *Fibres & Textiles in Eastern Europe 17*, 34-37.

Hwang, S; Sunghoon, J. (2011) Electrospun nano composites of poly(vinyl pyrrolidone)/nanosilver for antibacterial materials. *Journal of Nanoscience and Nanotechnology 11*, 610-613.

Ignatova, M; Manolova, N; Rashkov, I. (2007) Electrospinning of poly(vinyl pyrrolidone)-iodine complex and poly(ethylene oxide)/poly(vinyl pyrrolidone)-iodine complex – a prospective route to antimicrobial wound dressing materials. *Macromolecular Nanotechnology 43*, 1609-1623.

Ignatova, M; Manolova, N; Rashkov, I. (2007) Novel antibacterial fibers of quaternized chitosan and poly(vinyl pyrrolidone) prepared by electrospinning. *European Polymer Journal 43*, 1112-1122.

Jadhav, SV; Nikam, DS; Khot, VM; Thorat, ND; Phadatare, MR; Ningthoujam, RS; Salunkhe, AB; Pawar, SH. (2013) Studies on colloidal stability of PVP- coated LSMO nanoparticles for magnetic fluid hyperthermia. *New Journal of Chemistry 37*, 3121-3130.

Jagur-Grodzinsk, J. (2006) Polymers for tissue engineering, medical devices, and regenerative medicine. Concise general review of recent studies. *Polymer Advanced Technology 17*, 395-418.

Jannesari, M; Varshosaz, J; Morshed, M; Zamani, M. (2011) Composite poly(vinyl alcohol)/(poly(vinyl acetate) electrospun nanofibrous mats as a novel wound dressing matrix for controlled release of drugs. *International Journal of Nanomedicine 6*, 993-1003.

Jayakumar, R; Prabaharan, M; Nair, SV; Tamura, H. (2010) Novel chitin and chitosan nanofibers in biomedical applications. *Biotechnology Advances 28*, 142–150.

Jeun, J-P; Jeon, Y-K; Nho, Y-C; Kang, P-H. (2009) Effects of gamma irradiation on the thermal and mechanical properties of chitosan/PVA nanofibrous mats. *Journal of Industrial and Engineering Chemistry 15*, 430-433.

Jiang, Y-N; Mo, H-Y; Yu, D-G. (2012) Electrospun drug-loaded core-sheath PVP/zein nanofibers for biphasic drug release. *International Journal of Pharmaceutics 438*, 232-239.

Jin, H-J; Fridrikh, SV; Rutledge, GC; Kaplan, DL. (2002) Electrospinning *Bombyx mori* silk with poly(ethylene oxide). *Biomacromolecules 3*, 1233-1239.

Kadajji, VG; Betageri, GV. (2011) Water Soluble Polymers for Pharmaceutical Applications. *Polymers 3*, 1972-2009.

Karthik, R; Meenakshi, S. (2015) Removal of Cr(VI) ions by adsorption onto sodium alginate-polyaniline nanofibers. *International Journal of Biological Macromolecules 72*, 711–717.

Khorshidi, S; Solouk, A; Mirzadeh, H; Mazinani, S; Lagaron, JM; Shari fi, S; Ramakrishna, S. (2016) A review of key challenges of electrospun scaffolds for tissue-engineering applications. *Journal of Tissue Engineering and Regenerative Medicine 10*, 715-738.

Kleinubing, SA; Seraphim, DC; Vieira, MGA; Canevesi, RLS; Silva, EA; César, CL; Mei, LHI. (2014) Gastro-resistant controlled release of OTC encapsulated in alginate/chitosan matrix coated with acryl-EZE ® MP in fluidized bed. *Journal of Applied Polymer Science 131*, 40444-40449.

Koosha, M; Mirzadeh, H; Shokrgozar, MA; Farokhi, M. (2015) Nanoclay-reinforced electrospun chitosan/PVA nanocomposite nanofibers for biomedical applications. *RSC Advances 5*, 10479-10487.

Koski, A, Yim, K, Shivkumar, S. (2004) Effect of molecular weight on fibrous pva produced by electrospinning. *Materials Letters 58*, 493-497.

Kriegel, C; Kit, KM; McClements, DJ; Weiss, J. (2009) Electrospinning of chitosan-poly(ethylene oxide) blend nanofibers in the presence of micellar surfactant solutions. *Polymer 50*, 189-200.

Leung, V; Ko, F. Biomedical applications of nanofibers. (2011) *Polymers for Advanced Technology 22*, 350–365.

Li, C; Fu, R; Yu, C; Li, Z; Guan, H; Hu, D; Zhao, D; Lu, L. (2013) Silver nanoparticle/chitosan oligosaccharide/poly(vinyl alcohol) nanofibers as wound dressing: a preclinical study. *International Journal of Nanomedicine 8*, 4131-4145.

Li, D; McCann, JT; Xia, Y. (2006) Electrospinning: A Simple and Versatile Technique for Producing Ceramic Nanofibers and Nanotubes. *Journal of the American Ceramic Society 89*, 1861–1869.

Li, D; Herricks, T; Xia, Y. (2003) Magnetic nanofibers of nickel ferrite prepared by electrospinning. *Applied Physics Letters 83*, 4586.

Li, D; Xia, Y. (2004) Electrospinning of nanofibers: reinventing the wheel?. *Advanced Materials 16*, 1151-1170.

Liechty, WB; Kryscio, DR; Slaughter, BV; Peppas, NA. (2010) Polymers for Drug Delivery Systems. *Annual Review of Chemical and Biomolecular Engineering 1, 149–173.*

Lin, D; Wui, H; Zhang, R; Pan, W. (2007) Preparation of ZnS nanofibers via electrospinning. *Journal of the American Ceramic Society 90*, 3664-3666.

Lu, G; Li, S; Guo, Z; Farha, OK; Hauser, BG, Qi, X; Wang, Y; Wang, X; Han, S; Liu, X; DuChene, JS; Zhang, H; Zhang, Q; Chen, X; Ma, J; Loo, SCJ; Wei, WD; Yang, Y; Hupp, JT; Huo, F. (2012) Imparting functionality to a metal-organic framework material by controlled nanoparticle encapsulation. *Nature Chemistry 4*, 310-316.

Ma, G; Fang, D; Liu, Y; Zhu, X; Nie, J. (2012) Electrospun sodium alginate/poly(ethylene oxide) core–shell nanofibers scaffolds potential for tissue engineering applications. *Carbohydrate Polymers 87*, 737-743.

Meng, X; Tian, F; Yang, J; He, CN; Xing, N; Li, F. (2010) Chitosan and alginate polyelectrolyte complex membranes and their properties for wound dressing application. *Journal of Materials Science: Materials in Medicine 21*, 1751–1759.

Min, L; Yuan, Z; Zhong, L; Liu, Q; Wu, R; Zheng, Z. (2015) Preparation of chitosan based electrospun nanofiber membrane and its adsorptive removal of arsenate from aqueous solution. *Chemical Engineering Journal 267*, 132–141.

Moon, S; Lee, J. (2012) Electrospun Poly(ethylene oxide)/Hydrated Iron Oxide/Sodium Alginate Composite Nanofibers With Multi-Functional Properties. *Polymer Engineering & Science 53*, 1321-1326.

Nguyen, TTT; Park, JS. (2011) Fabrication of electrospun nonwoven mats of polyvinylidene fluoride/polyethylene glycol/fumed silica for use as energy storage materials. *Journal of Applied Polymer Science 121*, 3596-3603.

Nicknejad, ET; Ghoreishi, SM; Habibi, N. (2015) Electrospinning of Cross-Linked Magnetic Chitosan Nanofibers for Protein Release. *AAPS Pharm Sci Tech* 16, 1480-1486.

Nie, H; Ho, ML; Wang, CK; Wang, CW; Fu, YC. (2009) BMP-2 plasmid loaded PLGA/Hap composite scaffolds for treatment of bone defects in nude mice. *Biomaterials 30*, 892-901.

Nista, SVG; Bettini, J; Mei, LHI. (2015) Coaxial Nanofibers of Chitosan-Alginate-PEO polycomplex obtained by electrospinning. *Carbohydrate Polymers 127*, 222–228.

Nista, SVG; Peres, L; D'Ávila, MA; Schmidt, FL; Mei, LHI. (2012) Nanostructured Membranes Based on Cellulose Acetate Obtained by Electrospinning, Part 1: Study of the Best Solvents and Conditions by Design of Experiments. *Journal of Applied Polymer Science 126*, E70–E78.

Nonato, RC; Morales, AR; Vieira, AFM; Nista, SVG; Mei, LHI; Bonse, BC. (2016) Solution parameters in the manufacture of ceramic ZnO nanofibers made by electrospinning. *Applied Physics A 122*, 244.

Nonato, RC; Morales, AR; Rocha, MC; Nista, SVG; Mei, LHI; Bonse, BC. (2017) Process parameters in the manufacture of ceramic ZnO nanofibers made by electrospinning. *Applied Physics A 123*, 92.

Nunthanid, J; Luangtana-anan, M; Sriamornsak, P; Limmatvapirat, S; Huanbutta, K; Puttipipatkhachorn, S. (2009) Use of spray-dried chitosan acetate and ethylcellulose as compression coats for colonic drug delivery: Effect of swelling on triggering *in vitro* drug release. *European Journal of Pharmaceutics and Biopharmaceutics 71*, 356-361.

Peresin, MS; Habibi, Y; Zoppe, JO; Pawlak, JJ; Rojas, OJ. (2010) Nanofiber composites of polyvinyl alcohol and celulose nanocrystals: Manufacture and characterization. *Biomacromolecules 11*, 674-681.

Ramaseshan, R; Sundarrajan, S; Ramakrishna, RJ. (2007) Nanostructured ceramics by electrospinning. *Journal of Applied Physics 102*, 111101/1-111101/17.

Sambudi, NS; Sathyamurthy, M; Lee, GM; Park, SB. (2015) Electrospun chitosan/poly(vinyl alcohol) reinforced with CaCO 3 nanoparticles with enhanced mechanical properties and biocompatibility for cartilage tissue engineering. *Composites Science and Technology 106*, 76–84.

Sarhan, WA; Azzazy, HME. (2015) High concentration honey chitosan electrospun nanofibers: Biocompatibility and antibacterial effects. *Carbohydrate Polymers 122*, 135–143.

Sarmento, B; Ribeiro, A; Veiga, F; Ferreira, D; Neufeld, R. (2007) Oral bioavailability of insulin contained in polysaccharide nanoparticles, *Biomacromolecules 8:10*, 3054－3060.

Sell, SA; Wolfe, PS; Garg, K; McCool, JM; Rodriguez, IA; Bowlin, GL. (2010) The Use of Natural Polymers in Tissue Engineering: A Focus on Electrospun Extracellular Matrix Analogues. *Polymers 4*, 522-553.

Shalumon, KT; Anulekha, KH; Nair, SV; Chennazhi, KP; Jayakumar, R. (2011) Sodium alginate/poly(vinyl alcohol)/nano ZnO composite nanofibers for antibacterial wound dressings. *International Journal of Biological Macromolecules 49*, 247-254.

Shalumon, KT; Binulal, NS; Selvamurugan, N; Nair, SV; Menon, D; Furuike, T; Tamura, H; Jayakumar, R. (2009) Electrospinning of carboxymethyl chitin/poly(vinyl alcohol) nanofibrous scaffolds for tissue engineering applications. *Carbohydrate Polymers 77*, 863-869.

Sharma, A; Gupta, A; Rath, G; Goyal, A; Mathur, RB; Dhakate, SR. (2013) Electrospun composite nanofiber-based transmucosal patch for anti-diabetic drug delivery. *Journal of Materials Chemistry B 1*, 3410-3418.

Shao, C; Yang, X; Guan, H; Liu, Y; Gong, J. (2004) Electrospun nanofibers of NiO/ZnO composite. *Inorganic Chemistry Communications 7*, 625-627.

Shen, Q; Min, Q; Shi, J; Jiang, L; Zhang, J-R; Hou, W; Zhu, J-J. (2009) Morphology-controlled synthesis of palladium nanostructures by sonoelectrochemical method and their application in direct alcohol oxidation. *The Journal of Physical Chemistry C 113*, 1267-1273.

Simsek-Ege, FA; Bond, GM; Stringer, J. (2003) Polyelectrolye Complex Formation between Alginate and Chitosan as a Function of pH. *Journal of Applied Polymer Science 88*, 346–351.

Singh, SK; Yadav, M; Behrens, S; Roesky, PW. (2013) Au-based bimetallic nanoparticles for the intramolecular aminoalkene hydroamination. *Dalton Transactions 42*, 10404.

Song, X; Wang, Z; Liu, Y; Wang, C; Li, L. (2009) Ahighly sensitive ethanol sensor based on mesoporous ZnO-SnO_2 nanofibers. *Nanotechnology 20*, 075501.

Stotak, M; Ragusa, J; Gonzalez, D; Subramanian, A. (2011) Improved cellular infiltration into nanofibrous electrospun cross-linked gelatina scaffolds templated with micrometer-sized polyethylene glycol fibers. *Biomedical Materials 6*, 055012.

Sun, G; Teng, H; Zhang, C; Dou, Y; Li, Y. (2010) Preparation of Ultrafine Water-soluble Polymers Nanofiber Mats via Electrospinning. *Chemical Research in Chinese Universities 26*, 318-322.

Sun, Y; Xia, Y. (2002) Large-scale synthesis of uniform silver nanowires through a soft, self-seeding, polyol process. *Advanced Materials 14*, 833-837.

Sundaramurthi, D; Vasanthan, KS; Kuppan, P; Krishnan, UM; Sethuraman, S. (2012) Electrospun nanostructured chitosan-poly(vinyl alcohol) scaffolds: biomimetic extracellular matrix as dermal substitute. *Biomedical Materials 7*.

Taepaiboon, P; Rungsardthong, U; Supaphol, P. (2006) Drug-loaded electrospun mats of poly(vinyl alcohol) fibres and their release characteristics of four model drugs. *Nanotechnology 17*, 2317-2329.

Tang, Z; Wei, J; Yung, L; Ji, B; Ma, H; Qiu, C; Yoon, K; Wan, F; Fang, D.; Hsiao, BS; Chu, B. (2009) UV-Cured poly(vinyl alcohol) ultrafiltration nanofibrous membrane based on electrospun nanofiber scaffolds. *Journal of Membrane Science 328*, 1-5.

Tarun, K; Gobi, N. (2012) Calcium alginate/PVA blended nano fiber matrix for wound dressing. *Indian Journal of Fibre & Textile Research 37*, 127-132.

Tonsomboon, K; Oyen, ML. (2013) Composite electrospun gelatin fiber-alginate gel scaffolds for mechanically robust tissue engineered cornea. *Journal of the Mechanical Behavior of Biomedical Materials 21*, 185-194.

Totten, GE; Clinton, NA. (2008) Poly(ethylene Glycol) and derivatives as phase transfer catalysts. *Journal of Macromolecular Science Part C 38*, 77-142.

Verreck, G; Chun, I; Rosenblatt, J; Peeters, J; Dijck, AV; Mensch, J; Noppe, M; Brewster, ME. (2003) Incorporation of drugs in an amorphous state into electrospun nanofibers composed of a water-insoluble, nonbiodegradable polymer. *Journal of Controlled Release 92*, 349-360.

Yang, A; Tao, X; Pang, GKH; Siu, KGG. (2008) Preparation of Porous Tin Oxide Nanobelts Using the Electrospinning Technique. *Journal of the American Ceramic Society 91*, 257-262.

Yang, X; Shao, C; Liu, Y; Mu, R; Guan, H. (2005) Nanofibers of CeO_2 via an electrospinning technique. *Thin Solid Films 478*, 228-231.

Yang, X; Shao, C; Liu, Y. (2007) Fabrication of Cr2O3/Al2O3 composite nanofibers by electrospinning. *Journal of Materials Science 42*, 8470-8472.

Yao, L; Haas, TW; Guiseppi-Elie, A; Bowlin, GL; Simpson, DG; Wnek, GE. (2003) Electrospinning and stabilization of fully hydrolyzed poly(vinyl alcohol) fibers. *Chemistry of Materials 15*, 1860-1864.

Ye, F; Hu, W; Zhang, T; Yang, J; Ding, Y. (2012) Enhanced electrocatalytic activity of Pt-nanostructures prepared by electrodeposition using poly(vinyl pyrrolidone) as a shape-control agent. *Electrochimica Acta 83*, 383-386.

Wade, A, Weller, PJ. (Eds.) Handbook of Pharmaceutical Excipients. American Pharmaceutical Association, Washington, DC, 1994.

Wang, J; Yao, H-B; He, D; Zhang, C-L; Yu, S-H. (2012) Facile fabrication of gold nanoparticles-poly(vinyl alcohol) electrospun water-stable nanofibrous mats: Efficient substrate materials for biosensors. *Applied Materials & Interfaces 4*, 1963-1971.

Wang, Y; Chen, P; Liu, M. (2006) Synthesis of well-defined copper nanocubes by a one-pot solution process. *Nanotechnology 17*, 6000.

Wang, Y; Xie, S; Liu, J; Park, J; Huang, CCZ; Xia, Y. (2013) Shape-controlled synthesis of palladium nanocrystals: A mechanistic understanding of the evolution from octahedrons to tetrahedrons. *Nano Letters 13*, 2276-2281.

Wang, Z; Li, Z; Liu, L; Xu, X; Zhang, H; Wang, W; Zheng, W; Wang, C. (2010) A novel alcohol detector based on ZrO_2-doped SnO_2 electrospun nanofibers. *Journal of the American Ceramic Society 93*, 634-637.

Wei Lu, J; Zhu, Y; Guo, Z; Hu, P; Yu, J. (2006) Electrospinning of sodium alginate with poly(cthylcnc oxidc). *Polymer 47*, 8026-8031.

Wei, L; Cai, C; Lin, J; Wang, L; Zhang, X. (2011) Degradation controllable biomaterials constructed from lysozyme-loaded Ca-alginate microparticle/chitosan composites. *Polymer 52*, 5139-5148.

Wu, H; Pan, W; Lin, D; Li, H. (2012) Electrospinning of ceramic nanofibers: Fabrication, assembly and applications. *Journal of Advanced Ceramics 1*, 2-23.

Zeng, J; Aigner, A; Czubayko, F; Kissel, T; Wendorff, JH; Greiner, A. (2005) Poly(vinyl alcohol) nanofibers by electrospinning as a protein delivery system and the retardation of enzyme release by additional polymer coatings. *Biomacromolecules 6*, 1484-1488.

Zhang, H; Jin, M; Xia, Y. (2012) Enhancing the catalytic and electrocatalytic properties of Pt-based catalysts by forming bimetallic nanocrystals with Pd. *Chemical Society Reviews 41*, 8035.

Zhang, J-F; Yang, D-Z; Xu, F; Zhang, Z-P; Yin, R-X; Nie, J. (2009) Electrospun core-shell structure nanofibers from homogeneous solution of poly(ethylene oxide)/chitosan. *Macromolecules 42*, 5278-5284.

Zhang, Y; He, X; Li, J; Miao, Z; Huang, F. (2008) Fabrication and ethanol-sensing properties of micro gas sensor based on electrospun SnO_2 nanofibers. *Sensors and Actuators B: Chemical 132*, 67-73.

Zhang, Y-J; Yao, Q; Zhang, Y; Cui, T-Y; Li, D; Liu, W; Lawrence, W; Zhang, Z-D. (2008) Solvothermal synthesis of magnetic chains self-assembled by flowerlike cobalt submicrospheres. *Crystal Growth & Design 8*, 3206-3212.

Zheng, W; Li, Z; Zhang,H; Wang, W; Wang, Y; Wang, C. (2009) Electrospinning route for α-Fe_2O_3 ceramic nanofibers and their gas sensing properties. *Materials Research Bulletin 44*, 1432-1436.

Zhou, Y; Yang, D; Chen, X; Xu, Q; Lu, F; Nie, J. (2008) Electrospun water-soluble carboxyethyl chitosan/poly(vinyl alcohol) nanofibrous membrane as potential wound dressing for skin regeneration. *Biomacromolecules 9*, 349-354.

Zhou, W; Lin, L; Zhao, D; Guo, L. (2011) Synthesis of nickel bowl-like nanoparticles and their doping for inducing planar alignment of a nematic liquid Crystal. *Journal of the American Chemical Society 133*, 8389-8391.

Ziaei-Azad; H; Semagina, N. (2014) Bimetallic catalysts: Requirements for stabilizing PVP removal depend on the surface composition. *Applied Catalysis A: General 482*, 327-335.

Zong, X; Bien, H; Chung, C-Y; Yin, L; Fang, D; Hsiao, BS; Chu, B; Entcheva, E. (2005) Electrospun fine-textured scaffolds for heart tissue constructs. *Biomaterials 26*, 5330-5338.

In: Electrospinning and Electroplating
Editor: Toby Jacobs
ISBN: 978-1-53612-363-0

Chapter 3

DEVELOPMENTS IN TISSUE ENGINEERING SCAFFOLDING USING AN ELECTROSPINNING PROCESS

Nor Hasrul Akhmal Ngadiman[1], M. Y. Noordin[1], Ani Idris[2,*], Denni Kurniawan[3], Ehsan Fallahiarezoudar[1] and Izman Sudin[1]

[1]Faculty of Mechanical Engineering, Universiti Teknologi Malaysia, Johor Bahru, Johor, Malaysia

[2]Institute of Bioproduct Development, Faculty of Chemical and Energy Engineering Universiti Teknologi Malaysia, Johor Bahru, Johor, Malaysia

[3]Department of Mechanical Engineering, Curtin University, Sarawak, Malaysia

ABSTRACT

Electrospinning is a simple and efficient process in producing nanofibers. The use of an electrospinning process in fabricating tissue engineering scaffolds has received great attention in recent years due to its simplicity and ability to fabricate ultrafine nanofibers. Most of the recent progress in tissue engineering has embarked on the use of nanofibers as tissue engineering scaffolds. This is because nanofibers can replicate the structural design of natural human tissue at the nano-scale thus shortening the healing time. Although electrospinning is a simple process, there are still several parameters which need to be controlled or optimised in order to produce nanofibers with different

[*] Corresponding author: Emails: ani@cheme.utm.my, Tel: +607-5535603, Fax: +607-5588166.

characteristics. Different applications might require nanofibers with specific criteria to be produced. Hence, this review will reveal the fundamental working principles of electrospinning process and the effect of electrospinning process parameters towards the nanofibers morphology. Various polymeric materials and their composites/blends have been successfully electrospun for tissue engineering (TE) scaffolds and they have been tabulated. In many cases, secondary processes are also integrated with the electrospinning process so as to develop 3D TE scaffolds and overcome limitations in term of the nanofiber thickness.

1. Electrospinning Process

Electrospinning is a novel and efficient method by which fibers with diameters in nanometer scale namely nanofibers can be produced. The diameter of the nanofiber formed is in the range of 100-500 nm. Nanofibers have found their applications in biomedical field such as tissue engineering [1]–[9], drug delivery [10], [11] and wound dressing [12], [13]. They are also used in protective clothing [14], filtration [15], reinforcement in composite materials [16], [17] and micro-electronics such as battery [18], supercapacitors [19], transistor [20], sensors [21] and display devices [22].

During electrospinning the syringe pump injects the solution within the set up flow rate and the solution then flows through the tube until it reaches the nozzle which has a voltage supply connected to it. Upon reaching the nozzle, the body of solution becomes charged due to the sufficiently high voltage thus creating repulsive interactions between oppositely charged solution and collector. The tensile forces on the liquid triggered the pendant drop to elongate at the tip of the capillary. The droplet is stretched when the electrostatic forces balance out the surface tension due to the increase in electric field strength. At this critical point, the Taylor cone is formed due to the eruption of the liquid at the surface [23]. Stream breakup will not occur when the molecular cohesion of the liquid is sufficiently high and a charged liquid jet is formed when the droplets are electro sprayed. By the trashing process, the jet will be elongated at small bend in the fiber due to the electrostatic repulsion before depositing on the collector. The fiber formed will be in nanometer-scale diameters [24]. There are two main types of collector; static and rotating collector. Randomly oriented fiber mat is usually formed on the static collector while aligned fiber mat is formed with rotating collector. Figure 1 shows the electrospinning equipment with a rotating collector.

2. Process Parameter

Although electrospinning is a relatively easy process, there are several parameter settings that can greatly influence the diameter of nanofibers. The parameters concerned are solution concentration, collector rotating speed, distance between collector drum and needle, applied voltage and volume flow rate.

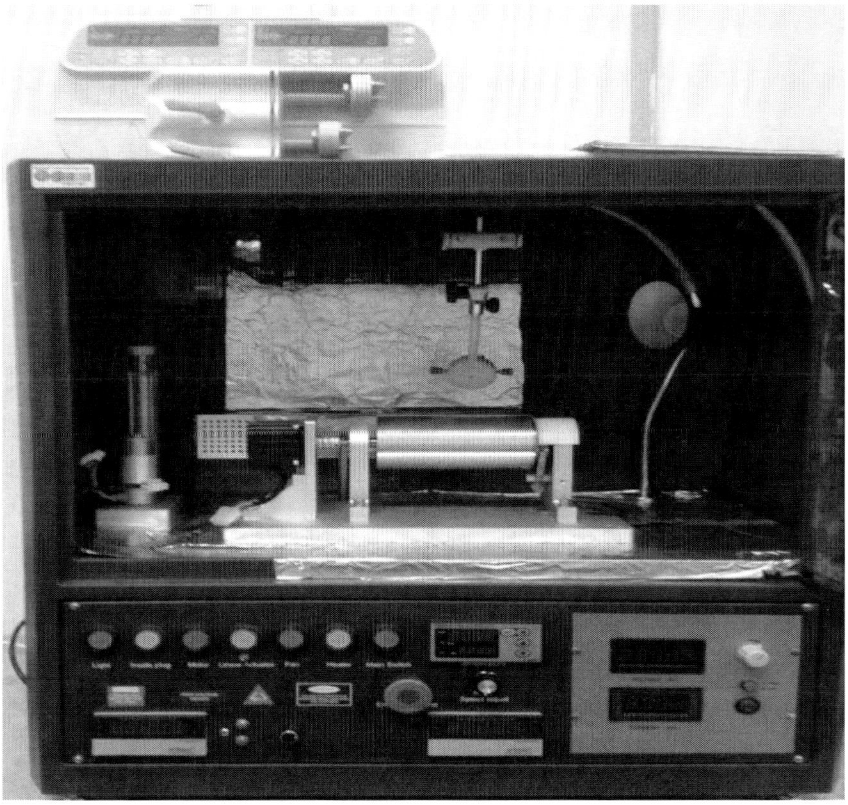

Figure 1. Electrospinning Machine.

2.1. The Effect of Polymer Concentration and Material with Fiber Diameter

There are many studies have been carried out to investigate the effect of material and solution concentration on fiber diameter during electrospinning process. Previous studies have reported that solution concentration is directly proportional with the diameter of nanofibers produced [25], [26], [1], [27]–[33]. Lower concentration polymer produced nanofibers with smaller diameter due to the large amount of solvent present in the solution. The solvent present will evaporate during spinning thus leaving the polymer. In addition, longer distance between needle and collector provided more time to stretch the jet in the electric field and also to evaporate the solvent. This will further promote thinner fiber formation.

However several studies have reported contradictory results where the increase in the concentration of solution produces thinner nanofiber diameter [34], [35]. Such phenomenon can occur due to the increase in the conductivity of the solution as a result of the increase in the concentration. If the electrical conductivity of the electrospinning precursor solution is higher, the diameter of electrospun polymer fiber is thinner [4].

Solution concentration is not the only factor that affects the diameter of fiber formation. The interaction of solvent concentration with the distance between needle and collector will also influence the diameter of nanofiber formation. Such interactions between various factors are reported by Haghi and Akbari [36] in their research. Their findings have revealed that solution concentration has two way interactions between the spinning distance, applied voltage and flow rate for the diameter of fiber formation.

2.2. The Effect of Spinning Distance with Fiber Diameter

Theoretically, spinning distance is inversely proportional with the fiber diameter. This is because the longer spinning distance will provide more time for the jet to stretch in the electric field before it is deposited onto the collector. At the same time, solvents will require longer time to evaporate resulting the formation of nanofibers on the collector to become thinner. According to the equation $E = V/d$, it is illustrated that the increase in spinning distance will decrease the electric field strength and also decrease the speed. As a result, thicker nanofibers are formed.

Different findings have been reported by several researchers regarding the influence of distance between needle and collector on nanofiber diameter. Some findings reported that increasing the spinning distance will decrease the fiber diameter [37] while others revealed that increasing the spinning distance will increase the nanofiber diameter [38]–[40]. Also, there are findings reported that spinning distance has no effect to the nanofiber diameter [41], [42].

2.3. The Effect of Applied Voltage with Fiber Diameter

Applied voltage is also known to have an effect on the nanofiber diameter. An increase in the applied voltage may decrease the nanofiber diameter [3], [7], [43] or an increase in the applied voltage is said to increase the fiber diameter [28], [38], [40], [41], [44], [45]. On the other hand, findings have also revealed that applied voltage do not seem to have an effect to the fiber diameter [37], [42].

Fiber diameter can be decreased by increasing the applied voltage because the electric field strength will increase and electrostatic stretching force will become larger. Such conditions will cause the jet to accelerate more in the electric field thus forming thinner nanofibers.

However, it is also believed that the increase in the voltage creates more surface charges on the jet which will subsequently increase the mass flow rate from the needle tip to the collector. Such phenomena will result in rapid drawing of solution from the tip of the needle causing the nanofiber diameter to increase.

2.4. The Effect of Volume Flow Rate with Fiber Diameter

According to Zong et al. (2002), a minimum value for the solution flow rate is required to form the drop of polymer at the tip of the needle to maintain a stable Taylor Cone [46]. His finding has clearly shown that flow rate could affect the fiber diameter. The increase in the volume flow rate will result in the increasing amount of solution delivered to the tip of needle. Hence, larger diameter nanofibers will be formed as revealed by many studies [37], [44]–[46].

3. Tissue Engineering

The shortage of organs for transplant is the main cause of death today [47]. The current solution to these problems lies in the current technology which offers bio-artificial tissues, organs and mechanical appliances which are the only options available to lead a normal life [48]. This contributes to the need for tissue engineered blood vessels [49], heart valves [50], bladders [51], dialyzer for haemodialysis [52], and xenografts techniques [53]. Regenerative medicine can be defined as transplant of cells, organs, or tissues with the purpose of restoring or replacing damaged or lost organs and body parts which brings hope for patients who are suffering from congenital defects or malfunction of vital organs [54]. Tissue engineering has a good potential to replace traditional therapeutic methods in terms of treatment for organ loss or failure but it needs to ultimately achieve the goals of harvesting organs or human tissues *in vitro* cultivation [55].

Tissue engineering is a new field that combines several areas and applies the principles of engineering sciences, biological and chemical in order to regenerate tissues which are lost or damage [56]. The science of design and fabrication of new tissues for the purpose of restoring functional impaired organs and replacing lost parts due to cancer, disease and trauma is defined as tissue engineering.

The principle of tissue engineering is to develop a three dimensional living construct that is architecturally functional and mechanically equivalent to or better than the tissue that needs to be replaced. This can be done by the combination of living cells with synthetic or natural support or scaffolds that is biodegradable [57]. The four key components that need to be carefully selected when developing a construct are scaffold, growth factors, extracellular matrix (ECM), and cells [58].

4. NANOFIBER

Most of the recent progress in tissue engineering have started to use nanofibers as scaffolds because they can potentially imitate the architecture of natural human tissue at the nano-scale [59]. Nanofibers can provide all the highly desired properties of the scaffold materials such as high surface volume ratio and microporous structure which favours cell adhesion, proliferation, migration, and differentiation [60]. Thus, current research trend in this field is very much dedicated on characterization, biocompatibility evaluation, fabrication, and nanofiber-based systems applications as scaffolds in tissue engineering [61].

5. VARIOUS MATERIALS FOR ELECTROSPUN TISSUE ENGINEERING SCAFFOLDS

One of the most challenging aspects in developing scaffolds is the complexity of recreating microenvironments similar to those found in the tissue of interest. As the case for many medical devices, the biomaterials for TE scaffold are taken from the pool of available materials. Many materials are selected and tested in order to find the biocompatible materials which can fulfil most of the requirements for TE scaffolds. Research on better and more robust materials or combination of materials which have the potential to become an ideal material for development of scaffolds is still ongoing.

Naturally occurring materials are used to mimic the extracellular structure for TE scaffolds. Biopolymers have various natural functions, such as having the capability of intracellular communication and storage. They also possess proteins that make up the structural materials and catalysts as well as contain polysaccharides in cell membranes [62].

Natural occurring biopolymers such as starch or chitosan are known to be biodegradable, biocompatible and have tailorable degradation rates [63]. However, they have drawbacks such as the limited mechanical properties and process ability or variation between different batches. Some common biopolymers which are used to produce scaffolds are collagen, alginate, chitosan and silk. These polymers can be combined with other synthetic materials to improve their process ability and mechanical properties. Combinations with hydroxyapatite (HA), aliphatic polyesters, or composites of different natural polymers can also improve the properties of the scaffolds.

Synthetic polymer such as poly (vinyl alcohol) (PVA), polycaprolactone (PCL), poly (L-lactide-co-caprolactone) (PLLACL), poly (lactic-co-glycolic Acid) (PLGA) and others have also become choices in the development of scaffolds. The list of materials that has been studied for the development of scaffolds is compiled in Table 1. PCL and PVA are the two most attractive materials which are used with various fillers or additives.

Pure polymers on their own are rarely used as TE scaffolds. In most cases, fillers are added to enhance the properties of the polymers itself. Some fillers/additives such as chitosan [64] and hydroxyapatite [1], [33]–[35], [65]–[68] are natural and commonly used to improve the biocompatibility characteristics of the polymers and to enhance the cell growth rate. Other fillers/additives such as nanoclay [69], bioactive glass [70], magnetite [64] have been reported to improve the mechanical properties of the polymer. Thus, by selecting a good combination of polymers and fillers/additives will improve the properties of TE scaffolds in terms of biocompatibility and strength.

Table 1 illustrates the use of various fillers for different polymers. The amount and type of fillers used are influenced by the diameter of the nanofiber. They also affect the mechanical properties such as the young modulus, tensile strength and strain of electrospun TE scaffolds. In some cases, the increase in the filler concentration will increase the fiber diameter of the nanofibers. The adding of fillers or additives to the main materials in developing TE scaffolds does not ensure that the fiber diameter and mechanical properties will improve. In some cases, it has an adverse effect.

Abdal-hay et al. (2013) [1] has investigated about hydroxyapatite which is added in calcium phosphate coated with nylon 6 at various concentration. It has revealed that the increase in the hydroxyapatite concentration will increase the fiber diameter [1]. The electrospun fiber diameter increased from 175 ± 40 nm for 0% HA to the 450 ± 55 nm for 5% HA and 850 ± 80 nm for 10% HA. The Young's modulus of the scaffold has also increased when increasing the filler concentration; from 9.8 MPa to 19.2 MPa and finally to 35. 7 MPa for 0%, 5% and 10% filler concentrations, respectively. However, the increase in tensile strength is not directly proportional with the fiber diameter and Young's modulus increment. Tensile strength has remained constant at 19.5 MPa when filler concentration is increased from 0% to 5%. A further increase to 10% has resulted in only a small increment in tensile strength to 20.3 MPa. In addition, the scaffold elongation will decrease with the increasing of HA concentration. It has been reported that the scaffold is becoming more brittle as the HA concentration loading is increased.

In another study, poly(lactic-co-glycolic acid) (PLGA) has been used as the main polymer while multiwalled carbon nanotubes (MWNTs) are used as the filler [32]. The results have revealed that the increasing in the loading of MWNTs will increase the fiber diameter from 727 nm, 1257 nm and 1400 nm for 0%, 0.25% and 0.5% MWNTs loading respectively. The increase in Young's modulus is also followed by an increase in the tensile strength.

Table 1. Mechanical Properties of Electrospun TE Scaffolds of Various Materials

Main Material	Filler/Additive	Particle Loading	Fiber Diameter (nm)	Young's Modulus (MPa)	Tensile Strength (MPa)	Tensile Srain (%)	Breaking Elongation (%)	Ref
Polycaprolactone (PCL)	NanoClay (NC)	0% NC	210	3.5	1.25			[69]
		1% NC	250	4.5	0.75			
		2% NC	250	4.5	1.00			
		4% NC	380	4.5	2.50			
		6% NC	480	4.75	3.25			
	Hydroxyapatite (HA)/b-Tricalcium Phosphate (TCP)	PCL	286 ± 136	1.50 ± 0.24	0.91 ± 0.12		139.07 ± 13	[71]
		PCL-HA	649.9 ± 111	2.81 ± 0.28	1.40 ± 0.29		64.41 ± 11.0	
		PCL-HA/TCP	868.7 ± 180	2.46 ± 0.10	1.31 ± 0.15		52.54 ± 85	
	Hydroxyapatite (HA) & Collagen I	PCL		14.63 ± 0.85	6.50 ± 0.74	73.96 ± 3.5		[67]
		PCL/HA		9.14 ± 1.15	3.99 ± 0.31	93.82 ± 8.3		
		PCL/COL/HA		13.93 ± 4.94	4.67 ± 0.82	70.64 ± 7.98		
	Hydroxyapatite (HA) & Calcium Carbonate ($CaCO_3$)	12% PCL	950 ± 0.02		2.84 ± 0.45			[68]
		12% PCL/0.5% $CaCO_3$	1020 ± 0.03		3.63 ± 0.50			
		12% PCL/1.0% $CaCO_3$	1120 ± 0.03		3.76 ± 0.94			
		12% PCL/0.5% HA	1240 ± 0.03		3.77 ± 0.14			
		12% PCL/1.0% HA	1260 ± 0.03		3.93 ± 0.05			
		10% PCL/0.83% HA	420 ± 0.02		n/a			
		8%PCL/0.67% HA	280 ± 0.02		n/a			

Table 1. (Continued)

Main Material	Filler/Additive	Particle Loading	Fiber Diameter (nm)	Young's Modulus (MPa)	Tensile Strength (MPa)	Tensile Srain (%)	Breaking Elongation (%)	Ref
Poly(Vinyl Alcohol) (PVA)	Hydroxyapatite (HA)/Type I Cellagen	PVA		2.67 ± 0.78	0.22 ± 0.09		41 ± 6.64	[65]
		PVA/Col		4.97 ± 2.41	0.62 ± 0.13		109 ± 11.34	
		PVA/Col/ 5% HA		11.10 ± 3.38	1.03 ± 0.17		135 ± 14.25	
		PVA/Col/ 10% HA		3.10 ± 0.94	0.17 ± 0.05		51 ± 6.95	
	Gelatin (GE)	PVA/GE (0/10)	50 ± 10		3.70 ± 0.5	15.0 ± 3		[72]
		PVA/GE (2/8)	90 ± 10		3.55 ± 0.5	19 ± 3		
		PVA/GE (6/4)	120 ± 20		3.10 ± 0.8	23 ± 5		
		PVA/GE (8/2)	130 ± 10		1.2 ± 0.4	30 ± 5		
		PVA/GE (10/0)	150 ± 20		0.85 ± 0.6	98 ± 5		
	Bioactive Glass (BG)	PVA	286 ± 14	126 ± 5	18 ± 2		94 ± 4	[70]
		PVA/BG	318 ± 36	275 ± 8	21 ± 2		64 ± 5	
	Gelatin (GE)	PVA	250 ± 20		0.85 ± 0.6	98.0 ± 5		[73]
		GE	50 ± 10		3.70 ± 0.5	15.0 ± 3.0		
		PVA/GE	100 ± 10		3.55 ± 0.5	19.0 ± 3.0		
		Crosslink PVA-GE	150 ± 10		4.20 ± 0.4	31.0 ± 5.0		
	Graphene Oxide (GO)	0% GO	300-500 decrease ↓		4.6 decrease ↓			[4]
		1% GO						
		3% GO						
		5%GO						
	Magnetite (Fe_3O_4)/ Chitosan (CS)	1% Fe_3O_4	286 ± 35	52.0 ± 3.9	3.9 ± 1.3	38.1 ± 2.3		[64]
		3% Fe_3O_4	280 ± 36	56.9 ± 2.6	3.8 ± 1.1	37.5 ± 4.1		
		5% Fe_3O_4	290 ± 43	58.4 ± 3.7	3.6 ± 1.3	36.6 ± 3.7		
	Maghemite	5% γ-Fe_20_3	286 ± 61	139 ± 15				[9]

Main Material	Filler/Additive	Particle Loading	Fiber Diameter (nm)	Young's Modulus (MPa)	Tensile Strength (MPa)	Tensile Srain (%)	Breaking Elongation (%)	Ref
Silk Fibroin	Hydroxyapatite (HA)	0% HAp	95 ± 17		0.43 ± 0.21		6.87 ± 2.77	[66]
		5% HAp	277 ± 46		0.54 ± 0.21		4.53 ± 0.98	
		10% HAp	234 ± 36		0.65 ± 0.03		6.08 ± 1.43	
		15% HAp	285± 55		0.91 ± 0.38		3.60 ± 1.20	
		30% Hap	582 ± 99		1.17 ± 0.04		6.55 ± 1.95	
Polyacrylonitrile (PAN)	Hydroxyapatite (HA)	0% HAp	393 ± 136		1.42			[34]
		5% HAp	260 ± 73		1.00			
		10% HAp	238 ± 84		0.65			
Calcium Phosphate (CaP) coating with Nylon 6 (N6)	Hydroxyapatite (HA)	0% HAp	175 ± 40	9.774	19.54		85	[1]
		5% HAp	450 ± 55	19.23	19.45		62	
		10% HAp	850 ± 80	35.67	20.32		59	
Poly(ε-caprolactone) (PCL)/Polydopamine (PDA)	Hydroxyapatite (HA)	HAp/ (PDA-PCL) (24h- $NaHCO_3$)	1200	459				[35]
		HAp/ (PDA-PCL) (48h- $NaHCO_3$)	>1200	768				
Poly(L-lactide-co-caprolactone) (PLLACL)	Collagen/Bone morphogenetic protein 2 (BMP2) and dexamethasone (DEX)	PLLACL	859.3		3.96±0.446			[74]
		PLLACL-Collagen (1:1)	365.4		2.19 ± 0.28			
		PLLACL-Collagen (3:1)	336.8		3.79 ± 0.31			
Poly (Lactic-co-Glycolic Acid) (PLGA)	Multiwalled Carbon Nanotubes (MWNTs)	0% MWNTs	727	163.53	5.88			[32]
		0.25% MWNTs	1257	176.83	9.08			
		0.5% MWNTs	1430	303.52	7.52			

On the other hand, it is also shown that the increasing of the concentration of fillers will decrease the properties of scaffolds. In the case of using polyacrylonitrile (PAN) as the main polymer, and hydroxyapatite (HA) as a filler [34], the fiber diameter decreases. Adding the concentration of HA by 5% and 10% will decrease the fiber diameter to 260 ± 73 nm and 238 ± 84 nm, from 393 ± 136 nm respectively. The tensile strength decreased from an initial value of 1.4 MPa to 1.0 MPa and 0.6 MPa for 5% and 10% of HA, respectively. This occurred due to the agglomeration of nano hydroapatite during mixing resulting in limited interfacial bonding. Therefore, this has proven that the combination of PAN and HA does not improve the characteristic of PAN itself.

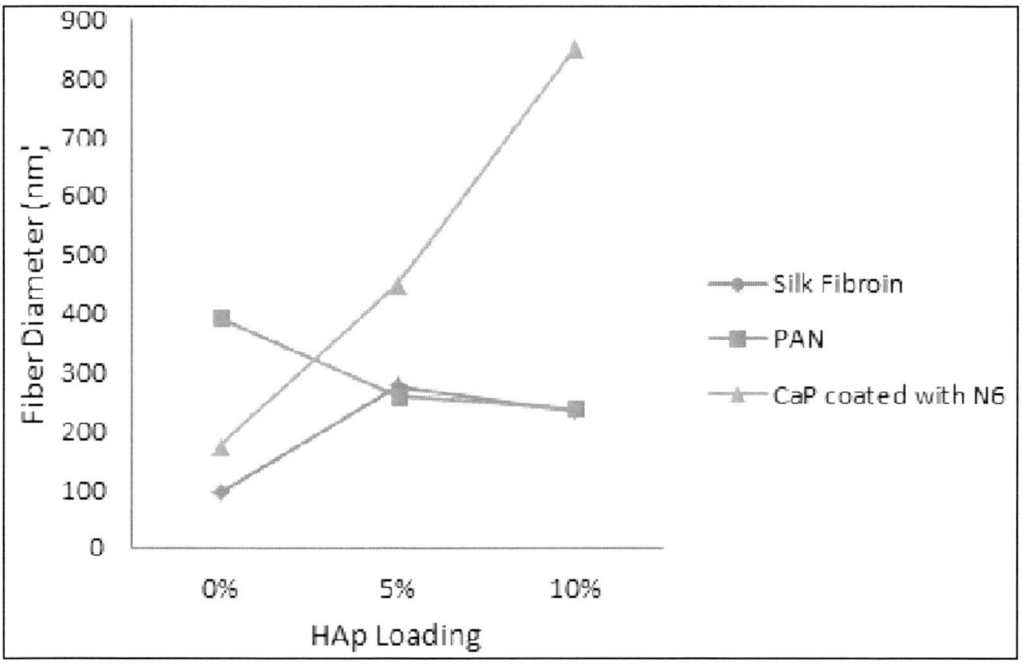

Figure 2. Influence of HAp Loading on Fiber Diameter for Various Polymer [1], [34], [66].

The combination of silk fibroin and HA has been experimented too [66]. At 0% HA loading, the fiber diameter obtained is 95 ± 17 nm. Increasing the concentration of HA loading to 5% has increased the fiber diameter to 277 ± 46 nm. Further increase of the filler concentration to 10% has reduced the fiber diameter to 234 ± 36 nm. When the researchers further increased the concentration of HA to 15% and 30%, it is found that the fiber diameter has increased again to 285 ± 55 nm and 582 ± 99 nm respectively. Due to the increase in fiber diameter size, the tensile strength has increased directly proportional with the concentration of HA. The presence of HA has improved the mechanical properties of silk fibrous scaffolds. However, the fiber diameter must be maintained to a reasonable diameter to provide an appropriate surface to volume ratio to promote cell growth.

Figure 2 and 3 show the influence of HA loading on fiber diameter and tensile strength respectively on different materials. It is obvious that there is no clear cut trend explaining the influence of additives and fillers on the fiber diameter and tensile strength. Some additives increase the properties of the polymeric materials while some have opposite effect. In cases like polyacrylonitrile (PAN), when it is combined with hydroxyapatite, its tensile strength is reduced. Thus, the selection of the polymeric materials and additives for bone scaffolds requires a careful and in depth study on the concentrations used with respect to the response variables.

Table 1 shows a compilation of data for polycaprolactone (PCL) from several studies [35], [67]–[69], [71], [75] for bone scaffolds. Polycaprolactone (PCL) is biodegradable polyester and it has attracted much interest due to numerous advantages over other biopolymers in used. PCL has good water, oil, solvent, chlorine resistance, low melting-point (59-60°C) and low viscosity. PCL has a tailorable degradation kinetic, good mechanical properties and is also easy to process. Its suitable pore size is favourable to tissue proliferation, and the controlled delivery of drugs is contained within its matrix. The chemical structure of PCL allows functional groups to be attached to render the polymer to be more hydrophilic, adhesive, and biocompatible which enables favourable cell responses. Due to the fact that PCL degrades at a slower rate than polyglycolide (PGA), poly d,l-lactide (PDLA) thus its copolymers is originally used in drug-delivery devices and slowly degrading suture materials [76].

Figure 4 shows the thickness of fiber diameter produced from the PCL nanofiber containing various additives/fillers. A combination of 12% w/v PCL mixture with 1% hydroxyapatite, produced nanofibers with large diameters. However, when PCL is combined with 1% and 2% nanoclays and also 0.83% of hydroxyapatite, it produced nanofibers with small diameters. One of the requirements of a good bone scaffold is to have nanofibers with fine diameters so as to imitate the extra cellular matrix (ECM) structures of bone.

In terms of mechanical properties, a combination of PCL with collagen and hydroxyapatite exhibits the highest young modulus and tensile strength as depicted in Figures 5 and 6 simultaneously. The mechanical properties of the various combination of PCL and other additives are also illustrated in these two graphs.

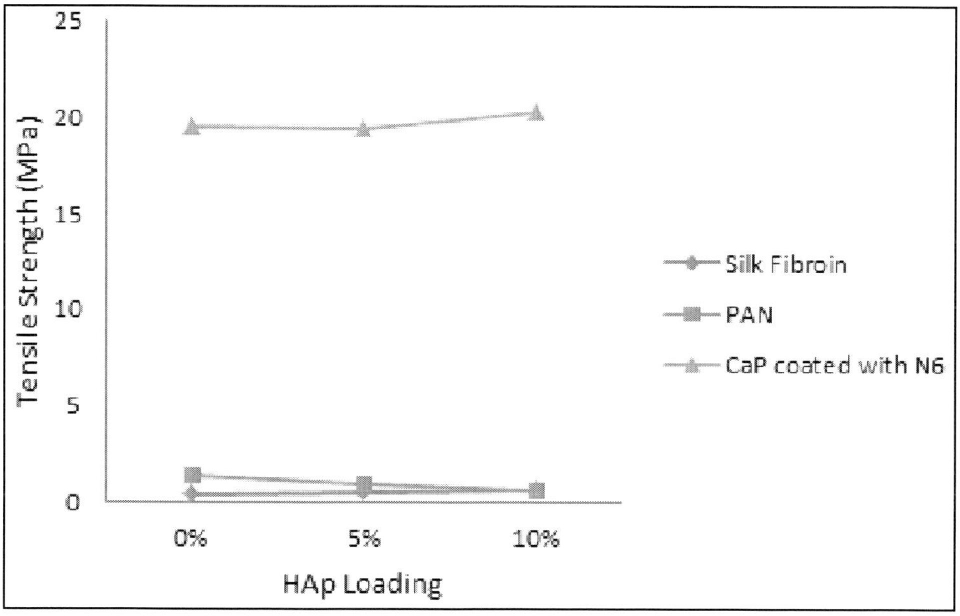

Figure 3. Influence of HA Loading Towards Tensile Strength for Various Polymer [1], [34], [66].

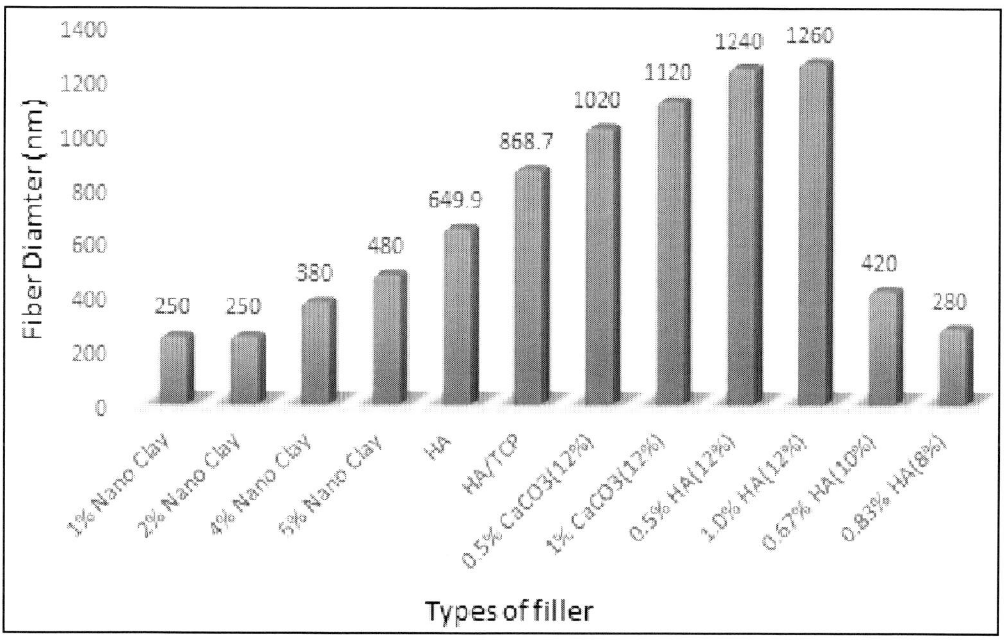

Figure 4. Influence of additives/fillers on fiber diameter of PCL nanofiber [68], [69], [71].

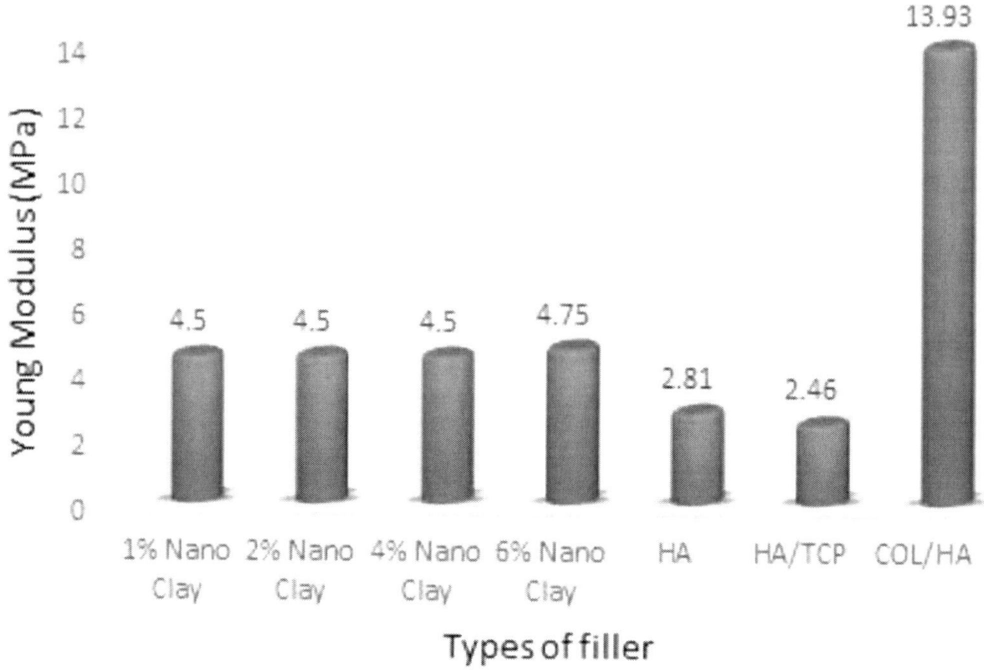

Figure 5. Effect of Young Modulus for PCL Nanofiber with various additives [69], [71].

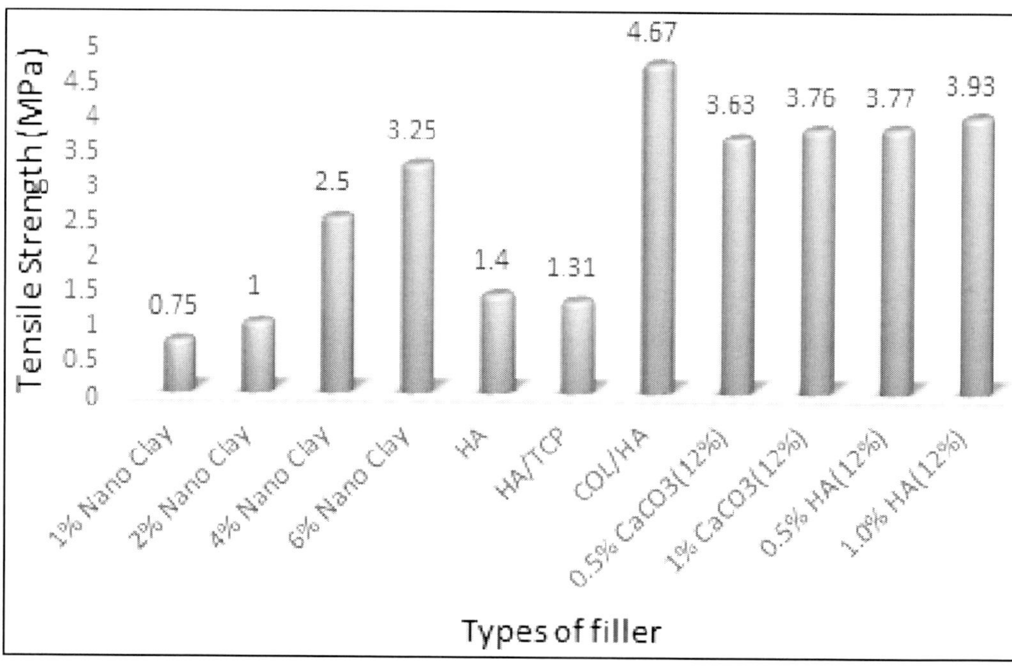

Figure 6. Effect Tensile Strength for PCL Nanofiber with various additives [67]–[69], [71].

Polyvinyl alcohol (PVA) is another material that is fast becoming attractive in development of TE scaffolds. PVA is nontoxic, inexpensive and robust synthetic polymer. Its uncomplicated chemical structure allows it to be modified by performing simple chemical reactions. PVA is a semi-crystalline polymer that possesses good chemical and thermal stability [15]. The synthetic polymer is soluble in water, nontoxic, biocompatible, and biodegradable. PVA has been extensively used in applications such as drug delivery devices, soft contact lenses, temporary skin covers or burn dressings, cartilage implants, and artificial organs [77]–[79]. Studies [80], [81] have proven that PVA can provide mechanical stability and flexibility as compared to conventional scaffolds, which are made from natural polymers. In spite of its potential use in TE application, its poor bioactivity and poor assimilation with host bone have narrowed its application as a scaffold material for bone repair [82]. Similar to other polymeric biomaterials, PVA is often combined with fillers to make blends or composites.

A study on PVA/Fe_3O_4/chitosan (CS) nanofiber fabricated using electrospinning method has been reported [64]. The influence of polymer concentration, applied voltage, and also filler (Fe_3O_4 nanoparticles) loading on the formation of magnetic nanofibers are also investigated. The MG63 human osteoblast like cells is seeded on the magnetic nanofibrous membranes to explore the potential application of the magnetic PVA/Fe_3O_4/CS nanofibrous membranes in bone regeneration. Cell adhesion and proliferation are examined to inspect the cell growth dynamics and results have proven that they are promising materials for bone scaffolds [64].

Magnetic nanoparticles have recently been used in the development of tissue engineering scaffold. Ngadiman et al. (2015) [9] have proven that by using very fine magnetic nanoparticles called maghemite (γ-Fe_2O_3), the mechanical properties of the developed electrospun nanofibrous membranes can be improved. These very fine sized nanoparticles have high surface area per volume ratio thus they have stronger magnetic field which can enhance the rate of cell adhesion, migration, differentiation and proliferation.

In another development, scaffold is prepared using a facile method where bioactive glass (BG) with the desirable structure is combined with nanofibrous biodegradable polymer. In this method, the electrospun PVA fibers are layered with sol–gel-derived BG coating and tests showed that the electrospun PVA scaffolds coated with BG exhibited improved response to mechanical loading and cell growth *in vitro* when compared with the uncoated PVA scaffolds [70]. A study on nano-structured scaffolds of PVA/gelatin (GE) is also performed where such blends are fabricated via electrospinning and further analysed *in vitro*. The influence of cross-linking the PVA/GE blends is evaluated in terms of its mechanical strength, physical and chemical properties. The biocompatibility of the nano-structured scaffolds is then assessed *in vitro* in terms of cellular adhesion, osteoblast cell growth, toxicity and proliferation using osteoblast like MG-63 cell line. It has been reported that the PVA/GE blends can be promising materials for bone scaffolds [73].

Table 1 shows several studies performed on PVA with different combinations of materials [4], [64], [65], [70], [72], [73], [75]. Figure 7 illustrates the compilation of results for fiber diameter produced when PVA nanofibers are combined with other materials. The figure clearly shows that PVA produced nanofibers with large diameters when combined with PCL. However, when it is combined with gelatin (GE) in the ratio of 2:8 it produced more nanofibers with small diameters. Thus a combination of PVA with gelatin in any proportions will produce nanofibers with small diameters which is an excellent characteristic for bone scaffolds.

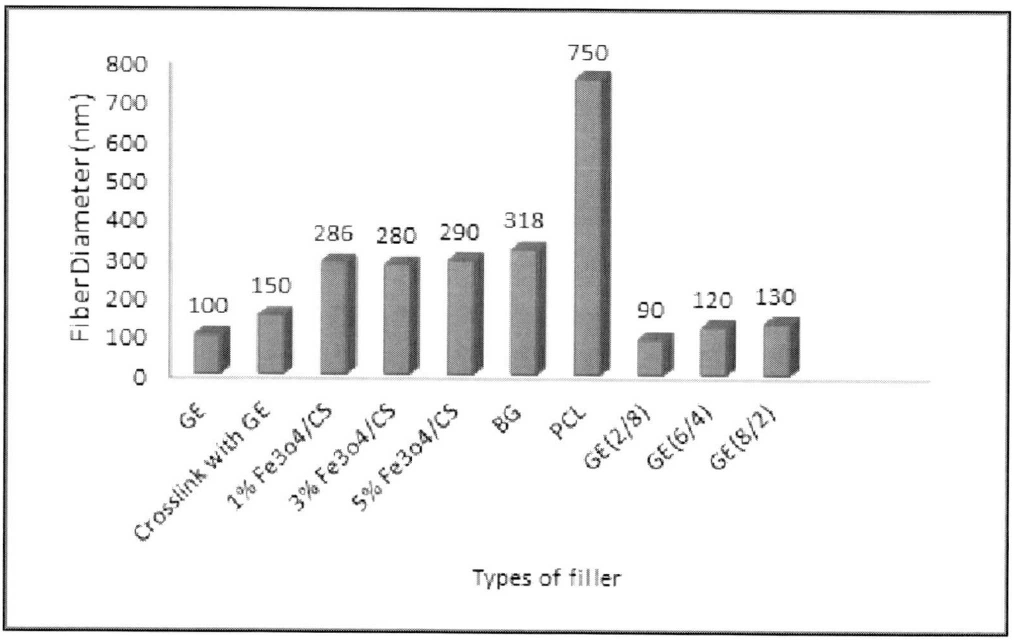

Figure 7. Effect of Fiber diameter for PVA Nanofiber with various additives [64], [70], [72], [73], [75].

Figures 8-11 show the mechanical properties for PVA nanofiber with different combination of additives. Among all the materials, the combination of PVA with bioactive glass shows the best result in terms of its mechanical properties with the highest values for young modulus and tensile strength.

The combination of PVA with the Fe_3O_4 exhibits good tensile strength at any percentage of particle loading. Crosslinking with gelatin in the ratio of 8/2 also shows good tensile strain. On the other hand, for breaking elongation, the combination of PVA with collagen and 5% of hydroxyapatite has a higher percentage of breaking elongation. However, when the percentage of hydroxyapatite is further increased to 10% the contrary occurred probably due to the agglomeration of hydroxyapatite caused by excessive loading of hydroxyapatite.

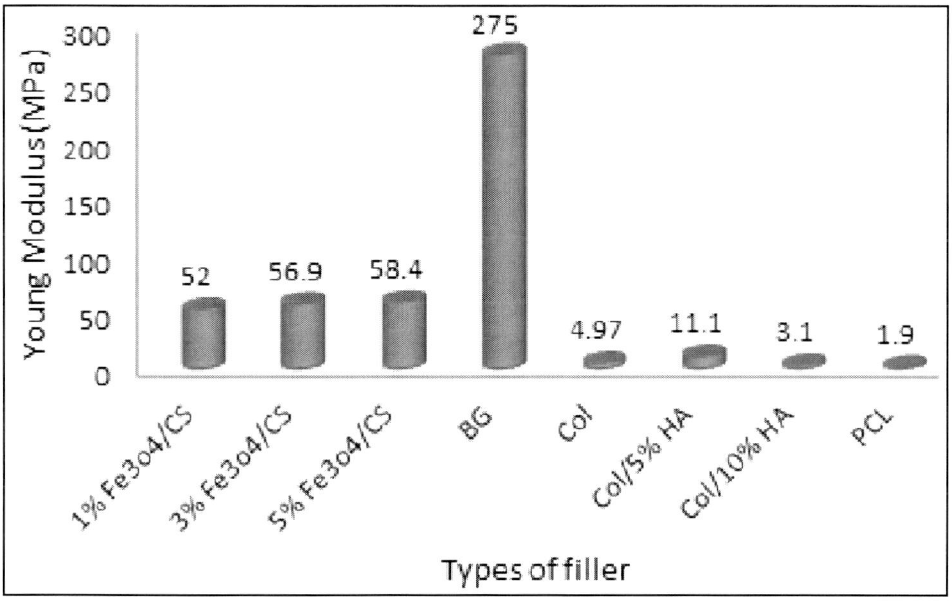

Figure 8. Influence of PVA Nanofiber with various additives towards Young Modulus [64], [65], [70], [75].

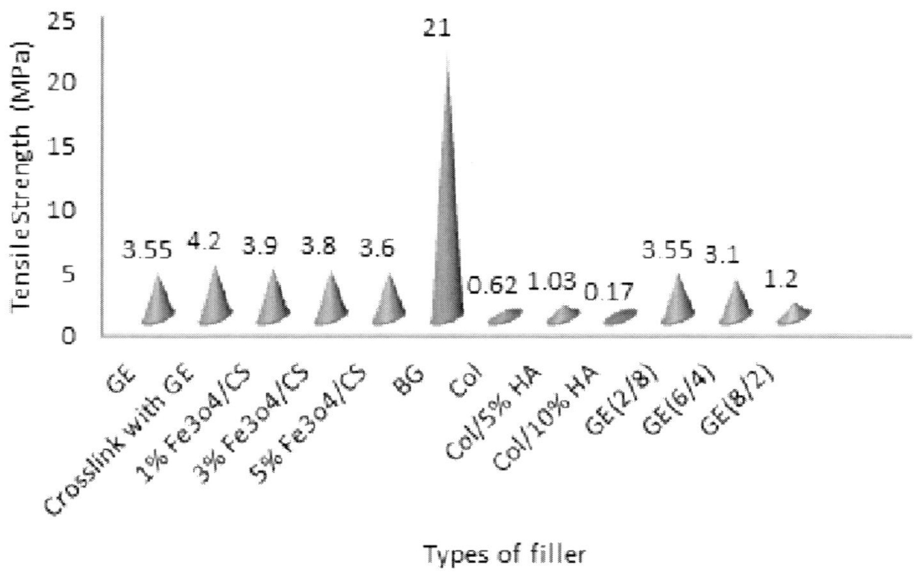

Figure 9. Influence of PVA Nanofiber with various additives on Tensile Strength [64], [65], [70], [72], [73].

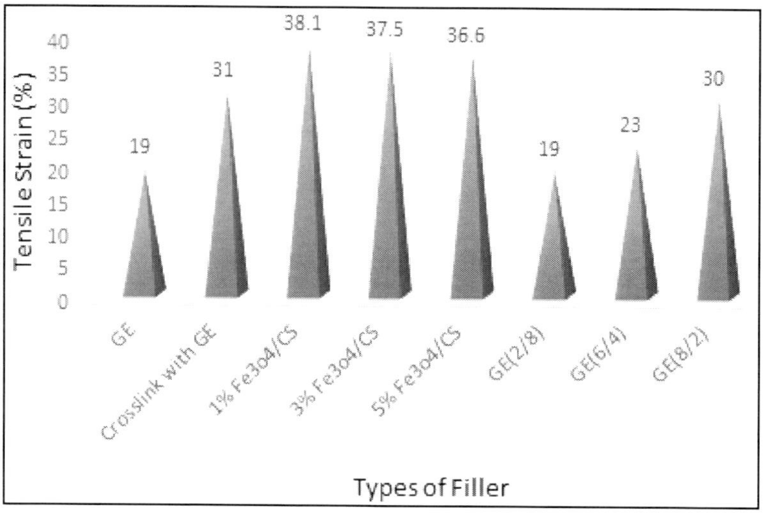

Figure 10. Influence of PVA Nanofiber with various additives on Tensile Strain [64], [72], [73].

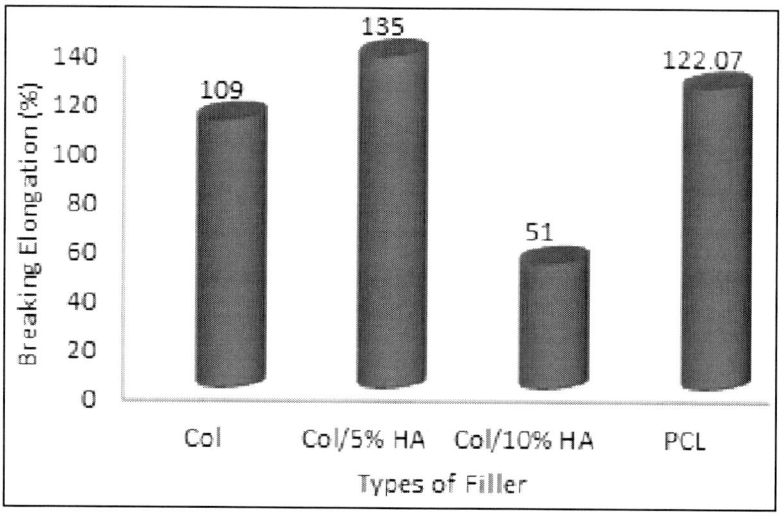

Figure 11. Influence of PVA Nanofiber with various additives on Breaking Elongation [65], [75].

6. FABRICATION OF 3D TISSUE ENGINEERING SCAFFOLDS

Although electrospinning is a feasible technique for TE scaffolds which can mimic the native ECM structure, it has limitation as it can only fabricate nanofibrous mat which is very thin; effectively a 2D construct [83], [84]. Up until now, most of the TE scaffolds are not yet ready for clinical use and are still in the research and development stage. Researchers are exploring the fabrication of 3D electrospun tissue engineering scaffolds by making modifications on the elecrospinning process. Some of the approaches are listed as follows.

6.1. Redesigned Electrospinning Collector

One of the methods to develop 3D electrospun TE scaffolds is by redesigning the electrospinning collector. In a study performed by Subramanian et al. (2011) [85], an insulating gap is installed at the rotating collector as depicted in Figure 12A. The insulating gap between the collectors will act as an auxiliary electrode so as to allow the fiber to deposit longitudinally on it. Hence, such modification allows tubular scaffolds to be developed from the collector. The 3D electrospun nerve TE scaffold shown in Figure 2B has been successfully developed by redesigning the collector of electrospinning process.

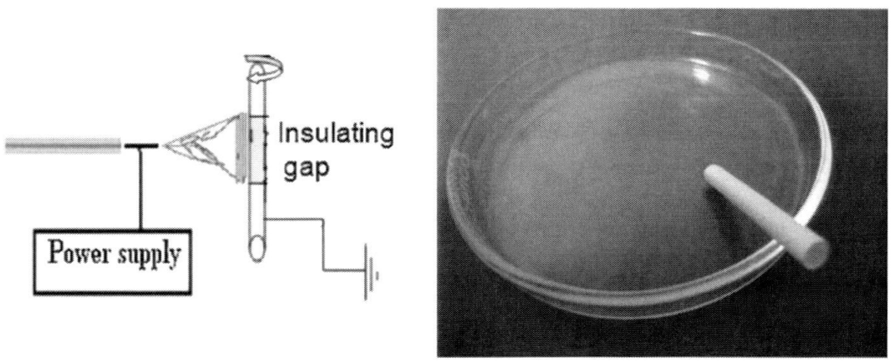

(A) (B)

Figure 12. (A) Electrospinning setup used for the fabrication of the longitudinally oriented tubular scaffold. (B) Developed 3D electrospun nerve TE scaffold [85].

(A) (B)

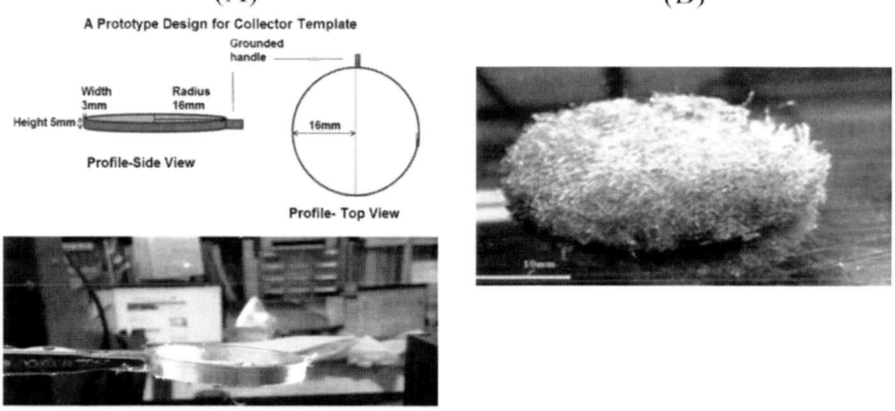

Figure 13. (A) Collector template and (B) Developed 3D electrospun TE scaffolds [86].

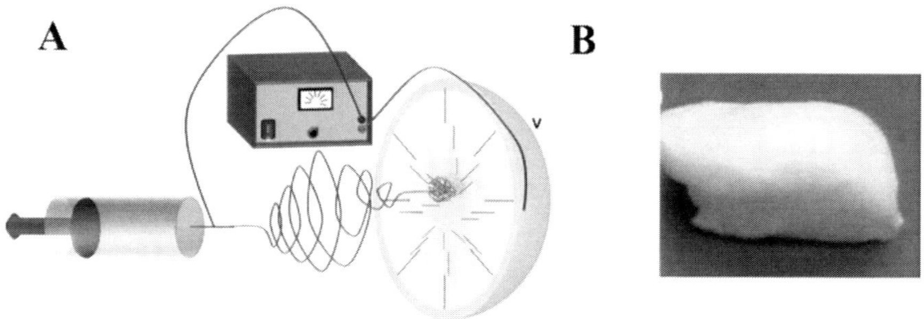

Figure 14. (A) Schematic diagram of electrospinning setup using spherical dish collector and (B) Developed 3D electrospun ultrafine fibers [87].

Park et al. (2013) [86], have also redesigned the collector of the electrospinning process by inventing a new type of collector to produce 3D electrospun TE scaffolds. Figure 13 shows the prototype of collector used in the development of 3D TE scaffolds. The collector which is 5 mm in thickness is rotated 180° so as to distribute the electrospun fiber uniformly during the process. Hence, the electrospun fibers filled the collector and formed a 3D shape The final product is shown in Figure 13.

Blakeney et al. (2011) [87] have modified the electrospinning setup by changing and replacing the collector with a spherical dish. The developed spherical foam dish is 8 inches in diameter and 0.125 inches in shell thickness backed by a stainless steel lining to provide an electrical ground. The needles are placed at 2 inch intervals radiating from the centre of the dish in five equidistant directions. Then the ultrafine fibers embedded to the spherical dish will be in the 3D form as shown in the Figure 14.

6.2. Modification of Electrospinning Process

Another method to develop 3D electrospun scaffolds is by modifying the electrospinning process. Dinis et al. (2015) [88] have developed 3D electrospun nerve TE scaffolds by rolling up the electrospun mats (Figure 15). Initially the 2D electrospun mats are produced from simple electrospinning process as depicted in 15A. These electrospun mats are then rolled up onto the Teflon stand shown in Figure 15B and the procedure is repeated for 50 sticks. The rest of the mats are then rolled up around the structure initially created forming the final 3D product illustrated in Figure 5G.

Ahn et al. (2015) [89] and Liu et al. (2015) [90] have used a similar technique as in Figure 15A to develop the 2D electrospun mats and then rolled up onto the teflon stands. However, the rolled up electrospun mats are then allowed to undergo amination of phosphate glass microfibers (PGF), followed by crossliking of CNT to PGF, undergoing another amination layering as depicted in Figures 6B, C, and D. Finally the rolled up electrospun mats are assembled using an electrospun aligned ultrafine fibers PLDLA wrapper [89]. In the case of Liu et al. (2015), co-culture cell mats are used to wrap the developed electrospun fibers as shown in Figure 17.

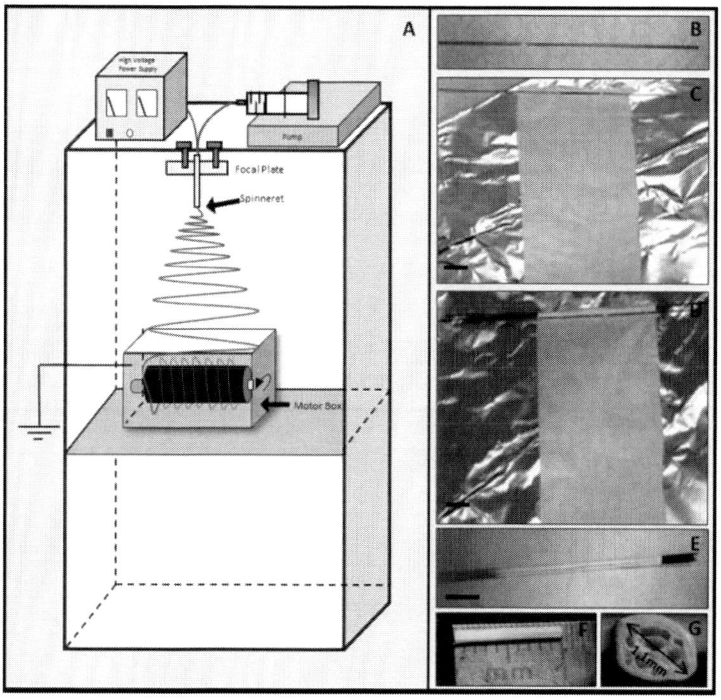

Figure 15. (A) Schematic of the electrospinning process to create 2D electrospun mats. (B) Teflon sticks (C) Roll up the electrospun mat. (D) The process is repeated. (E) The rest of electrospun mats are rolled up around the structure created. (F) The length of fabricated sticks (G) The final product of 3D electrospun nerve TE scaffolds [88].

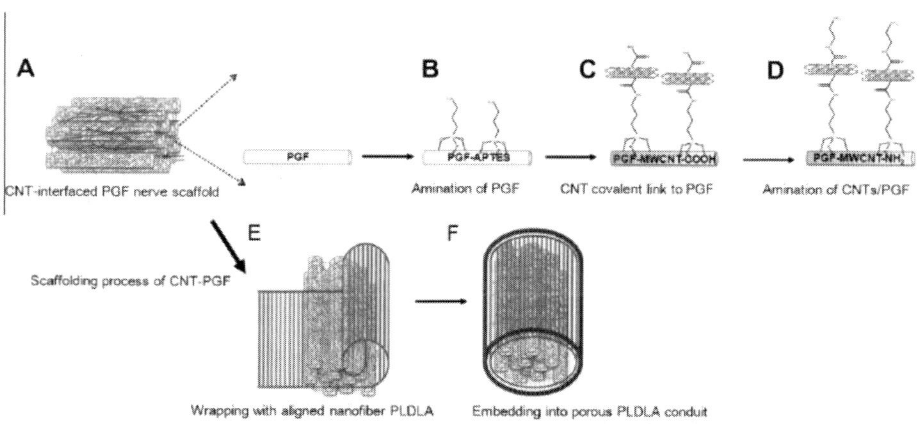

Figure 16. Schematics of the wrapping process by Ahn et al. (2015). (B), (C), and (D) are the processes to develop electrospun mats shown on (A), (E) is the wrapping process, and (F) is the final product [89].

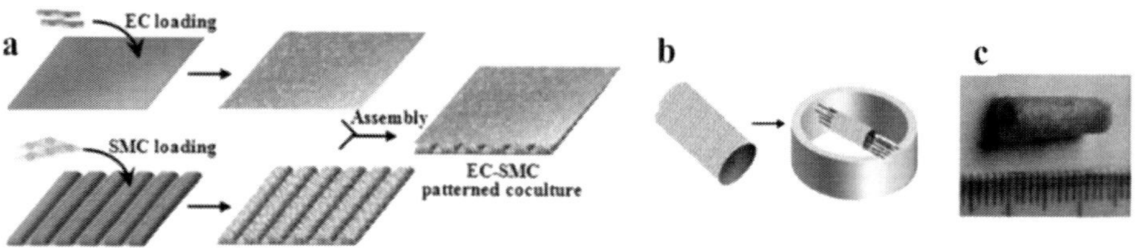

Figure 17. Schematics of the wrapping process using co-culture cell mat. (**A**) Process to develop co-culture cell mat, (B) wrapping of the electrospun ultrafine fibers using co-culture cell mat, and (C) final product [90].

Wright et al. (2010) [91] have developed 3D electrospun TE scaffold using vapor sintering process for poly(d,l-lactide) and poly(l-lactide) (PDLA/PLLA). Electrospun strips are overlapped, placed in the sintering chamber, and exposed to tetrahydrofuran (THF) vapor at 240°C for 10 min as shown in the process schematic diagram (Figure 18A). Then, electrospun cylinders are built by cutting strips at 1 cm tall and wrapping the strip around a 20-gauge blunt tip needle until the diameter is 0.5 cm. Figure 8B shows the final 3D electrospun TE scaffolds.

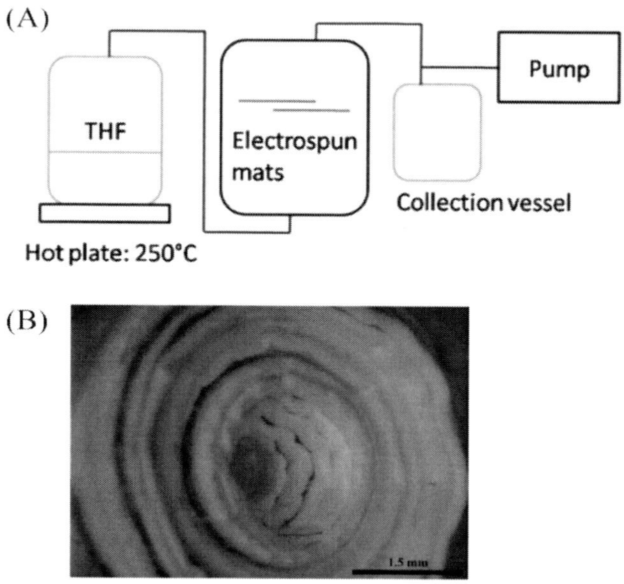

Figure 18. (A) Schematic diagram of vapor sintering electrospinning process and (B) developed 3D electrospun TE scaffolds [91].

Besides using vapor sintering which involves a high temperature process, 3D electrospun TE scaffold is also developed using a low temperature process. Faheem et al. (2015) [92] developed the 3D electrospun TE scaffold using a cold plate collector at -90°C. The solution is pumped using a syringe at the set flow rate and spun onto the cold plate collector. The polymer solidified during the electrospinning process due to solvent evaporation and is collected on a cold plate. Ice crystals formed on the cold plate due to rapid condensation and freezing of water vapour, creating pores in the fibrous mat. The layer is then stacked one over another. After the process, the developed 3D electrospun scaffold is immediately freeze dried. Figure 19 shows the cold plate electrospinning process and the final product.

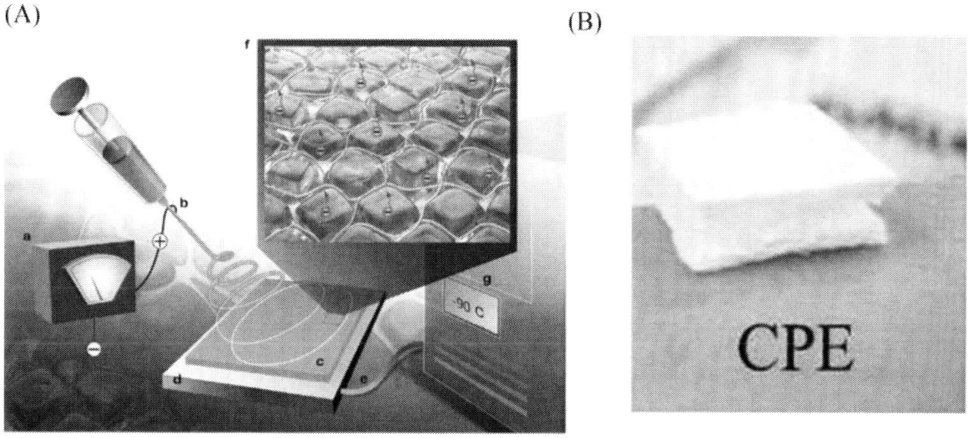

Figure 19. (A) Process overview of cold plate electrospinning (CPE) and (B) developed 3D electrospun TE scaffold [92].

6.3. Combination of Processes

3D electrospun TE scaffolds can also be developed by combining the electrospinning process with other methods. Vaquatte and Cooper (2013) [93], combined the thermal induced phase separation (TIPS) method with electrospinning method in order to make 3D electrospun TE scaffolds. Such combination of processes has proven that the morphology and structure of electrospun ultrafine fibers are maintained although they are in 3D form. This method is performed by stacking the electrospun disc with one another and they are adhered together by another polymer before freeze drying. Figure 20 shows the process and final product of 3D electrospun scaffolds.

Another technique reported is the combination of 3D bioprinting and electrospinning processes [94]–[96]. The process is performed by electrospinning the fibers onto the fabricated 3D bioprinting scaffolds in order to obtain the morphology of electrospun fibers inside the fabricated scaffolds. The developed 3D printed scaffolds are located on the collector of electrospinning setup. The ultrafine fibers are then sprayed onto it. This process is carried out layer-by-layer until the required thickness is achieved. The 3D bioprinted scaffold will provide good strength while electrospun ultrafine fibers will enhance the biocompatibility of the scaffolds. Such combination of processes can enhance the properties of the fabricated scaffolds. Figure 21 illustrates the process and final 3D electrospun TE scaffolds fabricated using these combined methods.

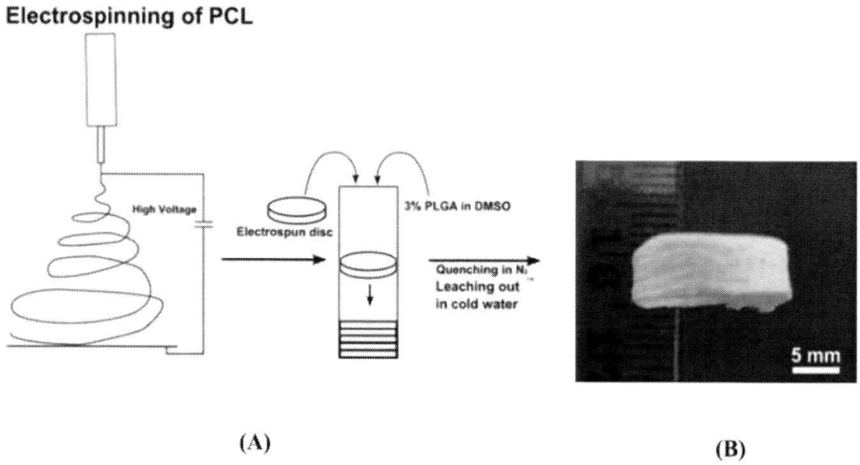

Figure 20. (A) Overview of combination of electrospinning and TIPS process and (B) developed 3D electrospun TE scaffold [93].

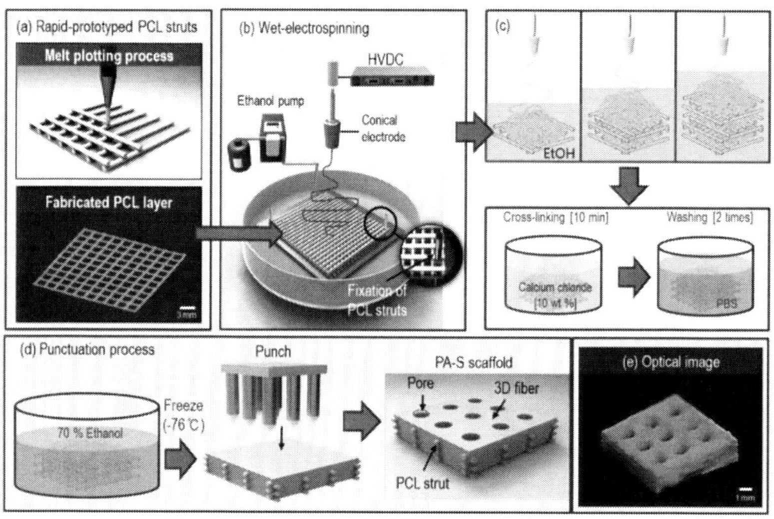

Figure 21. Overview of the combined rapid-prototyping and electrospinning process with the developed 3D TE scaffold [95].

7. Properties of 3D Electrospun Tissue Engineering Scaffold

In order to demonstrate the feasibility of the 3D electrospun TE scaffolds, *in vitro* cellular activities, including cell viability and proliferation are characterised and the results have revealed outstanding cell viability and proliferation [85], [86], [88], [91], [92], [94], [95], [97]–[99]. Thus, the electrospun scaffolds in 3D form can still maintain the biocompatibility characteristics.

Table 2 shows the materials, process and the properties of the 3D scaffolds. It can be observed that the fiber diameter does not influence the mechanical properties of the 3D TE scaffolds, but the type of process combination determines the strength of the 3D scaffolds. Although fiber diameter does not influence the mechanical properties of the 3D TE scaffolds, it has an influence on the profileration rate of cell growth, adhesion and differentiation within the construct.

Table 2. Fiber diameter and mechanical properties of the developed 3D TE scaffolds

No.	Materials	Process	Fiber Diameter	Mechanical Properties	Ref
1	Poly(lactide-co-glycolide) (PLGA)	Redesign Electrospinning Collector	197 ± 72 nm	• 2.6 ± 0.3 MPa (Tensile Strength) • 134.5 ± 22.7 MPa (Young's Modulus)	[85]
2	Silk fibroin	Roll the Electrospun Mats	792 ± 97 nm	• 183.57 MPa (Young's Modulus)	[88]
3	Poly(dl-lactide)–poly(ethylene glycol)	Wrapping Mats into Cylindrical Tube	0.85 ± 0.23 µm	• 2.35 MPa (Young's Modulus)	[90]
4	Poly(d,l-lactide)/ Poly(l-lactide) (PDLA/PLLA)	Vapor Sintering	766 - 1081 µm	• 72.3 MPa (Young's Modulus) • 6.69 MPa (Compressive Modulus) • 1.36 MPa (Compressive Yields)	[91]
5	Polycaprolactone (PCL)/Alginate	Rapid Prototype + Electrospinning	2.16 ± 0.33 µm	• 729 ± 41 kPa (Tensile Strength) • 4.3 ± 0.6 MPa (Young's Modulus)	[95]
6	Cell-Laden/Poly(e-caprolactone)	Layer-By-Layer	57 ± 28 µm	• 1.2 ± 0.3 MPa (Young's Modulus)	[96]
7	Polycaprolactone (PCL)/β-Tricalcium phosphate (TCP)	Modified Wet-Electrospinning Supplemented with Femtosecond Laser	-	• 0.36 ± 0.06 MPa (Young's Modulus)	[98]
8	Silk Fibroin (SF)/Poly(llactide-co-caprolactone) (P(LLA-CL)	Two-Collector Electrospinning System	30.56 ± 6.32 µm	• 24.25 ± 0.76 MPa (Tensile Strength) • 288.95 ± 13.26 MPa (Young's Modulus)	[100]
9	Gelatin (Gel) modified with Calcium Phosphate Nanoparticles (SG5) and Polycaprolactone (PCL)	Bi-layer	10.2 – 11.3 µm	• 0.4 MPa (Tensile Strength)	[101]
10	Collagen coated Poly(L-lactide-co-ε-caprolactone) (ccPLCL)	Custom Spinning Apparatus	5.6 ± 0.70 µm	• 8.3 ± 0.67 kPa (Young's Modulus)	[102]

8. CONCLUSION

After about two decades, there are still very few tissue engineered products that are in clinical use. The development of TE scaffolds is facing significant challenges in its ability to exhibit structural, mechanical, and biological properties to regenerate the defective tissues. Despite witnessing tremendous development in electrospinning, there is still room for further improvement in the process to produce ultrafine fibers for TE scaffolds especially with improved porosity, and mechanical properties. At this stage, the selection of materials is also limited; thus there is a need to search for new materials and enhance techniques to produce different types and properties of TE scaffolds. Besides that, more *in vivo* studies need to be performed to ensure the produced scaffolds can function efficiently in the biological systems. There is no doubt that electrospinning will be the technique of choice for TE scaffolds but its 2D mats produced and its limitations has further opened another dimension of generating 3D scaffolds. The emergence of the 3D electrospun scaffolds is made possible due to the modification of the electrospinning process itself or combining it with some other methods which can maintain the structure of electrospinning TE scaffolds. As mentioned previously, there are still limited studies on the development of 3D electrospun scaffolds. The future direction for ultrafine fibers in tissue engineering is to pursue the development of TE scaffolds in 3D form using a combination of several processes such as electrospinning and 3D bioprinting, electrospinning and rapid-prototyping, stacking, layering, and many more. The capabilities of established material processing techniques can be greatly exploited and enhanced by combining them with electrospinning. The transformation of 2D electrospun mats into 3D scaffolds promises TE scaffolds which are not only biocompatible but also possess sufficient mechanical strength to ensure functionality in their applications. Thus, the replacement and regeneration of damaged tissues and organs would be made possible and turned into reality with ease.

REFERENCES

[1] Abdal-hay, A; Tijing, LD; Lim, JK. "Characterization of the surface biocompatibility of an electrospun nylon 6/CaP nanofiber scaffold using osteoblasts," *Chem. Eng. J.*, vol. 215–216, pp. 57–64, Jan, 2013.

[2] Yu, CC; Chang, JJ; Lee, YH; Lin, YC; Wu, MH; Yang, MC; Chien, CT. "Electrospun scaffolds composing of alginate, chitosan, collagen and hydroxyapatite for applying in bone tissue engineering," *Mater. Lett.*, vol. 93, pp. 133–136, Feb, 2013.

[3] Ha, YM; Amna, T; Kim, MH; Kim, HC; Hassan, MS; Khil, MS. "Novel silicificated PVAc/POSS composite nanofibrous mat via facile electrospinning technique: potential scaffold for hard tissue engineering.," *Colloids Surf. B. Biointerfaces*, vol. 102, pp. 795–802, Mar, 2013.
[4] Qi, YY; Tai, ZX; Sun, DF; Chen, JT; Ma, HB; Yan, XB; Liu, B; Xue, QJ. "Fabrication and characterization of poly(vinyl alcohol)/graphene oxide nanofibrous biocomposite scaffolds," *J. Appl. Polym. Sci.*, vol. 127, no. 3, pp. 1885–1894, Feb. 2013.
[5] Meng, ZX; Li, HF; Sun, ZZ; Zheng, W; Zheng, YF. "Fabrication of mineralized electrospun PLGA and PLGA/gelatin nanofibers and their potential in bone tissue engineering," *Mater. Sci. Eng. C*, vol. 33, no. 2, pp. 699–706, Mar, 2013.
[6] Wang, XL; Xie, XH; Zhang, G; Chen, SH; Yao, D; He, K; Wang, XH; Yao, XS; Leng, Y; Fung, KP; Leung, KS; Qin, L. "Exogenous phytoestrogenic molecule icaritin incorporated into a porous scaffold for enhancing bone defect repair.," *J. Orthop. Res.*, vol. 31, no. 1, pp. 164–72, Jan, 2013.
[7] Abdal-hay, A; a Sheikh, F; Lim, JK. "Air jet spinning of hydroxyapatite/poly(lactic acid) hybrid nanocomposite membrane mats for bone tissue engineering.," *Colloids Surf. B. Biointerfaces*, vol. 102, pp. 635–43, Mar, 2013.
[8] Gao, C; Gao, Q; Li, Y; Rahaman, MN; Teramoto, A; Abe, K. "*In vitro* evaluation of electrospun gelatin-bioactive glass hybrid scaffolds for bone regeneration," *J. Appl. Polym. Sci.*, vol. 127, no. 4, pp. 2588–2599, Feb, 2013.
[9] Ngadiman, NHA; Idris, A; Irfan, M; Kurniawan, D; Yusof, NM; Nasiri, R. "γ-Fe2O3 nanoparticles filled polyvinyl alcohol as potential biomaterial for tissue engineering scaffold," *J. Mech. Behav. Biomed. Mater.*, vol. 49, pp. 90–104, 2015.
[10] Zeng, J; Yang, L; Liang, Q; Zhang, X; Guan, H; Xu, X; Chen, X; Jing, X. "Influence of the drug compatibility with polymer solution on the release kinetics of electrospun fiber formulation," *J. Control. release*, vol. 105, no. 1, pp. 43–51, 2005.
[11] Kenawy, ER; Bowlin, GL; Mansfield, K; Layman, J; Simpson, DG; Sanders, EH; Wnek, GE. "Release of tetracycline hydrochloride from electrospun poly (ethylene-co-vinylacetate), poly (lactic acid), and a blend," *J. Control. release*, vol. 81, no. 1, pp. 57–64, 2002.
[12] Khil, MS; Cha, DI; Kim, HY; Kim, IS; Bhattarai, N. "Electrospun nanofibrous polyurethane membrane as wound dressing," *J. Biomed. Mater. Res. Part B Appl. Biomater.*, vol. 67, no. 2, pp. 675–679, 2003.
[13] Min, BM; Lee, G; Kim, SH; Nam, YS; Lee, TS; Park, WH. "Electrospinning of silk fibroin nanofibers and its effect on the adhesion and spreading of normal human keratinocytes and fibroblasts *in vitro*," *Biomaterials*, vol. 25, no. 7, pp. 1289–1297, 2004.

[14] Gibson, PW; Schreuder-Gibson, HL; Rivin, D. "Electrospun fiber mats: transport properties," *AIChE J.*, vol. 45, no. 1, pp. 190–195, 1999.

[15] Qin, XH; Wang, SY. "Filtration properties of electrospinning nanofibers," *J. Appl. Polym. Sci.*, vol. 102, no. 2, pp. 1285–1290, 2006.

[16] Kim, JS; Reneker, DH. "Polybenzimidazole nanofiber produced by electrospinning," *Polym. Eng. Sci.*, vol. 39, no. 5, pp. 849–854, 1999.

[17] Huang, ZM; Zhang, YZ; Kotaki, M; Ramakrishna, S. "A review on polymer nanofibers by electrospinning and their applications in nanocomposites," *Compos. Sci. Technol.*, vol. 63, no. 15, pp. 2223–2253, 2003.

[18] Lee, SW; Choi, SW; Jo, SM; Chin, BD; Kim, DY; Lee, KY. "Electrochemical properties and cycle performance of electrospun poly (vinylidene fluoride)-based fibrous membrane electrolytes for Li-ion polymer battery," *J. Power Sources*, vol. 163, no. 1, pp. 41–46, 2006.

[19] Kim, C. "Electrochemical characterization of electrospun activated carbon nanofibres as an electrode in supercapacitors," *J. Power Sources*, vol. 142, no. 1, pp. 382–388, 2005.

[20] Pinto, NJ; Johnson, AT; MacDiarmid, AG; Mueller, CH; Theofylaktos, N; Robinson, DC; Miranda, FA. "Electrospun polyaniline/polyethylene oxide nanofiber field-effect transistor," *Appl. Phys. Lett.*, vol. 83, no. 20, pp. 4244–4246, 2003.

[21] Aussawasathien, D; Dong, JH; Dai, L. "Electrospun polymer nanofiber sensors," *Synth. Met.*, vol. 154, no. 1, pp. 37–40, 2005.

[22] Jang, SY; Seshadri, V; Khil, MS; Kumar, A; Marquez, M; Mather, PT; Sotzing, GA. "Welded electrochromic conductive polymer nanofibers by electrostatic spinning," *Adv. Mater.*, vol. 17, no. 18, pp. 2177–2180, 2005.

[23] NHA; Ngadiman, A; Yusof, NM; Idris, A; Kurniawan, D. "Characterisation of Electrospun Magnetic Nanoparticle," *Proc. NAMRI/SME*, vol. 42, pp. 2–6, 2014.

[24] Li, D; Xia, Y. "Electrospinning of nanofibers: reinventing the wheel?," *Adv. Mater.*, vol. 16, no. 14, pp. 1151–1170, 2004.

[25] Chen, L; Zhu, C; Fan, D; Liu, B; Ma, X; Duan, Z; Zhou, Y. "A human-like collagen/chitosan electrospun nanofibrous scaffold from aqueous solution: electrospun mechanism and biocompatibility.," *J. Biomed. Mater. Res. A*, vol. 99, no. 3, pp. 395–409, Dec, 2011.

[26] Deng, M; Kumbar, SG; Nair, LS; Weikel, AL; Allcock, HR; Laurencin, CT. "Biomimetic Structures: Biological Implications of Dipeptide-Substituted Polyphosphazene-Polyester Blend Nanofiber Matrices for Load-Bearing Bone Regeneration," *Adv. Funct. Mater.*, vol. 21, no. 14, pp. 2641–2651, Jul. 2011.

[27] Wang, C; Wang, M. "Dual-source dual-power electrospinning and characteristics of multifunctional scaffolds for bone tissue engineering.," *J. Mater. Sci. Mater. Med.*, vol. 23, no. 10, pp. 2381–97, Oct, 2012.

[28] Zhang, H. "Effects of electrospinning parameters on morphology and diameter of electrospun PLGA/MWNTs fibers and cytocompatibility *in vitro*," *J. Bioact. Compat. Polym.*, vol. 26, no. 6, pp. 590–606, Oct, 2011.

[29] Wang, X; Gittens, Ra; Song, R; Tannenbaum, R; Olivares-Navarrete, R; Schwartz, Z; Chen, H; Boyan, BD. "Effects of structural properties of electrospun TiO2 nanofiber meshes on their osteogenic potential.," *Acta Biomater.*, vol. 8, no. 2, pp. 878–85, Mar, 2012.

[30] Nie, H; Shen, X; Zhou, Z; Jiang, Q; Chen, Y; Xie, A; Wang, Y; Han, CC. "Electrospinning and characterization of konjac glucomannan/chitosan nanofibrous scaffolds favoring the growth of bone mesenchymal stem cells," *Carbohydr. Polym.*, vol. 85, no. 3, pp. 681–686, Jun. 2011.

[31] Fischer, RL; McCoy, MG; Grant, Sa. "Electrospinning collagen and hyaluronic acid nanofiber meshes.," *J. Mater. Sci. Mater. Med.*, vol. 23, no. 7, pp. 1645–54, Jul, 2012.

[32] Zhang, H. "Electrospun poly (lactic-co-glycolic acid)/multiwalled carbon nanotubes composite scaffolds for guided bone tissue regeneration," *J. Bioact. Compat. Polym.*, vol. 26, no. 4, pp. 347–362, Jun, 2011.

[33] Ravichandran, R; Venugopal, JR; Sundarrajan, S; Mukherjee, S; Ramakrishna, S. "Precipitation of nanohydroxyapatite on PLLA/PBLG/Collagen nanofibrous structures for the differentiation of adipose derived stem cells to osteogenic lineage.," *Biomaterials*, vol. 33, no. 3, pp. 846–55, Jan. 2012.

[34] Rajzer, I; Kwiatkowski, R; Piekarczyk, W; Biniaś, W; Janicki, J. "Carbon nanofibers produced from modified electrospun PAN/hydroxyapatite precursors as scaffolds for bone tissue engineering," *Mater. Sci. Eng. C*, vol. 32, no. 8, pp. 2562–2569, Dec, 2012.

[35] Xie, J; Zhong, S; Ma, B; Shuler, FD; Lim, CT. "Controlled biomineralization of electrospun poly(ε-caprolactone) fibers to enhance their mechanical properties.," *Acta Biomater.*, vol. 9, no. 3, pp. 5698–707, Mar, 2013.

[36] Haghi, AK; Akbari, M. "Trends in electrospinning of natural nanofibers," *Phys. status solidi*, vol. 204, no. 6, pp. 1830–1834, 2007.

[37] Wang, T; Kumar, S. "Electrospinning of polyacrylonitrile nanofibers," *J. Appl. Polym. Sci.*, vol. 102, no. 2, pp. 1023–1029, 2006.

[38] Jia, Z; Li, Q; Liu, J; Yang, Y; Wang, L; Guan, Z. "Preparation and properties of poly (vinyl alcohol) nanofibers by electrospinning," *J. Polym. Eng.*, vol. 28, no. 1–2, pp. 87–100, 2008.

[39] Jarusuwannapoom, T; Hongrojjanawiwat, W; Jitjaicham, S; Wannatong, L; Nithitanakul, M; Pattamaprom, C; Koombhongse, P; Rangkupan, R; Supaphol, P. "Effect of solvents on electro-spinnability of polystyrene solutions and morphological appearance of resulting electrospun polystyrene fibers," *Eur. Polym. J.*, vol. 41, no. 3, pp. 409–421, 2005.

[40] Baker, SC; Atkin, N; Gunning, PA; Granville, N; Wilson, K; Wilson, D; Southgate, J. "Characterisation of electrospun polystyrene scaffolds for three-dimensional *in vitro* biological studies," *Biomaterials*, vol. 27, no. 16, pp. 3136–3146, 2006.

[41] Zhang, C; Yuan, X; Wu, L; Han, Y; Sheng, J. "Study on morphology of electrospun poly (vinyl alcohol) mats," *Eur. Polym. J.*, vol. 41, no. 3, pp. 423–432, 2005.

[42] Sukigara, S; Gandhi, M; Ayutsede, J; Micklus, M; Ko, F. "Regeneration of Bombyx mori silk by electrospinning part 1: processing parameters and geometric properties," *Polymer (Guildf).*, vol. 44, no. 19, pp. 5721–5727, 2003.

[43] Yang, C; Li, Y; Nan, K. "Biologically inspired growth of hydroxyapatite crystals on bio-organics-defined scaffolds," *Mater. Res. Bull.*, vol. 48, no. 3, pp. 1128–1131, Mar, 2013.

[44] Salifu, A; Nury, BD; Lekakou, C. "Electrospinning of nanocomposite fibrillar tubular and flat scaffolds with controlled fiber orientation.," *Ann. Biomed. Eng.*, vol. 39, no. 10, pp. 2510–20, Oct. 2011.

[45] Jaiswal, AK; Kadam, SS; Soni, VP; Bellare, JR. "Improved functionalization of electrospun PLLA/gelatin scaffold by alternate soaking method for bone tissue engineering," *Appl. Surf. Sci.*, vol. 268, pp. 477–488, Mar, 2013.

[46] Zong, X; Kim, K; Fang, D; Ran, S; Hsiao, BS; Chu, B. "Structure and process relationship of electrospun bioabsorbable nanofiber membranes," *Polymer (Guildf).*, vol. 43, no. 16, pp. 4403–4412, 2002.

[47] Baumann, A; Audibert, G; Lafaye, CG; Puybasset, L; Mertes, PM; Claudot, F. "Elective non-therapeutic intensive care and the four principles of medical ethics," *J. Med. Ethics*, vol. 39, no. 3, pp. 139–142, 2013.

[48] Yang, S; Leong, KF; Du, Z; Chua, CK. "The design of scaffolds for use in tissue engineering. Part II. Rapid prototyping techniques," *Tissue Eng.*, vol. 8, no. 1, pp. 1–11, 2002.

[49] L'Heureux, N; Dusserre, N; Konig, G; Victor, B; Keire, P; Wight, TN; Chronos, NAF; Kyles, AE; Gregory, CR; Hoyt, G. others, "Human tissue-engineered blood vessels for adult arterial revascularization," *Nat. Med.*, vol. 12, no. 3, pp. 361–365, 2006.

[50] Sacks, MS; Schoen, FJ; Mayer, Jr. JE. "Bioengineering challenges for heart valve tissue engineering," *Annu. Rev. Biomed. Eng.*, vol. 11, pp. 289–313, 2009.

[51] Atala, A; Bauer, SB; Soker, S; Yoo, JJ; Retik, AB. "Tissue-engineered autologous bladders for patients needing cystoplasty," *Lancet*, vol. 367, no. 9518, pp. 1241–1246, 2006.

[52] Lee, K; Jeong, JH; Mun, CH; Lee, SR; Yoo, KJ; Park, YW; Won, YS; Min, BG. "Convection-enhanced High-Flux Hemodialysis," *Artif. Organs*, vol. 31, no. 8, pp. 653–658, 2007.

[53] Kvist, M; Sondell, M; Kanje, M; Dahlin, LB. "Regeneration in, and properties of, extracted peripheral nerve allografts and xenografts," *J. Plast. Surg. Hand Surg.*, vol. 45, no. 3, pp. 122–128, 2011.

[54] Kim, MS; Kim, JH; Min, BH; Chun, HJ; Han, DK; Lee, HB. "Polymeric scaffolds for regenerative medicine," *Polym. Rev.*, vol. 51, no. 1, pp. 23–52, 2011.

[55] Tyson, T; Finne-Wistrand, A; Albertsson, AC. "Degradable porous scaffolds from various L-lactide and trimethylene carbonate copolymers obtained by a simple and effective method," *Biomacromolecules*, vol. 10, no. 1, pp. 149–154, 2008.

[56] Hoerstrup, SP; Vacanti, JP. "Overview of tissue engineering," *Biomater. Sci. an Introd. to Mater. Med. 2nd ed. San Diego Elsevier Acad. Pr. p*, pp. 712–727, 2004.

[57] Stock, UA; Vacanti, JP. "Tissue engineering: current state and prospects," *Annu. Rev. Med.*, vol. 52, no. 1, pp. 443–451, 2001.

[58] Knight, MAF; Evans, GRD. "Tissue engineering: progress and challenges," *Plast. Reconstr. Surg.*, vol. 114, no. 2, p. 26e--37e, 2004.

[59] Ngadiman, NHA; Yusof, NM; Idris, A; Kurniawan, D. "Mechanical properties and biocompatibility of co-axially electrospun polyvinyl alcohol/maghemite," *Proc. Inst. Mech. Eng. Part H J. Eng. Med.*, p. 954411916649632, 2016.

[60] Bhattarai, SR; Bhattarai, N; Yi, HK; Hwang, PH; Cha, DIl; Kim, HY. "Novel biodegradable electrospun membrane: scaffold for tissue engineering," *Biomaterials*, vol. 25, no. 13, pp. 2595–2602, 2004.

[61] Li, WJ; Laurencin, CT; Caterson, EJ; Tuan, RS; Ko, FK. "Electrospun nanofibrous structure: a novel scaffold for tissue engineering," *J. Biomed. Mater. Res.*, vol. 60, no. 4, pp. 613–621, 2002.

[62] Kaplan, DL. *Biopolymers from renewable resources*. Springer, 1998.

[63] Vårum, KM; Myhr, MM; Hjerde, RJN; Smidsrød, O. "*In vitro* degradation rates of partially< i> N</i>-acetylated chitosans in human serum," *Carbohydr. Res.*, vol. 299, no. 1, pp. 99–101, 1997.

[64] Wei, Y; Zhang, X; Song, Y; Han, B; Hu, X; Wang, X; Lin, Y; Deng, X. "Magnetic biodegradable Fe3O4/CS/PVA nanofibrous membranes for bone regeneration.," *Biomed. Mater.*, vol. 6, no. 5, p. 55008, Oct, 2011.

[65] Asran, AS; Henning, S; Michler, GH. "Polyvinyl alcohol–collagen–hydroxyapatite biocomposite nanofibrous scaffold: Mimicking the key features of natural bone at the nanoscale level," *Polymer (Guildf).*, vol. 51, no. 4, pp. 868–876, Feb. 2010.

[66] Ming, J; Zuo, B. "A novel electrospun silk fibroin/hydroxyapatite hybrid nanofibers," *Mater. Chem. Phys.*, vol. 137, no. 1, pp. 421–427, Nov, 2012.

[67] Phipps, MC; Clem, WC; Catledge, Sa; Xu, Y; Hennessy, KM; Thomas, V; Jablonsky, MJ; Chowdhury, S; Stanishevsky, AV; Vohra, YK; Bellis, SL. "Mesenchymal stem cell responses to bone-mimetic electrospun matrices composed of polycaprolactone, collagen I and nanoparticulate hydroxyapatite.," *PLoS One*, vol. 6, no. 2, p. e16813, Jan, 2011.

[68] Wutticharoenmongkol, P; Sanchavanakit, N; Pavasant, P; Supaphol, P. "Preparation and characterization of novel bone scaffolds based on electrospun polycaprolactone fibers filled with nanoparticles.," *Macromol. Biosci.*, vol. 6, no. 1, pp. 70–7, Jan, 2006.

[69] Nitya, G; Nair, GT; Mony, U; Chennazhi, KP; Nair, SV. "*In vitro* evaluation of electrospun PCL/nanoclay composite scaffold for bone tissue engineering.," *J. Mater. Sci. Mater. Med.*, vol. 23, no. 7, pp. 1749–61, Jul, 2012.

[70] Gao, C; Gao, Q; Li, Y; Rahaman, MN; Teramoto, A; Abe, K. "Preparation and *in vitro* characterization of electrospun PVA scaffolds coated with bioactive glass for bone regeneration," *J. Biomed. Mater. Res. Part A*, vol. 100, no. 5, pp. 1324–1334, 2012.

[71] Nelson, MT; Keith, JP; Li, BB; Stocum, DL; Li, J. "Electrospun composite polycaprolactone scaffolds for optimized tissue regeneration," *Proc. Inst. Mech. Eng. Part N J. Nanoeng. Nanosyst.*, vol. 226, no. 3, pp. 111–121, Jul, 2012.

[72] Linh, NTB; Min, YK; Song, HY; Lee, BT. "Fabrication of polyvinyl alcohol/gelatin nanofiber composites and evaluation of their material properties.," *J. Biomed. Mater. Res. B. Appl. Biomater.*, vol. 95, no. 1, pp. 184–91, Oct, 2010.

[73] Linh, NTB; Lee, BT. "Electrospinning of polyvinyl alcohol/gelatin nanofiber composites and cross-linking for bone tissue engineering application," *J. Biomater. Appl.*, vol. 27, no. 3, pp. 255–266, 2012.

[74] Su, Y; Su, Q; Liu, W; Lim, M; Venugopal, JR; Mo, X; Ramakrishna, S; Al-Deyab, SS; El-Newehy, M. "Controlled release of bone morphogenetic protein 2 and dexamethasone loaded in core-shell PLLACL-collagen fibers for use in bone tissue engineering.," *Acta Biomater.*, vol. 8, no. 2, pp. 763–71, Mar, 2012.

[75] Shafiee, A; Soleimani, M; Chamheidari, GA; Seyedjafari, E; Dodel, M; Atashi, A; Gheisari, Y. "Electrospun nanofiber-based regeneration of cartilage enhanced by mesenchymal stem cells.," *J. Biomed. Mater. Res. A*, vol. 99, no. 3, pp. 467–78, Dec, 2011.

[76] Woodruff, MA; Hutmacher, DW. "The return of a forgotten polymer—Polycaprolactone in the 21st century," *Prog. Polym. Sci.*, vol. 35, no. 10, pp. 1217–1256, Oct. 2010.

[77] Fundueanu, G; Constantin, M; Ascenzi, P. "Poly (vinyl alcohol) microspheres with pH-and thermosensitive properties as temperature-controlled drug delivery," *Acta Biomater.*, vol. 6, no. 10, pp. 3899–3907, 2010.

[78] Matsumura, K; Hayami, T; Hyon, SH; Tsutsumi, S. "Control of proliferation and differentiation of osteoblasts on apatite-coated poly (vinyl alcohol) hydrogel as an artificial articular cartilage material," *J. Biomed. Mater. Res. Part A*, vol. 92, no. 4, pp. 1225–1232, 2010.

[79] Kang, YO; Yoon, IS; Lee, SY; Kim, DD; Lee, SJ; Park, WH; Hudson, SM. "Chitosan-coated poly (vinyl alcohol) nanofibers for wound dressings," *J. Biomed. Mater. Res. Part B Appl. Biomater.*, vol. 92, no. 2, pp. 568–576, 2010.

[80] Sailaja, GS; Sreenivasan, K; Yokogawa, Y; Kumary, TV; Varma, HK. "Bioinspired mineralization and cell adhesion on surface functionalized poly (vinyl alcohol) films," *Acta Biomater.*, vol. 5, no. 5, pp. 1647–1655, 2009.

[81] Schmedlen, RH; Masters, KS; West, JL. "Photocrosslinkable polyvinyl alcohol hydrogels that can be modified with cell adhesion peptides for use in tissue engineering," *Biomaterials*, vol. 23, no. 22, pp. 4325–4332, 2002.

[82] Sheikh, FA; Barakat, NAM; Kanjwal, MA; Park, SJ; Park, DK; Kim, HY. "Synthesis of poly (vinyl alcohol)(PVA) nanofibers incorporating hydroxyapatite nanoparticles as future implant materials," *Macromol. Res.*, vol. 18, no. 1, pp. 59–66, 2010.

[83] Zhang, X; Baughman, CB; Kaplan, DL. "*In vitro* evaluation of electrospun silk fibroin scaffolds for vascular cell growth," *Biomaterials*, vol. 29, no. 14, pp. 2217–2227, 2008.

[84] Zhang, X; Reagan, MR; Kaplan, DL. "Electrospun silk biomaterial scaffolds for regenerative medicine," *Adv. Drug Deliv. Rev.*, vol. 61, no. 12, pp. 988–1006, 2009.

[85] Subramanian, A; Krishnan, UM; Sethuraman, S. "Fabrication of uniaxially aligned 3D electrospun scaffolds for neural regeneration.," *Biomed. Mater.*, vol. 6, p. 25004, 2011.

[86] Park, KY; Ramaraj, B; Choi, WS; Yoon, KR. "Fabrication and metallization of 3D electrospun nanofiberous architecture with gold and silver coating for applications related to electrochemical supercapacitors," *Mater. Chem. Phys.*, vol. 142, pp. 600–607, 2013.

[87] Blakeney, BA; Tambralli, A; Anderson, JM; Andukuri, A; Lim, D; Dean, DR; Jun, H. "Cell infiltration and growth in a low density, uncompressed three-dimensional electrospun nano fi brous scaffold," *Biomaterials*, vol. 32, no. 6, pp. 1583–1590, 2011.

[88] Dinis, TM; Elia, R; Vidal, G; Dermigny, Q; Denoeud, C; Kaplan, DL; Egles, C; Marin, F. "3D multi-channel bi-functionalized silk electrospun conduits for peripheral nerve regeneration," *J. Mech. Behav. Biomed. Mater.*, vol. 41, pp. 43–55, 2015.

[89] Ahn, H; Hwang, J; Soo, M; Lee, J; Kim, J; Kim, H; Sang, U; Knowles, JC; Kim, H; Keun, J. "Carbon-nanotube-interfaced glass fiber scaffold for regeneration of transected sciatic nerve," *Acta Biomater.*, vol. 13, pp. 324–334, 2015.

[90] Liu, Y; Lu, J; Li, H; Wei, J; Li, X. "Engineering blood vessels through micropatterned co-culture of vascular endothelial and smooth muscle cells on bilayered electrospun fibrous mats with pDNA inoculation," *Acta Biomater.*, vol. 11, pp. 114–125, 2015.

[91] Wright, LD; Young, RT; Andric, T; Freeman, JW. "Fabrication and mechanical characterization of 3D electrospun scaffolds for tissue engineering.," *Biomed. Mater.*, vol. 5, p. 55006, 2010.

[92] Sheikh, Fa; Ju, HW; Lee, JM; Moon, BM; Park, HJ; Lee, OJ; Kim, JH; Kim, DK; Park, CH. "3D electrospun silk fibroin nanofibers for fabrication of artificial skin," *Nanomedicine Nanotechnology, Biol. Med.*, vol. 11, no. 3, pp. 681–691, 2015.

[93] Vaquette, C; Cooper-White, J. "A simple method for fabricating 3-D multilayered composite scaffolds.," *Acta Biomater.*, vol. 9, no. 1, pp. 4599–608, Jan, 2013.

[94] Moroni, L; Schotel, R; Hamann, D; De Wijn, JR; Van Blitterswijk, Ca. "3D fiber-deposited electrospun integrated scaffolds enhance cartilage tissue formation," *Adv. Funct. Mater.*, vol. 18, pp. 53–60, 2008.

[95] Kim, MS; Kim, G. "Three-dimensional electrospun polycaprolactone (PCL)/alginate hybrid composite scaffolds," vol. 114, pp. 213–221, 2014.

[96] Yeo, M; Kim, G. "Fabrication of cell-laden electrospun hybrid scaffolds of alginate-based bioink and PCL microstructures for tissue regeneration," *Chem. Eng. J.*, vol. 275, pp. 27–35, 2015.

[97] Yohe, ST; Herrera, VLM; Colson, YL; Grinstaff, MW. "3D superhydrophobic electrospun meshes as reinforcement materials for sustained local drug delivery against colorectal cancer cells," *J. Control. Release*, vol. 162, no. 2012, pp. 92–101, 2012.

[98] Kim, MS; Kim, GH. "Highly porous electrospun 3D polycaprolactone/β-TCP biocomposites for tissue regeneration," *Mater. Lett.*, vol. 120, pp. 246–250, 2014.

[99] Gao, S; Calcagni, M; Welti, M; Hemmi, S; Hild, N; Stark, WJ; Meier Bürgisser, G; Wanner, Ga; Cinelli, P; Buschmann, J. "Proliferation of ASC-derived endothelial cells in a 3D electrospun mesh: Impact of bone-biomimetic nanocomposite and co-culture with ASC-derived osteoblasts," *Injury*, vol. 45, pp. 974–980, 2014.

[100] Yang, C; Deng, G; Chen, W; Ye, X; Mo, X. "A novel electrospun-aligned nanoyarn-reinforced nanofibrous scaffold for tendon tissue engineering," *Colloids Surfaces B Biointerfaces*, vol. 122, pp. 270–276, 2014.

[101] Rajzer, I; Menaszek, E; Kwiatkowski, R; Planell, Ja; Castano, O. "Electrospun gelatin/poly(ε-caprolactone) fibrous scaffold modified with calcium phosphate for bone tissue engineering," *Mater. Sci. Eng. C*, vol. 44, pp. 183–190, 2014.

[102] Lorden, ER; Miller, KJ; Bashirov, L; Ibrahim, MM; Hammett, E; Jung, Y; Medina, Ma; Rastegarpour, A; Selim, Ma; Leong, KW; Levinson, H. "Mitigation of hypertrophic scar contraction via an elastomeric biodegradable scaffold.," *Biomaterials*, vol. 43, pp. 61–70, 2015.

About the Author

Prof. Dr. Ani Idris is currently a Professor in the Department of Bioprocess Engineering and fellow in Institute of Bioproduct, Faculty of Chemical Engineering at Universiti Teknologi Malaysia. She obtained her first degree in Chemical Engineering in Universiti Teknologi Malaysia in 1988 and Masters the following year from University College London, UK. She obtained her Phd in Bioprocess Engineering in Universiti Teknologi Malaysia. She is a Chartered Chemical Engineer and her research areas are: 1) Materials and nanotechnology 2) Membrane technology involves: making of reverse osmosis, dialysis and ultrafiltration membranes; 3) Bioprocessing; Converting agricultural waste to higher value added products 3) Microalgae cultivation and bioprocessing into biodiesel. She has published many papers relating to her research area, obtained over 1600 citations, H- index 21 and has 5 patents granted.

She has secured many government grants; FRGS, ERGS, EsciFunds, Cradle Funds, MOA Technofund and L2M Grants. The government grants secured for the university in total within 5 years are worth RM 2,284,000 in which she is the leader to all these projects. She has also established a spinoff company named MEMTEC PLT, a manufacturing plant to produce the prototype membranes ready to be commercialised in line with the university and government mission to see successful research products that can be commercialised. She was recently awarded Malaysian Top research Scientist in 2015. She is currently appointed as a Research Fellow in the Institute of Bioproduct Development, Universiti Teknologi Malaysia.

Publications in the Last 3 Years:

2017

[1] Ngadiman, N.H.A., Yusof, N.M., Idris, A., Misran, E., Kurniawan, D. Development of highly porous biodegradable γ-Fe_2O_3/polyvinyl alcohol nanofiber mats using electrospinning process for biomedical application. Materials Science and Engineering C. 70, 520-534

[2] Fulazzaky, M.A., Majidnia, Z., Idris, A. Mass transfer kinetics of Cd(II) ions adsorption by titania polyvinylalcohol-alginate beads from aqueous solution. Chemical Engineering Journal. 308, 700-709.

[3] Zawawi, N.M., Hamzah, F., Sarif, M.[b], Manaf, S.F.A., Idris, A. Characterization of activated carbon using chemical activation via microwave ultrasonic system. Malaysian Journal of Analytical Sciences. 21 (1) 159-165.

[4] Chee Loong, T., Idris, A. One step transesterification of biodiesel production using simultaneous cooling and microwave heating. Journal of Cleaner Production. (146) 57-62.

[5] Fallahiarezoudar, E., Ahmadipourroudposht, M., Idris, A., Yusof, N.M., Optimization and development of Maghemite (γ-Fe_2O_3) filled poly-L-lactic acid (PLLA)/thermoplastic polyurethane (TPU) electrospun nanofibers using Taguchi orthogonal array for tissue engineering heart valve. Materials Science and Engineering C. 76, 616-627.

2016

[6] Mahtab Nasiri, Sayed Ali Hassanzadeh Tabrizi, Javad Hamzehhalipour Almaki, Rozita Nasiri, Ani Idris, Shadad Dabagh, Synthesisi, functionalization, characterization and in vitro evaluation of robust pH-sensitive CFNs-PA-$CaCO_3$, (2016) 87 RSC Advances

[7] Madiha Atta, Attaullah Bukhari, Ani Idris, Enhanced lipid selective extraction from *Chlorella vulgaris* without cell sacrifice. (2016). Algal Research, 20, 7- 15.

[8] Nasiri, R, Hamzehhalipour Almaki, J., Idris, A., Abdul Majid, F.A., Nasiri, M., Irfan, M., Amini, N., Maribaigi, M., *In vitro* evaluation of actively targetable superparamagnetic nanoparticles to the folate receptor positive cancer cells, Materials Science Engineering C., 69, 1147- 1158.

[9] Teo Chee Loong, Ani Idris, One step transesterification of biodiesel production using simultaneous cooling and microwave heating. Journal of Cleaner Production.xxx (2016) 1-6.

[10] Lai, L.W., Idris, A. Comparison of steam alkali-chemical and microwave alkali pretreatment for enhancing the enzymatic saccharafication of oil palm trunk. Renewable Energy. 99, 738 -746.

[11] Shaarani, S.M., Jahim, J.M., Rahman, R.A., Murad, A.M.A., Illias, R.M., Silanized maghemite for cross-linked enzyme aggregates of recombinant xylanase from Trichoderma resei. Journal of Molecular Catalysis B: Enzymatic. 133, 65-78.

[12] Othman, N., Harruddin, N., Idris, A., Ooi, Z.-Y., Fatiha, N., Raja Sulaiman, R.N, (2016). Fabrication of polypropylene membrane via thermally induced phase separation as a support matrix of tridodecylamine supported liquid membrane for Red 3BS dye removal. Desalination and Water Treatment. (2016), 57 (26) 12287-12301.

[13] Hassan, N., Idris, A. (2016) Simultaneous saccharification and fermentation of lactic acid from empty fruit bunch at high solids loading. Bioresources, 11(2) 3799 – 3812.

[14] Wahidin, S.'Idris, A., Shaleh, S.R.M. (2016). Ionic liquid as a promising biobased green solvent in combination with microwave irradiation for direct biodiesel production. Bioresource Technology. 206, 150-154.

[15] Idris, A., Majidnia, Z, Nor Kamarudin, K.S.B. (2016.) Photocatalyst treatment for lead (II) using titanium oxide nanoparticles embedded in PVA-alginate beads. Desalination and Water Treatment. 57, (11), 5035-5044.

[16] Almaki, J.H., Nasiri, R.,Idris, A.,Majid, F.A.A.,Salouti, M.,Wong, T.S., Dabagh, S., Marvibaigi, M., Amini, N. (2016) Synthesis, characterization and in vitro evaluation of exquisite targeting SPIONs-PEG-HER in HER2+ human breast cancer cells. Nanotechnology. 27(10) 105601.

[17] Leong, S.A.N., Mohd Samin, P., Idris, A., Mazlan, S.A., Rahman, A.H.A. (2016) Synthesis, characterization and magnetorheological properties of carbonyl iron suspension with superparamagnetic nanoparticles as an additive. Smart Materials and Structures. (25), 2, 025025.

[18] Wong, E.T., Chan, K.H., Irfan, M., Idris, A, (2016) Investigation of Cu(II) removal by cobalt-doped iron oxide captured in PVA-alginate beads. Desalination and Water Treatment. (57), 5, 2052-2063

[19] Majidnia, Z, Idris, A., Majid, M. Zin, R., Ponraj, M.(2016). Efficiency of barium removal from radioactive waste water using the combination of maghemite and titania nanoparticles in PVA and alginate beads. Applied Radiation and Isotopes (105), 2015, 105-113.

[20] Irfan, M., Idris, A., Khairuddin, N.F.M. (2015) Removal of heavy metal ions from its low concentrated lake water via LiBr/PES hollow fiber membrane module system. Desalination and Water Treatment. 7 November 2015, (Online).

[21] Zohreh Majidnia, Ani Idris, Synergistic effect of maghemite and titania nanoparticles in PVA-alginate encapsulated beads for photocatalytic reduction of Pb (II). *Chemical Engineering Communications.* 203,(4) 2016, 425-434

[22] Ehsan Fallahiarezoudar, Mohaddeseh Ahmadipourroudposht, Noordin Mohd Yusof & Ani Idris Characterization of maghemite (γ-Fe_2O_3) loaded poly L-lactic acid/thermoplastic polyurethane electrospun mats for soft tissue engineering. Journal of Material Science, 51(18) 8361-8381.

[23] Azura Hanis A. Rahman, Chee Loong Teo, Ani Idris, Efaliza Misran, Siti Asma' Nikmat Leong Polyvinyl alcohol alginate ferrophoto gels for mercury II removal. Journal of Industrial and Engineering Chemistry. 33.190-196.

2015

[24] Ngadiman, N.H.A., Idris, A., Irfan, M., Kurniawan, D., Yusof, N.M., Nasiri, R. (2015) γ-Fe2O3 nanoparticles filled polyvinyl alcohol as potential biomaterial for tissue engineering scaffold. Journal of the Mechanical Behaviour of Biomedical Materials. 49, 90 -104.

[25] Akhtar, J, Teo, C.L., Lai, L.W., Hassan, N, Ani Idris, and Ramlan Abd. Aziz. Factors Affecting Delignification of Oil Palm Empty Fruit Bunch by Microwave-assisted Dilute Acid/Alkali Pretreatment Bioresources. 10(1)588-596 (IF 1.59).

[26] Ehsan Fallahiarezoudar, Mohaddeseh Ahmadipourroudposht, Noordin Mohd Yusof & Ani Idris (2015) Fabrication (Ferrofluid/Polyvinyl Alcohol) Magnetic Nanofibers via Co-Axial Electrospinning, Journal of Dispersion Science and Technology, 36, (1), 28-31

[27] Ehsan Fallahiarezoudar, Mohaddeseh Ahmadipourroudposht, Noordin Mohd Yusof & Ani Idris (2015) Influence of Process Factors on Diameter of Core (γ-Fe2O3)/Shell (Polyvinyl Alcohol) Structure Magnetic Nanofibers during Co-Axial Electrospinning, International Journal of Polymeric Materials and Polymeric Biomaterials, Volume 64, Issue 1, pages 15-24.

[28] Ahmadipourroudposht, M., Fallahiarezoudar, E., Yusof, N.M, Ani Idris. Application of response surface methodology in optimization of electrospinning process to fabricate (ferrofluid/PVA) magnetic nanofibers. Materials Science and Engineering C, 50, 234-241.

[29] Ehsan Fallahiarezoudar, Mohaddeseh Ahmadipourroudposht, Ani Idris, Noordin Mohd Yusof, A review of: Application of synthetic scaffold in tissue engineering heart valves, Materials Science and Engineering: C, (48) 556-56.

[30] Zohreh Majidnia, Ani Idris, Evaluation of cesium removal from radioactive waste water using maghemite PVA - alginate beads *Chemical Engineering Journal*, *262*, *372-382*

[31] Kian Hwa Chan, Ee Ting Wong, Muhammad Irfan, Ani Idris, Noordin Mohd Yusof. Enhanced Cu(II) rejection and fouling reduction through fabrication of PEG-PES nanocomposite ultrafiltration membrane with PEG-coated cobalt doped iron oxide nanoparticle. *Journal of the Taiwan Institute of Chemical Engineers*, *47. 50-58*

[32] Kian Hwa Chan, Ee Ting Wong, Ani Idris, Noordin Mohd Yusof, Modification of PES membrane by PEG-coated cobalt doped iron oxide for improved Cu(II) removal. Journal of Industrial and Engineering Chemistry, 27, 283-290 (IF 2.063)

[33] Ee Ting Wong, Kian Hwa Chan, Ani Idris, Kinetic and equilibrium investigation of Cu(II) removal by Co(II)-doped iron oxide nanoparticle-immobilized in PVA-alginate recyclable adsorbent under dark and photo condition. Chemical Engineering Journal, 268, 311 -324.

[34] Ani Idris, Zohreh Majidna, (2015). Evaluation of the Cd removal efficacy from aqueous solutions using titania PVA-alginate beads. Desalination and Water Treatment 56(1) 266-273

[35] Zohreh Majidna, Ani Idris, (2015). Photocatalytic reduction of iodine in radioactive waste water using maghemite and titania nanoparticles in PVA-alginate beads. Journal of Taiwan Institute of Chemical Engineers. 54, 137-144

[36] Zohreh Majidnia, Ani Idris, Combination of maghemite and titanium oxide nanoparticles in polyvinyl alcohol-alginate encapsulated beads for cadmium ions removal. Korean Journal of Chemical Engineering. 32(6) 1094-1100.

[37] Wan-Ping Voo, Boon-Beng Lee, Ani Idris, Aminul Islam, Beng-Ti Tey, Eng-Seng Chan Production of ultra-high concentration calcium alginate beads with prolonged dissolution profile. RSC Advances, 5, (46) 36687-36695.

[38] Zohreh Majidnia, Ani Idris, Removal of barium from radioactive aqueous solution by PVA - alginate encapsulatd titanium oxide using sunlight and other light types. RSC Advances. 5 (78) 63588-63595

[39] R. Jusoh, A. A. Jalil*, S. Triwahyono, A. Idris, M. Y. Noordin Photodegradation of 2-chlorophenol over colloidal <alpha>-FeOOH supported mesostructured silica nanoparticles: Influence of a pore expander and reaction optimization. Separation and Purification Technology, 149, 55-64.

In: Electrospinning and Electroplating
Editor: Toby Jacobs
ISBN: 978-1-53612-363-0

Chapter 4

An Introduction to Electrospun Nanofibers for Tissue Engineering Heart Valves

Ehsan Fallahiarezoudar[1], Noordin Mohd Yusof, *
Ani Idris[2] and Nor Hasrul Akmal Ngadiman[1]
[1]Department of Materials, Manufacturing & Industrial Engineering,
Faculty of Mechanical Engineering, Universiti Teknologi Malaysia,
Skudai, Johor Bahru, Malaysia
[2]Department of Bioprocess Engineering, Faculty of Chemical Engineering,
Universiti Teknologi Malaysia, Skudai, Johor Bahru, Malaysia

Abstract

In recent years, the application of natural/synthetic based nanofibers in different industries such as textile, environmental engineering, biomedical engineering, energy and electronics have been the subject of many researches. This is particularly due to their unique properties (particularly high surface-to-volume ratio that is approximately 1,000 times more than that of human hair). Electrospinning is a straightforward and promising technique used to fabricate ultrafine quality of continuous nanofibers within a diameter range of 20-1000 nm. As a customary setup for electrospinning, a high potential electrical field is applied to the emerging solution at the spinneret nozzle tip for transforming the jet into the nanofibers. Electrospinning can be employed in a laboratory as well as in industries when expanded. Obviously, the process/system parameters involved influence the structural and mechanical properties of electrospun nanofibers. The microstructure of nanofibers and subsequently the macro-properties of electrospun mats can be modified by varying the parameters involved in electrospinning process. The fabricated electrospun mats are interconnected, non-woven nanofibers deposited over the collector surface. High

* Corresponding Author Email: noordin@fkm.utm.my.

porosity, remarkable mechanical properties such as an elastic modulus within the MPa/GPa range and capacity to be formed into a variety of shapes are the other properties of electrospun nanofibers. Co-axial electrospinning is an advanced method of electrospinning where a dual nozzle spinneret is used for fabricating a core/shell structure of nanofibers. Any conductive polymer solution can be used as the shell for any other conductive polymer solution or nanoparticles depending on the application. This review of an electrospinning technique provides detailed information on the background of electrospinning, fundamental principles and theory, investigation on parameters involved in nanofibers' structural/ biological/mechanical characteristics, advantages of superb properties and biomedical applications of electrospun nanofibers, particularly in tissue engineering heart valves. In addition, the reasons for common instabilities, which result in the failure of Taylor cone formation and subsequently the failure of fiber production, are also explained.

Keywords: electrospinning, nanofiber, Taylor cone, morphology, elastic modulus, tissue engineering

INTRODUCTION

Over the past few decades, polymer based nanotechnology has attracted a lot of interests due to its unique chemical, mechanical and biological properties of the objects within the size of 1-1000 nm [1, 2]. The science towards nanotechnology has been dominant as the current frontier in materials science and indeed will be one of the enabling sciences in the next century. The importance of polymers application in various fields such as electronics, energy, filtration, biomedicine, drug encapsulation and military industries has been increasing. Nano-structuring is an advanced approach in enhancing the mechanical modulus, heat resistance, thermal stability and permeability as well as decreasing the flammability and thermal expansion [3, 4]. Electrospinning is a straightforward nanofabricating process that is widely used in different industries.

FUNDAMENTALS AND THEORY OF ELECTROSPINNING

Electrospinning (also known as electro-spraying and electrostatic spinning) is the simplest, fascinating and affordable process for fabricating the polymeric/natural-based nanofibers within the range of 20-1000 nm [5, 6]. Ultrafine quality of continuous electrospun nanofibers as well as high surface to volume ratio and their correspondingly high porosity has attracted the interest of the industries and researchers, unlike other fabrication techniques [7]. Table 1 presents the pros and cons of various nanofabrication techniques.

Table 1. Comparison between different techniques of nanofiber fabrication

No.	Method	Advantage	Disadvantage
1	Phase separation	Simple procedure, No complexity in terms of equipment	Difficult to control the fibers size, Time consuming, applicable in particular types of polymers
2	Self-assembly	Nanofiber with smaller size can be fabricated	No capacity for continuous fiber, time consuming process
3	Drawing	Single nanofibers are fabricated using a simple instruments	Highly dependent to operator, no control on fibers size, time consuming
4	Template synthesis	Continuous fiber can be obtained, capacity to control the fiber diameter, easy to shape in various forms	Not applicable in mass production, template replacement is required
5	Electro-spinning	Low cost, simple equipment, uniform ultrafine nanofibers, high porous fiber, no need for expensive purification,	Expert operator is required, high electrical consumption, highly dependent on the experimental parameter

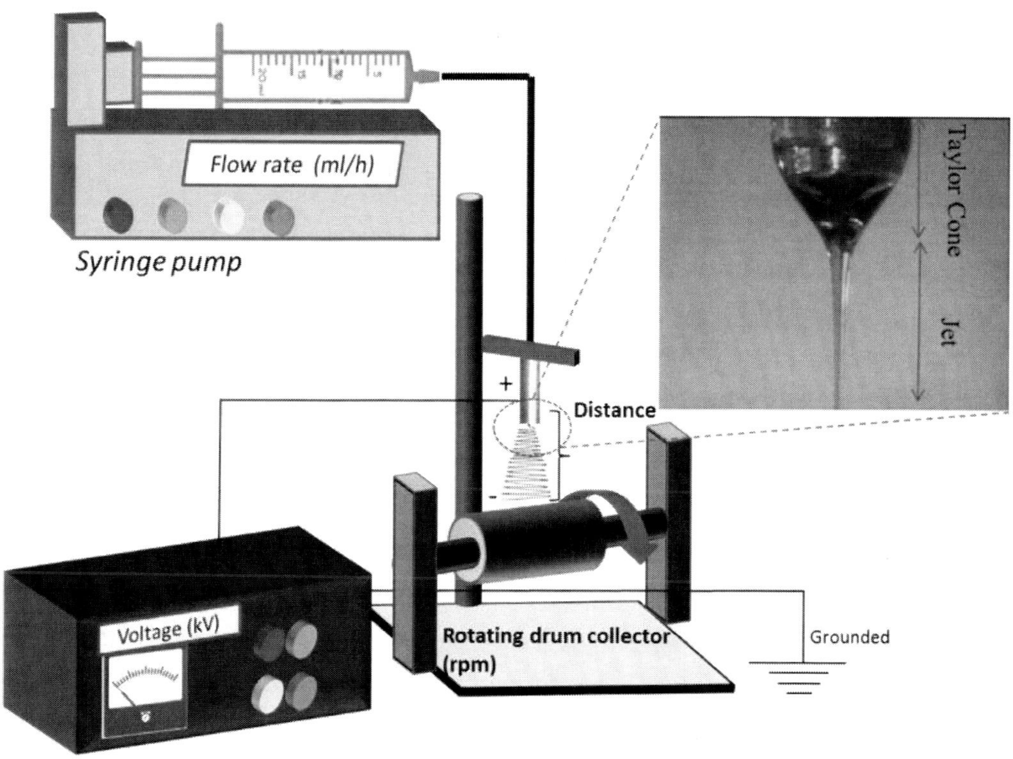

Figure 1. Schematic of electrospinning setup and Taylor cone.

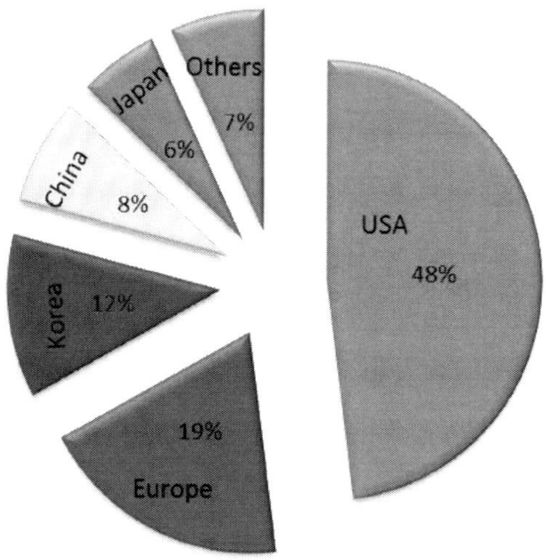

Figure 2. Analysis of publications percentage based on electrospinning keyword by the year 2015.

As a customary setup for electrospinning, a high electrostatic field is applied to the raw materials supplied through a syringe pump and transformed the emerging jet at the nozzle spinneret tip into the nanofibers [8, 9]. The nanofibers are then deposited over the collector surface and the electrospun mat is formed. Commonly, the high molecular polymer is preferred where the surface charge of polymer solution and the potential electrical field have direct relationships [10]. The electrospinning comprises of four main parts including: High voltage DC supplier, syringe pump to control the flow rate of the solution, spinneret nozzle (simple or dual) and collector (rotating/static) which is grounded. Figure 1 illustrates the schematic of electrospinning apparatus. The distance between the nozzle and the collector is an important factor that has effect on the fibers morphology and diameter [11, 12]. The distance can be adjusted with respect to the type of solvent which is used for polymer solution preparation. The solvent evaporation before the deposition will improve the quality of fabricated nanofibers [13, 14]. The applied voltage creates an electrical field between the nozzle (positive terminal) and the collector (negative terminal). The emerging solution at the nozzle tip is held due to the surface tension. As soon as the created electrical field reaches the threshold of the polymer surface tension, the Taylor cone is formed and the fiber formation initiates [15].

In 1960s, the studies on the jet forming and Taylor cone were performed by Taylor. Since 1990s more than 34 types of polymers have been successfully reported as the raw materials for electrospinning [2, 3]. The history of electrospinning traced back as early as 1902 based on the studies of Morton [16] and Cooley [17]. They invented an apparatus for electrically dispersing fluids. In 1914 John Zeleny reported a mathematical model for liquid under electrical force [18]. In 1929 Hagiwara proposed a process for manufacturing of the artificial silk using the electrical field [19]. During 1930s-1940s Formhals made a significant progress in this area and registered more than 10 patents [20, 21]. Finally in

1944 he made an apparatus for spinning of the liquids for fiber production [22]. During 1964-1969, Taylor generated the theoretical fundamental of electrospinning and the 'Taylor cone' was named after him [23, 24]. The Taylor cone semivertical and apex angle of 49.3° and 98.6° was defined respectively [3, 25]. In his work the hopper form was modelled to upgrade the electrospinning [25]. In 1986, Groitzsch and Fahrbach fabricated multilayered microporous nonwoven polymer for biomedical application [26]. Reneker in 1990s applied high voltage to polyolefin polymer solution to fabricate fibers with diameter less than 5μm [27]. After that, many researches have been carried out to study the relationships between the process/system parameters on structural, mechanical and chemical properties of the fabricated fibers. The analysis of most active countries in this research field indicates that the United States of America dedicates 48% of the publication and after than Europe, Korea, China, Japan and other countries are the next. Figure 2 illustrates the plot of analysis based on the keyword of electrospinning by the year 2015 [3, 28, 29].

ELECTROSPINNING PARAMETERS

Two types of factors (process and system) are known to influence the characteristics of the fabricated nanofibers using electrospinning. The process factors include the apparatus parameters such as voltage, flow rate, needle-collector distance, rotating speed of the collector and ambient condition (temperature and humidity) [6, 12, 30]. On the contrary, the system factors revolve around the solution parameters such as viscosity, conductivity, molecular weight, type of solvent and amount of additive [31-33]. Electrospinning process is highly dependent on the parameters' setting. Previously, many experiments have been done to optimize the parameters involved. Lijima incorporated the carbon nanotubes (CNTs) into the electrospun nanofibers to enhance the conductivity as well as mechanical strength of the nanofibers [34]. In 1999, Fong investigated the formation of beads as the result of voltage variation during fabrication of poly(ethylene oxide) (PEO) electrospun nanofibers [35]. Deitzel et al. [36], investigated the effect of solution concentration and applied voltage on the structural properties of PEO electrospun mats. They reported that the fibers' diameter distribution and morphology had greatly changed when these parameters were adjusted. In 2004, Sundarary [37] developed polystyrene (PS) nanofiber using the dynamic/conductive needle and insulating drum collector where the thickness and porosity of the fabricated electrospun mats can be controlled. Milleret et al. [38], tuning electrospinning parameters for fabricating 3D Degrapol®-PLGA fiber in terms of diameter distribution and alignments to meet the requirements for scaffolding in tissue engineering principle. Their study showed that flow rate and working distance affect fiber diameter and alignment in an inverse relation. Recently, Fallahiarezoudar et al. [30], developed the core/shell structure of magnetic nanofibers using the ferrofluid/polyvinyl alcohol (PVA). They optimized the parameters settings using the systematic method as the design of experiments (DOE) to develop ultrafine quality of nanofibers with size of 245 nm. They found that the flow rate, voltage and drum collector rotating speed had significant effect on the diameter of the fibers. In addition, a reverse relationship between the diameter of the fibers and elastic modulus of the nanofibers was achieved. Systematic techniques such as DOE, Taguchi design, response surface methodology (RSM) are highly recommended instead on one-factor-at-a-time traditional approach [9, 12, 30].

In our very recent work [12], the Taguchi orthogonal array was used to optimize the elastic modulus of electrospun poly-L-lactic acid (PLLA)/thermoplastic polyurethane (TPU) nanofibers containing maghemite (γ-Fe_2O_3) nanoparticles as the potential for tissue engineering heart valves. The results indicated that the solution concentration had the most influence on elastic modulus while the voltage, maghemite percent in the content, flow rate and rotating speed were the next influential parameters. Furthermore, by controlling the microstructure of the fibers, the macro-properties of electrospun mats can be modified. For example, by varying the fibers' diameter, the porosity, surface roughness, hydrophilicity and tensile strength of the electrospun mats can also be modified. As a result, the biocompatibility properties of a fabricated scaffold may be affected [39, 40].

(a) Process Parameters

(i) Voltage: the proper applied voltage is the crucial factor in the electrospinning process. As the result of the applied voltage, the polymer solution gets charged and subsequently the Taylor cone is formed [40, 41]. The increase in the voltage has reverse relationship with the droplet volume. Rayleigh instability (which is a type of axisymmetric instability) can occur when the strength of the electrical field is too low or the viscosity of solution is below the optimum point [8]. Several researchers have also reported the reverse relationship between fiber diameter and applied voltage [3, 42]. Figure 3 indicates the field emission scanning electron microscopy (FE-SEM) images of electrospun nanofibers with and without beads formation.

(ii) Flow rate: the feed rate of the solution can significantly affect the fiber morphology and diameter. For a given voltage, an increase in the feed rate will also lead to the increase of the fibers' diameter which will produce the beads [40, 43]. When the flow rate is high than the voltage, the solution cannot be fully transformed into the fibers. As a result, the solution droplets are deposited all over the collector surface which known as defect [8]. Figure 4 depicts the deposition of solution droplets on the collector surface as a result of high feed rate of solution.

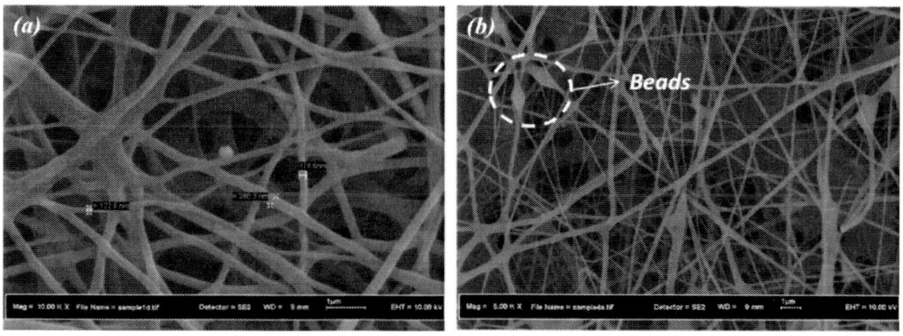

Figure 3. FE-SEM images of (a) well fabricated of PVA nanofibers (b) PVA nanofibers with beads formation.

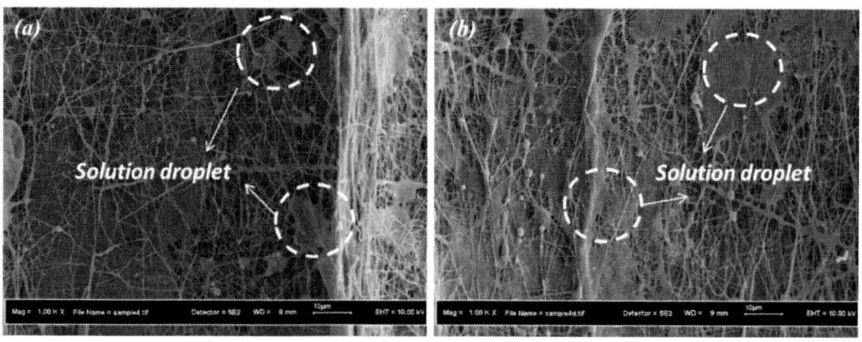

Figure 4. FE-SEM images of PVA nanofibers fabricated at voltage 20 kV and (a) flow rate of 3.5 ml/h (b) flow rate of 4.5 ml/h.

(iii) Needle-collector distance: the gap between the needle and collector can be adjusted to control the time for the evaporation of the solvent. Even though, the short distance may result in higher electrical field, the insufficient time for evaporation will lead to the formation of beads [44, 45]. For cases where evaporation of the solvent does not happen quickly, the distance seems to be neutral in fiber properties especially when water is the solvent of PVA [8, 30].

(iv) Collector geometry: the collector is the negative polarity of the electrical field. Commonly, the collector is covered with an aluminium foil for better conductivity [46]. The drum rotating collector is preferred than the plate collector because more aligned fibers can be fabricated [47]. Aligned fibers indicate higher tensile strength compare to random fibers [12, 30]. The rotating speed of the collector plays an important role in forming aligned pattern of the fibers. Figure 5 illustrates the FE-SEM images of fabricated nanofibers through drum collector with rotating speed and static plate collector. The aligned orders of fibers are visible in drum collector with rotating speed.

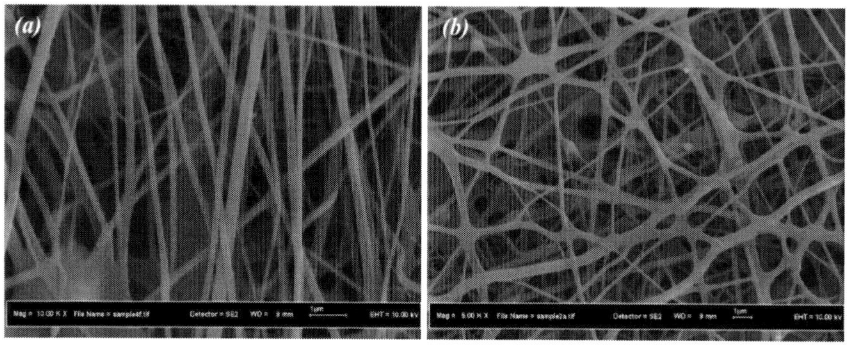

Figure 5. FE-SEM images of fabricated PVA nanofibers using (a) drum collector (b) plate collector.

(v) Ambient condition: the ambient condition such as temperature can affect the viscosity of the emerging solution and correspondingly affect the fibers' diameter. Higher temperature results in lower viscosity which reduces the diameter of the fibers [48, 49]. Furthermore, higher temperature also results in the evaporation of the solvent to be deposited over the collector surface [50]. Ambient condition in terms of humidity can affect the fibers morphology while the water droplets will condense in the fibers [51]. Commonly, humidity less than 25% results in smooth fibers, while greater humidity of 30-45% creates small pores on the surface of fibers. Higher humidity will lead to coalescence of the small pores [3, 52]. In addition, solvent evaporation will not occurr easily. Therefore, the humidity and temperature have to be adjusted accordingly.

(b) System Parameters

(i) Viscosity/Concentration: solution viscosity remarkably has an influence on the fibers' diameter and morphology. When the viscosity of a solution is below the optimum point, the Rayleigh instability and fiber breakage may happen during the spinning process [53, 54]. The low viscosity of solution also results in the formation of beads [55]. Based on the power law relationship, higher solution concentration will lead to larger fibers' diameter [3, 56]. Higher concentration also improves the polymer chain and correspondingly prevents the breakage of the fibers. The surface tension of the solution can be affected by the concentration as well. On the other hand, when the viscosity is very high due to high amount of the solvent, beads will form in the fibers [40, 57].

(ii) Conductivity: the spinning process involves applying the electric field to charge the solution droplet surface. The higher the conductivity of the solution, the thinner the fibers are fabricated [58, 59]. In some cases, in order to improve the conductivity, adding any conductive chemicals to the solution is recommended. The sizes of ions being produced can affect the fibers' diameter. Commonly, salt is added to the solution for better conductivity. Small ions can move faster than bigger size ions which shows that the size of ions can influence the diameter of fibers [60, 61].

(iii) Molecular weight: molecular weight of the polymers also affects the morphology of the fibers. At a fixed concentration, higher molecular weight of the polymer may improve its quality and prevent the formation of beads. However, above a certain solution concentration, the effect of molecular weight is neutral [62, 63].

(iv) Solvent type: dissolving is an inevitable step in electrospinning, thus, selection of a desirable solvent for full interaction between the solvent molecules and polymer chain is required. It has been reported in several cases that the solvent type has a significant influence on the morphology of fibers. [64, 65]. Similar to the application of fabricated electrospun mats, the type of solvent should be selected properly. For instance, in biomedical application, toxic solvent may not be appropriate as it may damage the cells. However, solvent that can be evaporated easily will be better preferred.

(v) Solution additives: examples of the additives can be nanoparticles or any other polymers. Additives can improve the characteristics of the solution in respective manner [66, 67]. For example, the PLLA nanofibers are too rigid. Hence, adding TPU into the PLLA axis will enhance the elasticity of the electrospun mats enabling it to be a potential material for soft tissue engineering. Furthermore, adding proper nanoparticles with respect to the application can influence the macro structure of the fibers [12, 59]. Previously, the addition of maghemite nanoparticles has resulted in higher tensile strength and better cell proliferation in the tissue engineering field [11].

Various Types Of Electrospinning Process

Several types of electrospinning processes have been carried out to fabricate the nanofibers for different applications. Despite the effect of parameters involved on the morphology and microstructure of the fibers, the type of process can also affect the characteristics and structural of the nanofabricated fibers [3]. Some of the common types of nanofiber fabrication processes are melt electrospinning, multichannel electrospinning, co-axial electrospinning, near field electrospinning, yarn electrospinning and centrifugal electrospinning. All these processes have the same fundamentalst. However, different types of spinneret nozzle or collector substrates differentiated the fabrication method. The following sections explain the types of electrospinning processes mentioned above.

(i) Melt electrospinning: in order to remove the dissolving steps which finally may require solvent evaporation, the melt electrospinning process is performed [68,

69]. In melt electrospinning, the molten polymer is pumped to the nozzle and the spinning takes place. A temperature controller and heater are attached to the polymer container which transforms the polymer into molten state. The high concentration of solution, low degradation rate and various melting temperature of amorphous and semicrystalline polymer are the drawbacks of this method, despite overcoming of polymer dissolution particularly in biomedical applications.

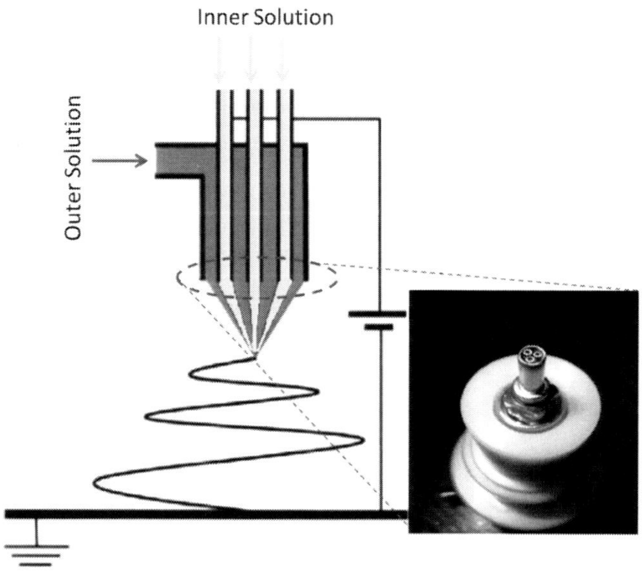

Figure 6. Schematic of multi-channel spinneret nozzle.

(ii) Multichannel electrospinning: this method can be considered as the application of a particular type of spinneret nozzle. The spinneret nozzle includes the multiple tubes inside the bigger tube as depicted in Figure 6. Two different solutions are pumped into the inner and outer nozzles to fabricate the nanofibers. The key to success when using this fabrication technique is the immiscibility of two polymer solutions [70, 71]. Removing the inner solution will lead to multichannel nanofibers.

(iii) Co-axial electrospinning: similar to the multichannel method, in co-axial electrospinning method, a particular type of spinneret nozzle is used where a smaller nozzle is connected to a bigger capillary [8, 30]. The coaxial method is used to fabricate the core/shell structure of nanofibers. The core solution is pumped into the inner capillary and the shell solution is pumped into the outer part. Figure 7 illustrates the coaxial spinneret nozzle and high resolution transmission electron microscopy (HR-TEM) image of ferrofluid/PVA nanofibers. Immiscibility of utilized polymer solution is the key factor for a successful result [8].

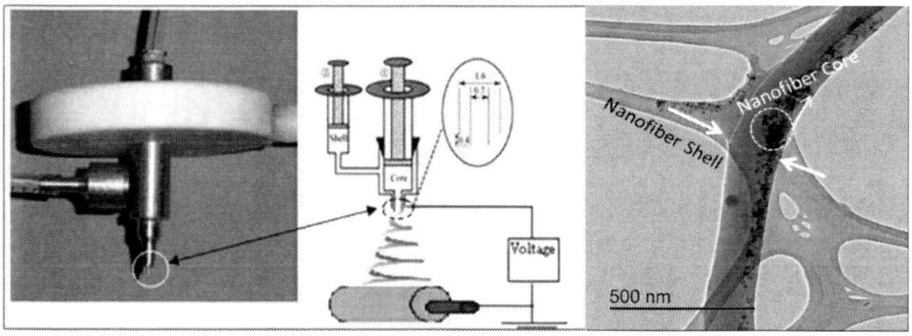

Figure 7. Schematic of Co-axial electrospinning and related spinneret nozzle as well as HR-TEM image of ferrofluid/PVA nanofibers.

(iv) Near-field electrospinning: this method is used to fabricate a single yarn of nanofibers. Usually the gap between the nozzle and collector is within 0.5-3 mm [72, 73]. In this method, the jet is deposited over the moving substrate before whipping. The motion speed of the collector greatly influences the quality and straight collection of the nanofibers [73].

(v) Yarn electrospinning: in this method, uniaxial bundle of nanofibers are fabricated using a liquid container as the collector. A metal plate is placed at the bottom of the container to create a negative pole for the electrical field. Initially, the fibers' yarn is drawn by the hand slowly, and attached to the rotating collector at slow speed (usually less than 16 Hz) [74, 75]. In this method, the fibers seem to be in micro dimension diameter, since they are difficult to be seen. Water is commonly used as the liquid container, which may help the solvent dissolves prior to the collection by rotating collector.

(vi) Centrifugal electrospinning: in this method, a rotating spinneret nozzle is attached over a nonconductive cylindrical chamber which is covered with aluminium plate. The chamber is also connected to a speed motor. The rotating speed of the cylindrical chamber will assist the electrospinning process to obtain an aligned orientation of nanofibers. By commencing the electrospinning, the centrifugal force assists the thinning of the emerging jet to be collected over the cylindrical chamber [76-78].

CHARACTERIZATION OF ELECTROSPUN NANOFIBERS

In order to characterize the different properties of nanofibers (either the macro or nano properties) various types of analytical methods have been developed. The structural, chemical, mechanical and biological properties of the fabricated electrospun mats with respect to the application are usually investigated [46, 59]. Structural properties such as the morphology, porosity, hierarchical structure and surface roughness are analysed using the FE-SEM/TEM analysis and atomic force microscopy (AFM), respectively.

In terms of chemical analysis properties, such as the hydrophilicity/ hydrophobicity, well distribution and formation of two polymers into the nanofiber matrix, chemical bond and crystallinity can be analysed. They are being measured using the water contact angle measurement, X-ray diffraction (XRD), energy-dispersive X-ray spectroscopy (EDX), Fourier transform infrared spectroscopy (FTIR) and differential scanning calorimetry (DSC), respectively [79].

Mechanical analysis such as the tensile stress, tensile strain and subsequently elastic modulus of either the electrospun mats or a single yarn of nanofibers can be measured. For this purpose, uniaxial tensile test, macro-indentation test, biaxial mechanical test and viscoelasticity test are some of the common tests for the macro analysis of electrospun mats. In addition, Nano-indentation test, which is connected to a microscope is developed in order to analyse the mechanical characteristic of a single yarn nanofiber. Various types of apparatus are available for mechanical testing of nanofibers, where the applicable load should be very low. The most famous machine is the dynamic mechanical analyser (DMA) which is widely used particularly in testing fabricated nanofibers for biomedical application [80, 81].

In terms of biological analysis, the degradation rate, biocompatibility of the electrospun mats through cytotoxicity test and desirable environment for cell attachment and proliferation is also being considered. The degradation rate of nanofibers can be investigated during the incubation time in a special environment to simulate the real condition [59, 82]. The MTT assay is a simple method to test the cytotoxicity of the electrospun mats. However, providing a proper environment for cell attachment and proliferation is highly dependent on the appropriate structure of nanofibers such as porosity.

Application Of Electrospun Nanofibers in Tissue Engineering Heart Valves

The fabricated nanofibers through electrospinning technique can be used in different industries. Recently, electrospun mats properties are characterized as a potential for scaffolding different engineered tissue. Scaffolding through electrospinning is advantageous due to its impressive properties of fabricated electrospun mats such as hierarchical structure (which mimic the extracellular matrix), high surface-to-volume ratio, desired biodegradability and remarkable mechanical properties [5, 59]. Hence, 3D biofabrication of poly-L-lactic acid (PLLA)/thermoplastic polyurethane (TPU) containing maghemite nanoparticles has been developed for tissue engineering heart valve.

The polymer solutions are prepared by dissolving the PLLA and TPU in dimethylformamide (DMF) and dichloromethane (DCM), respectively. Then, they are mixed in 50:50% (v/v) ratio until homogeneous solution is formed. In addition, the maghemite nanoparticles are synthesized in the laboratory as described in Fallahiarezoudar et al. [59]. The PLLA and TPU are two immiscible polymers which can be presented in the fibers axis as their characteristics can fulfill the requirements. Various techniques have been developed to transform the 2D electrospun mats into the 3D scaffold such as melt processing. The 3D scaffold is fabricated using templating the aortic heart valve and attached as the collector for electrospinning process. The fibers are collected over the template. Finally, by removing the template, the 3D scaffold of aortic the heart valve is obtained.

Table 2. Factors and levels for Taguchi experimental design

	No.	Factors/Levels	Level (1)	Level (2)
Controllable Factors	1	A-Flow rate (ml/h)	2	3
	2	B-Voltage (kV)	20	30
	3	C-Maghemite (w/v %)	1	3
	4	D-Concentration (wt. %)	10	15
	5	E-Rotating speed (rpm)	1000	2000
Noise Factors	6	F-Temperature (°C)	30	45
	7	G-Humidity (%)	30%	80%
	8	H-Nozzle type	Aluminium	Steel

In this case, in order to optimize the parameters involved, a series of controllable factors such as flow rate, voltage, rotating speed of collector, solution concentration and percent of maghemite in the solution content are investigated using the two-level Taguchi orthogonal array (L8 design). Temperature, humidity and nozzle type are considered as the noise factors in the experimental design. Table 2 summarizes the parameters involve and their levels for spinning process. The Taguchi design (the function of the bigger the better) is performed and the optimum parameters settings in terms of elastic modulus are achieved. Based on the analysis, the optimum elastic modulus is found to be approximately 28.459 MPa. At the same time, the flow rate, voltage, rotating speed, concentration and maghemite percent are fixed at 3 ml/h, 30 kV, 2000 rpm, 10 wt% and 3% (w/v) respectively. The obtained elastic modulus is approximately double the natural heart valve.

After finding the optimum parameters setting, the fabrication of 3D scaffold is carried out. For this purpose, aluminium foil is used to produce the aortic heart valve template. The aluminium foil is cut into three similar semicircular shapes to resemble the aortic valve leaflets. The leaflets are then fold from the free-edge length to form a closed position of the valve. Finally, the leaflets are attached to the top of a cylindrical tube to resemble the aortic root. The dimensions of the aortic valve are extracted from the literature [83, 84]. Figure 8 displays the steps for 3D template fabrication. The template is attached as the collector in the apparatus. Figure 9 illustrates the 3D electrospun scaffold fabricated through this technique.

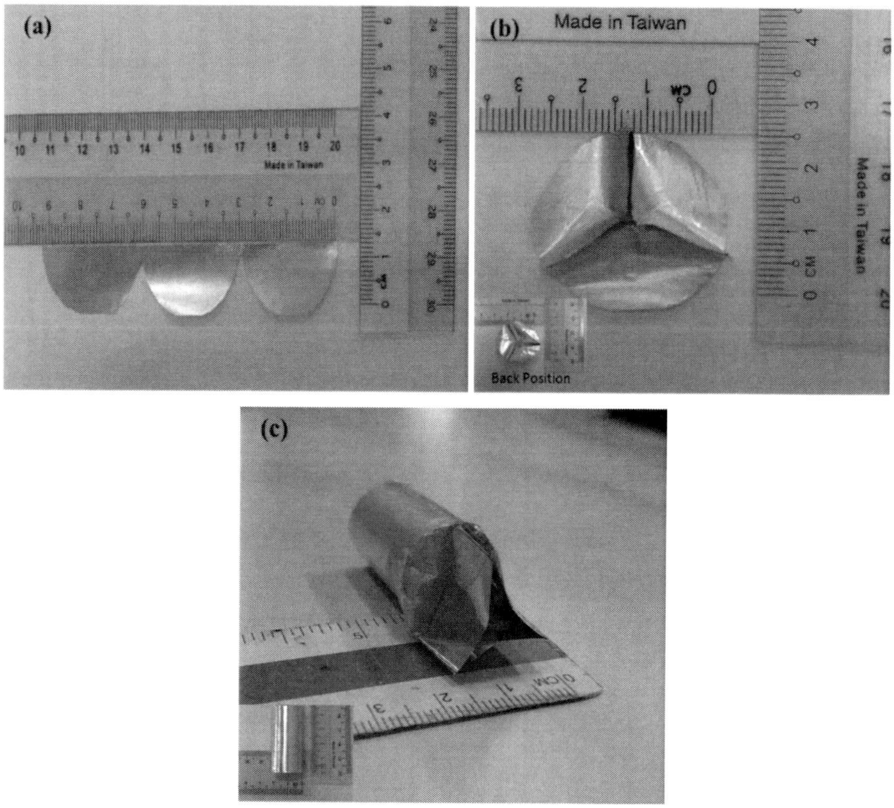

Figure 8. Procedure of 3D template fabrication of aortic heart valve.

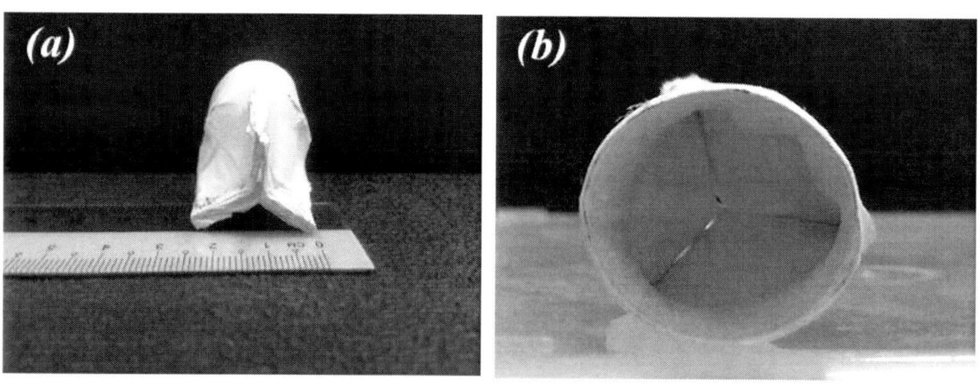

Figure 9. Images of (a) exterior and (b) interior of 3D electrospun scaffold.

STRUCTURAL AND CHEMICAL CHARACTERIZATION

The 3D fabricated scaffold is structurally and chemically characterized in terms of morphology, porosity properties, degradability and existence of all the polymers into the matrix through EDX. The morphology is investigated using FE-SEM microscopy (SUPRA, 35VP). The result indicates ultrafine quality of nanofibers with hierarchical structure which mimics the extracellular matrix. Figure 10(a) indicates the FE-SEM images of fabricated electrospun mats at the optimum parameters setting at an acceleration voltage of 10.00 KX. Furthermore, the surface roughness of electrospun mats is checked through AFM (Park XE-100). An area of 10 μm×10 μm is analysed and the average of surface roughness (R_a) is founded to be 578 nm. This shows that the higher the surface roughness, the better the cell attachment [59]. Figure 10(b) illustrates the 3D AFM image of the analysed area. Different colours represent different heights.

The porosity of 3D scaffold is obtained using liquid displacement technique. Generally, a certain volume of ethanol is filled into a gradual cylinder and then the 3D scaffold is immersed into it for a while. The change in the volume of ethanol is recorded. Later, the scaffold is removed from the ethanol and the new volume is recorded as well. Equation 1 is used to calculate the porosity of the 3D scaffold. The result indicates the porosity of the fabricated scaffold is approximately 83.33% which is very desirable for this purpose.

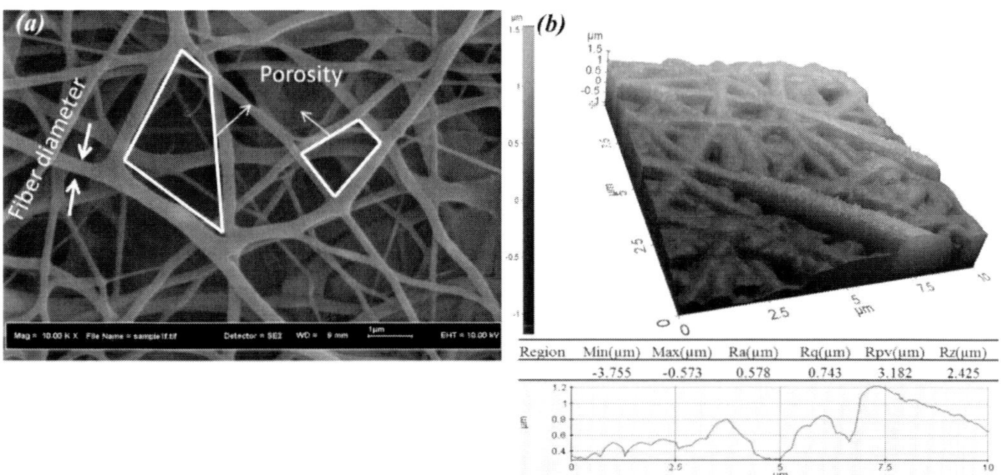

Figure 10. Surface morphology (a) FE-SEM image of PLLA/TPU-(γ-Fe_2O_3) electrospun mats (b) AFM image of surface roughness.

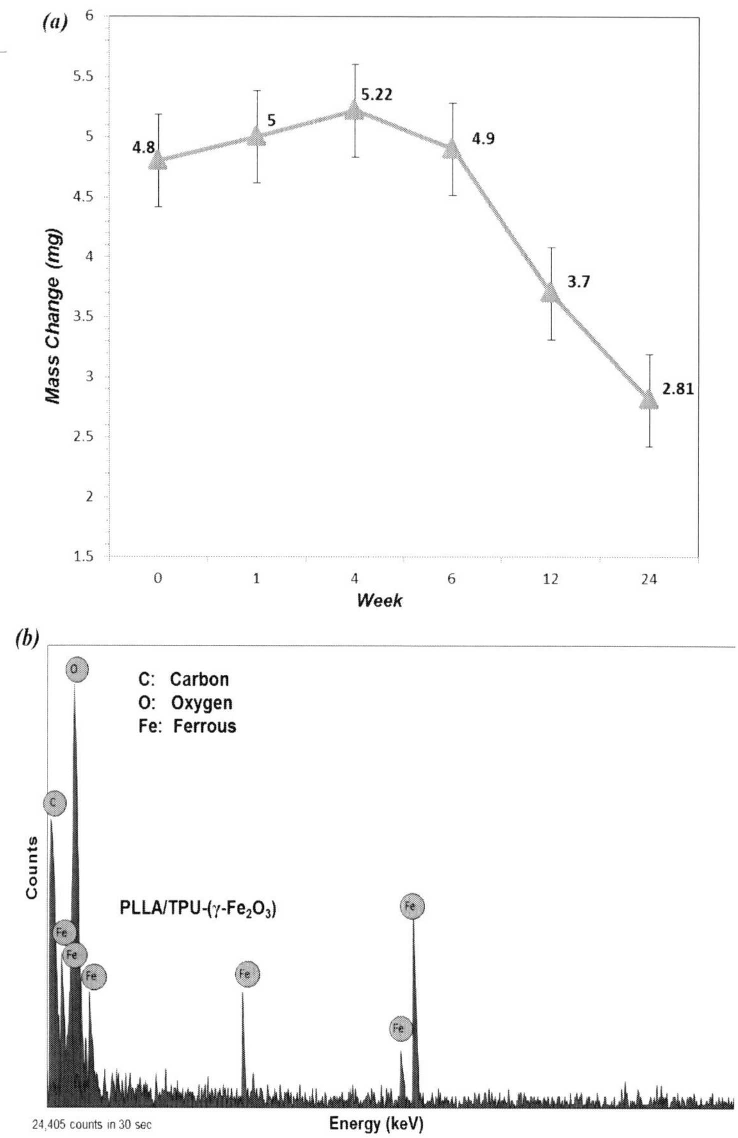

Figure 11. Degradation studies (a) plot of degradation rate in terms of mass change (b) EDX of PLLA/TPU-(γ-Fe2O3) electrospun mats.

$$\text{Porosity}(\%)=\left(\frac{V_1\text{-}V_3}{V_2\text{-}V_3}\right)\times 100 \tag{1}$$

where, the 'V_1' is the initial volume of ethanol,'V_2' is the volume of ethanol after scaffold immersion, 'V_3' is the volume of ethanol after scaffold removal.

The degradation rate of scaffold is characterized by incubating the scaffold into the simulated body fluid [85] during 1, 4, 6, 12 and 24 weeks. The result indicates a slow degradation rate during the first 4 weeks. After week 4th, a good degradation rate is observed and after week 24, almost 41.45% of the scaffold weight has reduced. Figure 11

(a) illustrates the degradation rate as a function of incubation time. Furthermore, in order to verify the existence of all the utilized chemical inside the matrix of the nanofibers, EDX is performed and the result indicates the presence of carbon and oxygen which are the main components of the PLLA and TPU as well as ferrous (Figure 11(b)). After fully degradation of the polymers, the nanoparticles will be dispersed into the blood and finally filtered by the kidney and spleen.

BIOLOGICAL PROPERTIES

The biological properties of the 3D scaffold in terms of cell attachment and proliferation have been investigated using the human aortic smooth muscles cell (HAOSMCs). For this purpose, the cells are cultured according to the normal procedure up to passage 7th [86]. Prior to the cell seeding, the 3D scaffold is incubated in Dulbecco's modified Eagle's medium (DMEM) for 6 days for better cell attachment. Later, suitable number of cells (5×10^4 cell/cm^2) are seeded over the scaffold surface and incubated at 37°C and 5% CO_2. The cell proliferation rate is investigated during 1, 3, 5 and 7 days of incubation using MTT (3-(4,5-dimethylthiazol-2-yl)-2,5-diphenyltetrazolium bromide) assay. Furthermore, the FE-SEM analysis is performed to verify the cell attachment to the scaffold surface properly. Figure 12 illustrates the proliferation rate (MTT analysis) plot as a function of incubation time. A uniform increasing rate in cell proliferation is visible. Figure 13 displays the FE-SEM images of cell attachment and migration within 7 days of incubation.

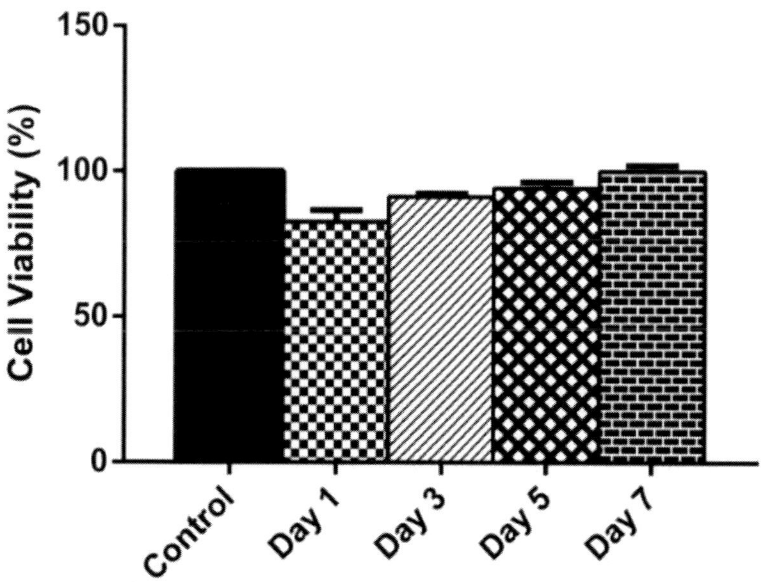

Figure 12. Bar plot of cell viability (%) as a function of incubation time.

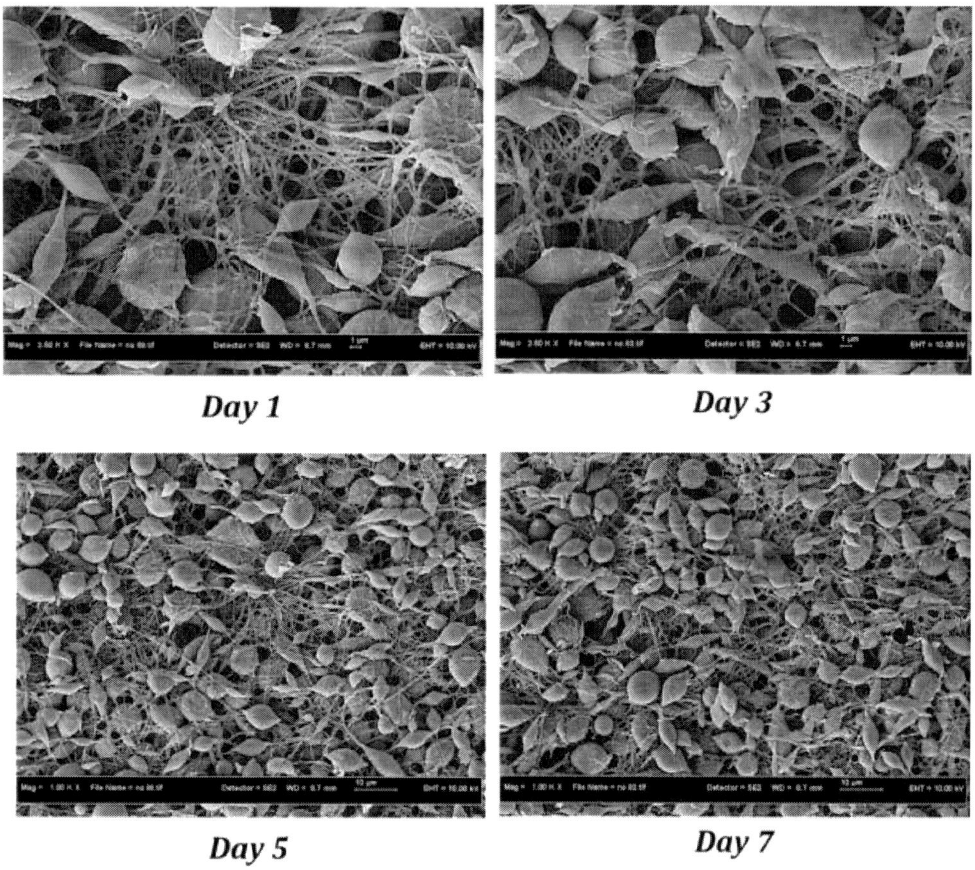

Figure 13. FE-SEM images of cell attachment and proliferation over the scaffold surface during 1, 3, 5 and 7 days of incubation at 37°C and 5% CO_2.

MECHANICAL CHRACTERIZAION

The electrospun nanofibers are mechanically characterized in terms of elastic modulus in order to optimize the parameters involved in the electrospinning process. Uniaxial tensile tester (Lloyd, LRX) is used to obtain the tensile stress ($\sigma_{(\varepsilon)}$), tensile strain (ε) and correspondingly elastic modulus (E_e). The tensile stress is defined as the applied force per cross sectional area. Furthermore, the tensile strain is defined as the change in the original length of the specimen as a function of applied force [11, 81]. The elastic modulus is achieved through the ratio of stress to strain. Therefore, the elastic modulus is calculated using Equation 2.

$$E_e = \frac{F/A_0}{\Delta L/L_0} \tag{2}$$

where, 'E_e' is the elastic modulus, 'F' is the applied force, 'A_0' is the cross sectional area, 'ΔL' is the change in the length and 'L_0' is the original length of the sample.

In this case, the 3D scaffold mechanical properties in terms of elastic modulus are investigated using the macro-indentation test. Macro-indentation flexural test through LF plus materials testing analyzer apparatus (Lloyd Tensile Tester, EZ) according to the standard ISO 14577-1 is performed to analyse the deformation and elastic modulus of 3D scaffold. The elastic modulus measurements via macro-indentation bending test is performed easily as compared to very small elongation in compressive or tensile load. In order to prepare sample for the test, the scaffold is cut from commissures and clamped over a round hole with diameter 21 mm with a ball probe (diameter 10 mm). Indentation force of 100N at quasi-static rate at a cross head speed of 10 mm/min is applied to leaflets until rupture occurred. In order to analyse the elastic modulus, the maximum load which can be applied to the leaflets before rupture (N) and maximum extension at break (indentation depth before rupture) need to be translated into stress and strain. The results are analysed by looking at the applied load versus the depth of indentation by NexygenPlus data analysis software. The tests are performed three times (n = 3) in two groups of wet and dried scaffolds.

The Hertz theory is used to analyze the force indentation data. Equations 3 and 4 represent the procedure for calculating the elastic modulus of scaffold. The relative elastic modulus 'E_r' is given by [87]:

$$E_r = \sqrt{\frac{9F^2}{16R_e\delta^3}} \tag{3}$$

where, 'F' represents the force applied, 'δ' is the depth of indentation, and 'R_e' is the contact surface area between ball probe and leaflet.

The elastic modulus of leaflets (electrospun nanofibers) E_e are calculated by:

$$E_e = E_r(1-V_f^2) \tag{4}$$

where, V_f is the Poisson's ratio of the nanofibers which is assumed to be 0.33 [88].

Figure 14 exhibits the load versus extension curve and related values. The obtained elastic modulus is around 28.11 ± 1.32 MPa which is more than that it is required. Since the heart valve requires a dynamic function during the cardiac cycling, the PLLA is too rigid to be used. Hence, TPU which is an elastic polymer, is used to enhance the elasticity. Furthermore, the presence of the maghemite nanoparticles in the latter's surface of the electrospun nanofibers has improved the tensile strength.

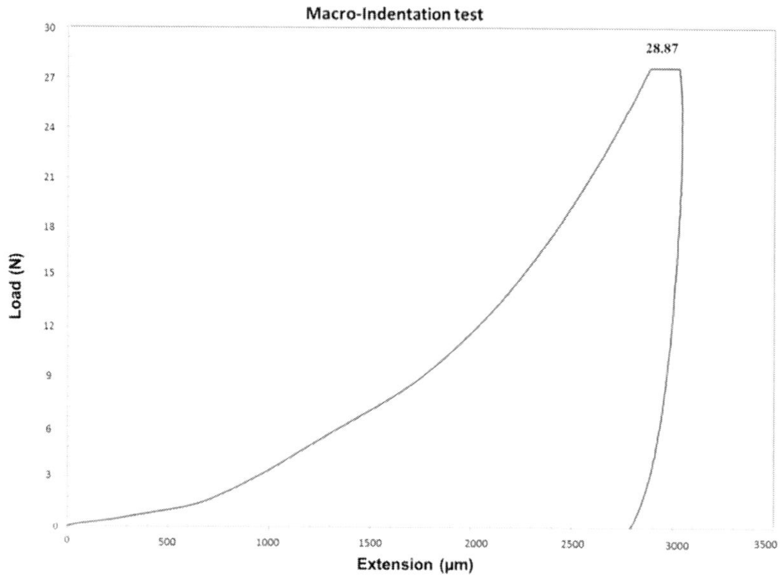

No.	Load (N)	Extension (µm)	Elastic modulus (MPa)
1	28.87±1.2	2870±34	28.11±1.32

Figure 14. Load versus extension curve of macro-indentation test.

CONCLUSION

The review presented provides some detailed information about electrospinning fundamentals and theory. The various types of electrospinning processes as well as the influence of parameters involved in fibers' morphology have been described too. In addition, a particular application of electrospun nanofibers in the tissue engineering field has been considered. The 3D aortic heart valve scaffold is developed using the electrospinning technique and has been characterized in terms of structural, chemical, biological and mechanical properties. For that purpose, the electrospinning parameters are optimized prior to the fabrication. The optimum parameters are used for developing the 3D scaffold and then characterizing it. The results indicate a high quality of porous electrospun mats which can resemble the extracellular matrix and provide good initial templates for cell growth. The mechanical properties of the scaffold are tested using the macro-indentation test, which indicates a remarkable elastic modulus (28.11 ± 1.32 MPa almost double that of a native heart valve 10-15 MPa). The electrospinning is an emerging technique that is widely used in different industries and the result is quite promising. The presence of maghemite nanoparticles in the solution improve the solution conductivity and act as additives on the latter's surface to improve the cell growth rate as well as the mechanical strength.

REFERENCES

[1] Ghorani, B. and N. Tucker, Fundamentals of electrospinning as a novel delivery vehicle for bioactive compounds in food nanotechnology. *Food Hydrocolloids,* 2015. 51: p. 227-240.

[2] Mitchell, G.R., K.-h. Ahn, and F.J. Davis, The potential of electrospinning in rapid manufacturing processes: The fundamentals of electrospinning, key process parameters, materials and potential application in rapid manufacturing are presented in this paper. *Virtual and Physical Prototyping,* 2011. 6(2): p. 63-77.

[3] Senthil, T., G. George, and A. Srinivasan, From Fundamentals to Applications. *Advances in Polymer Materials and Technology,* 2016.

[4] Pham, Q.P., U. Sharma, and A.G. Mikos, Electrospinning of polymeric nanofibers for tissue engineering applications: a review. *Tissue engineering,* 2006. 12(5): p. 1197-1211.

[5] Fallahiarezoudar, E., et al., A review of: application of synthetic scaffold in tissue engineering heart valves. *Materials Science and Engineering:* C, 2015. 48: p. 556-565.

[6] Fallahiarezoudar, E., et al., Performance Evaluation of Electrospinning Process to Fabricate Magnetic Nanofibers via DOE. Proceedings of NAMRI/SME, 2014. 42.

[7] Gilmore, C.M., Fundamentals and Applications of Micro-and Nanofibers. MRS BULLETIN, 2015. 40: p. 87-88.

[8] Fallahiarezoudar, E., et al., Fabrication (ferrofluid/polyvinyl alcohol) magnetic nanofibers via co-axial electrospinning. *Journal of Dispersion Science and Technology,* 2015. 36(1): p. 28-31.

[9] Ahmadipourroudposht, M., et al., Application of response surface methodology in optimization of electrospinning process to fabricate (ferrofluid/polyvinyl alcohol) magnetic nanofibers. *Materials Science and Engineering:* C, 2015. 50: p. 234-241.

[10] Mokhena, T., V. Jacobs, and A. Luyt, A review on electrospun bio-based polymers for water treatment. *Express Polym. Lett,* 2015. 9: p. 839-880.

[11] Ngadiman, N.H.A., et al., Fabricating high mechanical strength γ-Fe_2O_3 nanoparticles filled poly (vinyl alcohol) nanofiber using electrospinning process potentially for tissue engineering scaffold. *Journal of Bioactive and Compatible Polymers*, 2016: p. 0883911516681328.

[12] Fallahiarezoudar, E., et al., Optimization and development of Maghemite (γ-Fe_2O_3) filled poly-l-lactic acid (PLLA)/thermoplastic polyurethane (TPU) electrospun nanofibers using Taguchi orthogonal array for tissue engineering heart valve. *Materials Science and Engineering:* C, 2017.

[13] Casasola, R., et al., Electrospun poly lactic acid (PLA) fibres: effect of different solvent systems on fibre morphology and diameter. *Polymer,* 2014. 55(18): p. 4728-4737.

[14] Kara, M.O.P. and M.W. Frey, Effects of solvents on the morphology and conductivity of poly (3, 4-ethylenedioxythiophene): Poly (styrenesulfonate) nanofibers. *Journal of Applied Polymer Science,* 2014. 131(11).
[15] Sui, T., et al., Operando observation of the Taylor cone during electrospinning by multiple synchrotron X-ray techniques. *Materials & Design,* 2016. 110: p. 933-934.
[16] Morton, W.J., Method of dispersing fluids. 1902, Google Patents.
[17] Cooley, J.F., *Apparatus for electrically dispersing fluids.* 1902, Google Patents.
[18] Mirjalili, M. and S. Zohoori, Review for application of electrospinning and electrospun nanofibers technology in textile industry. *Journal of Nanostructure in Chemistry,* 2016. 6(3): p. 207-213.
[19] Hagiwara, K., Process for manufacturing artificial silk. 1927, Canada Patent.
[20] Formhals, A., Method and apparatus for spinning. US patent, 1939. **2**(160): p. 962.
[21] Formhals, A., *Electrospinning of submicron diameter polymer filaments.* 1940.
[22] Anton, F., *Method and apparatus for spinning.* 1944, Google Patents.
[23] Taylor, G. Disintegration of water drops in an electric field. in Proceedings of the Royal Society of London A: Mathematical, Physical and Engineering Sciences. 1964. The Royal Society.
[24] Taylor, G. The force exerted by an electric field on a long cylindrical conductor. in Proceedings of the Royal Society of London A: Mathematical, Physical and Engineering Sciences. 1966. The Royal Society.
[25] Taylor, G. Electrically driven jets. in Proceedings of the Royal Society of London A: Mathematical, Physical and Engineering Sciences. 1969. The Royal Society.
[26] Groitzsch, D. and E. Fahrbach, *Microporous multilayer nonwoven material for medical applications.* 1986, Google Patents.
[27] Reneker, D.H. and I. Chun, Nanometre diameter fibres of polymer, produced by electrospinning. *Nanotechnology,* 1996. **7**(3): p. 216.
[28] Kitsara, M., et al., Fibers for hearts: A critical review on electrospinning for cardiac tissue engineering. *Acta Biomaterialia,* 2016.
[29] Sarbatly, R., D. Krishnaiah, and Z. Kamin, A review of polymer nanofibres by electrospinning and their application in oil–water separation for cleaning up marine oil spills. *Marine pollution bulletin,* 2016. 106(1): p. 8-16.
[30] Fallahiarezoudar, E., et al., Influence of process factors on diameter of core (γ-Fe_2O_3)/shell (polyvinyl alcohol) structure magnetic nanofibers during co-axial electrospinning. *International Journal of Polymeric Materials and Polymeric Biomaterials,* 2015. 64(1): p. 15-24.
[31] Nezarati, R.M., M.B. Eifert, and E. Cosgriff-Hernandez, Effects of humidity and solution viscosity on electrospun fiber morphology. *Tissue Engineering Part C: Methods,* 2013. 19(10): p. 810-819.

[32] Nasouri, K., A. Shoushtari, and A. Kaflou, Investigation of polyacrylonitrile electrospun nanofibres morphology as a function of polymer concentration, viscosity and Berry number. *Micro & Nano Letters,* 2012. 7(5): p. 423-426.

[33] Rieger, K.A., N.P. Birch, and J.D. Schiffman, Electrospinning chitosan/poly (ethylene oxide) solutions with essential oils: Correlating solution rheology to nanofiber formation. *Carbohydrate polymers,* 2016. 139: p. 131-138.

[34] Bhat, M.A., et al., Nanotechnology, Metal Nanoparticles, and Biomedical Applications of Nanotechnology, in Nanotechnology Applications for Improvements in Energy Efficiency and Environmental Management. 2015, IGI Global. p. 116-155.

[35] Fong, H., I. Chun, and D. Reneker, Beaded nanofibers formed during electrospinning. *Polymer,* 1999. 40(16): p. 4585-4592.

[36] Deitzel, J.M., et al., The effect of processing variables on the morphology of electrospun nanofibers and textiles. *Polymer,* 2001. 42(1): p. 261-272.

[37] Sundaray, B., et al., Electrospinning of continuous aligned polymer fibers. *Applied physics letters,* 2004. 84(7): p. 1222-1224.

[38] Milleret, V., et al., Tuning electrospinning parameters for production of 3D-fiber-fleeces with increased porosity for soft tissue engineering applications. *Eur Cell Mater,* 2011. 21: p. 286-303.

[39] Liu, C., et al., Microporous CA/PVDF membranes based on electrospun nanofibers with controlled crosslinking induced by solvent vapor. *Journal of Membrane Science,* 2016. 512: p. 1-12.

[40] Pillay, V., et al., A review of the effect of processing variables on the fabrication of electrospun nanofibers for drug delivery applications. *Journal of Nanomaterials*, 2013. 2013.

[41] Dhanalakshmi, M., A.K. Lele, and J.P. Jog, Electrospinning of Nylon11: Effect of processing parameters on morphology and microstructure. *Materials Today Communications,* 2015. 3: p. 141-148.

[42] Ahmed, F.E., B.S. Lalia, and R. Hashaikeh, A review on electrospinning for membrane fabrication: challenges and applications. *Desalination,* 2015. 356: p. 15-30.

[43] Xia, X., et al., The effects of electrospinning parameters on coaxial Sn/C nanofibers: Morphology and lithium storage performance. *Electrochimica Acta,* 2014. 121: p. 345-351.

[44] Homayoni, H., S.A.H. Ravandi, and M. Valizadeh, Electrospinning of chitosan nanofibers: processing optimization. *Carbohydrate polymers,* 2009. 77(3): p. 656-661.

[45] Henriques, C., et al., A systematic study of solution and processing parameters on nanofiber morphology using a new electrospinning apparatus. *Journal of nanoscience and nanotechnology,* 2009. 9(6): p. 3535-3545.

[46] Huang, Z.-M., et al., A review on polymer nanofibers by electrospinning and their applications in nanocomposites. *Composites science and technology,* 2003. 63(15): p. 2223-2253.

[47] Subbiah, T., et al., Electrospinning of nanofibers. *Journal of Applied Polymer Science,* 2005. 96(2): p. 557-569.

[48] De Vrieze, S., et al., The effect of temperature and humidity on electrospinning. *Journal of materials science,* 2009. 44(5): p. 1357.

[49] Hajra, M., K. Mehta, and G. Chase, Effects of humidity, temperature, and nanofibers on drop coalescence in glass fiber media. *Separation and purification technology,* 2003. 30(1): p. 79-88.

[50] Tripatanasuwan, S., Z. Zhong, and D.H. Reneker, Effect of evaporation and solidification of the charged jet in electrospinning of poly (ethylene oxide) aqueous solution. *Polymer,* 2007. 48(19): p. 5742-5746.

[51] Thompson, C., et al., Effects of parameters on nanofiber diameter determined from electrospinning model. *Polymer,* 2007. 48(23): p. 6913-6922.

[52] Hardick, O., B. Stevens, and D.G. Bracewell, Nanofibre fabrication in a temperature and humidity controlled environment for improved fibre consistency. *Journal of materials science,* 2011. 46(11): p. 3890-3898.

[53] He, J.-H., Y.-Q. Wan, and J.-Y. Yu, Effect of concentration on electrospun polyacrylonitrile (PAN) nanofibers. *Fibers and Polymers,* 2008. 9(2): p. 140-142.

[54] Jia, Y.-T., et al., Fabrication and characterization of poly (vinyl alcohol)/chitosan blend nanofibers produced by electrospinning method. *Carbohydrate Polymers,* 2007. 67(3): p. 403-409.

[55] Min, B.-M., et al., Electrospinning of silk fibroin nanofibers and its effect on the adhesion and spreading of normal human keratinocytes and fibroblasts in vitro. *Biomaterials,* 2004. 25(7): p. 1289-1297.

[56] Ki, C.S., et al., Characterization of gelatin nanofiber prepared from gelatin–formic acid solution. *Polymer,* 2005. 46(14): p. 5094-5102.

[57] Sarhan, W.A. and H.M. Azzazy, High concentration honey chitosan electrospun nanofibers: Biocompatibility and antibacterial effects. *Carbohydrate polymers,* 2015. 122: p. 135-143.

[58] Chen, M.-C., Y.-C. Sun, and Y.-H. Chen, Electrically conductive nanofibers with highly oriented structures and their potential application in skeletal muscle tissue engineering. *Acta biomaterialia,* 2013. 9(3): p. 5562-5572.

[59] Fallahiarezoudar, E., et al., Characterization of maghemite (γ-Fe_2O_3)-loaded poly-l-lactic acid/thermoplastic polyurethane electrospun mats for soft tissue engineering. *Journal of Materials Science:* p. 1-21.

[60] Balint, R., N.J. Cassidy, and S.H. Cartmell, Conductive polymers: towards a smart biomaterial for tissue engineering. *Acta biomaterialia,* 2014. 10(6): p. 2341-2353.

[61] Zhong, Z., et al., Structure-induced enhancement of thermal conductivities in electrospun polymer nanofibers. *Nanoscale,* 2014. 6(14): p. 8283-8291.

[62] Essalhi, M. and M. Khayet, Self-sustained webs of polyvinylidene fluoride electrospun nano-fibers: Effects of polymer concentration and desalination by direct contact membrane distillation. *Journal of Membrane Science,* 2014. 454: p. 133-143.

[63] Sharma, R., et al., Recent advances in polymeric electrospun nanofibers for drug delivery. *Critical Reviews™ in Therapeutic Drug Carrier Systems,* 2014. 31(3).

[64] Jørgensen, L., K. Qvortrup, and I.S. Chronakis, Phospholipid electrospun nanofibers: effect of solvents and co-axial processing on morphology and fiber diameter. *RSC Advances,* 2015. 5(66): p. 53644-53652.

[65] Golecki, H.M., et al., Effect of Solvent Evaporation on Fiber Morphology in Rotary Jet-Spinning. *Langmuir: The ACS journal of surfaces and colloids,* 2014. 30(44): p. 13369.

[66] Guo, Z., et al., Electrospun nanofibers prepared using polystyrene (PS) with polymeric additives for the determination of nicotine in cigarette mainstream smoke. *Analytical Methods,* 2014. 6(14): p. 5120-5126.

[67] Liao, Y., R. Wang, and A.G. Fane, Fabrication of bioinspired composite nanofiber membranes with robust superhydrophobicity for direct contact membrane distillation. *Environmental science & technology,* 2014. 48(11): p. 6335-6341.

[68] Brown, T.D., P.D. Dalton, and D.W. Hutmacher, Melt electrospinning today: An opportune time for an emerging polymer process. *Progress in Polymer Science,* 2016. 56: p. 116-166.

[69] Farrugia, B.L., et al., Dermal fibroblast infiltration of poly (ε-caprolactone) scaffolds fabricated by melt electrospinning in a direct writing mode. *Biofabrication,* 2013. 5(2): p. 025001.

[70] Yu, Y., et al., Tin nanoparticles encapsulated in porous multichannel carbon microtubes: preparation by single-nozzle electrospinning and application as anode material for high-performance Li-based batteries. *Journal of the American Chemical Society,* 2009. 131(44): p. 15984-15985.

[71] Tang, K., et al., Multichannel hollow TiO_2 nanofibers fabricated by single-nozzle electrospinning and their application for fast lithium storage. *Electrochemistry Communications,* 2013. 28: p. 54-57.

[72] Sun, D., et al., Near-field electrospinning. *Nano letters,* 2006. 6(4): p. 839-842.

[73] Liu, Z., et al., Piezoelectric properties of PVDF/MWCNT nanofiber using near-field electrospinning. *Sensors and Actuators A: Physical,* 2013. 193: p. 13-24.

[74] Ali, U., et al., Direct electrospinning of highly twisted, continuous nanofiber yarns. *Journal of the Textile Institute,* 2012. 103(1): p. 80-88.

[75] Smit, E., U. Bűttner, and R.D. Sanderson, Continuous yarns from electrospun fibers. *Polymer,* 2005. 46(8): p. 2419-2423.

[76] Edmondson, D., et al., Centrifugal electrospinning of highly aligned polymer nanofibers over a large area. *Journal of Materials Chemistry,* 2012. 22(35): p. 18646-18652.

[77] Kancheva, M., et al., Advanced centrifugal electrospinning setup. *Materials Letters,* 2014. 136: p. 150-152.

[78] Liu, S.L., et al. Fabrication of Fluorescent Polymer Crossbar Arrays and Microropes via Centrifugal Electrospinning. In *Advanced Materials Research.* 2013. Trans Tech Publ.

[79] Kaur, S., et al., Review: the characterization of electrospun nanofibrous liquid filtration membranes. *Journal of Materials Science,* 2014. 49(18): p. 6143-6159.

[80] Pauly, H.M., et al., Mechanical properties and cellular response of novel electrospun nanofibers for ligament tissue engineering: Effects of orientation and geometry. *Journal of the mechanical behavior of biomedical materials,* 2016. 61: p. 258-270.

[81] Li, Y., C.T. Lim, and M. Kotaki, Study on structural and mechanical properties of porous PLA nanofibers electrospun by channel-based electrospinning system. *Polymer,* 2015. 56: p. 572-580.

[82] Yin, A., et al., Electrospinning collagen/chitosan/poly (L-lactic acid-co-ϵ-caprolactone) to form a vascular graft: Mechanical and biological characterization. *Journal of Biomedical Materials Research Part A,* 2013. 101(5): p. 1292-1301.

[83] Labrosse, M.R., et al., Geometric modeling of functional trileaflet aortic valves: development and clinical applications. *Journal of biomechanics,* 2006. 39(14): p. 2665-2672.

[84] Fallahiarezoudar, E., M. Ahmadipourroudposht, and N.M. Yusof, Geometric Modeling of Aortic Heart Valve. *Procedia Manufacturing,* 2015. 2: p. 135-140.

[85] Jamesh, M.I., et al., Electrochemical corrosion behavior of biodegradable Mg–Y–RE and Mg–Zn–Zr alloys in Ringer's solution and simulated body fluid. *Corrosion Science,* 2015. 91: p. 160-184.

[86] Willmer, E.N., *Cells and tissues in culture: methods, biology and physiology.* 2015: Elsevier.

[87] Fischer-Cripps, A.C., *Factors Affecting Nanoindentation Test Data.* 2000: Springer.

[88] Sung, Y.K., B.W. Ahn, and T.J. Kang, Magnetic nanofibers with core (Fe_3O_4 nanoparticle suspension)/sheath (poly ethylene terephthalate) structure fabricated by coaxial electrospinning. *Journal of magnetism and magnetic materials,* 2012. 324(6): p. 916-922.

In: Electrospinning and Electroplating
Editor: Toby Jacobs
ISBN: 978-1-53612-363-0

Chapter 5

FABRICATION AND CHARACTERIZATION OF ELECTROSPUN PVDF, PVDF/PLA AND PVDF/G MEMBRANES

Grissel Rodríguez-Roldán, Daniel Hernández-Rivera and Ernesto Suaste-Gómez
Department of Electrical Engineering, Section of Bioelectronics,
Center for Research and Advanced Studies of the National Polytechnic Institute,
Mexico City, Mexico

ABSTRACT

Electrospinning is a versatile technique for generating ultrathin fibers from a rich variety of materials, including polymers and ceramics. Polyvinylidene difluoride (PVDF) is a smart polymer which exhibits piezoelectricity and it is often combined with other materials in order to improve or modify its properties. This work was focused in the fabrication and characterization of electrospun PVDF, PVDF/PLA (50/50 wt %) and PVDF/G (99.5/0.5 wt %) membranes. Analyses of PVDF, PVDF/PLA and PVDF/G membranes were performed by scanning electron microscopy (SEM) and energy-dispersive x-ray micro-analysis. As a result, low porous flexible membranes were obtained with fiber diameters in a range from 50 nm to 700 nm. These membranes are a promising tool in fields such as biomedical engineering, robotics and electronics as scaffolds, sensors or actuators due to their ferroelectric nature.

Keywords: graphene, electrospinning, polylactic acid, polyvinylidene difluoride

1. INTRODUCTION

Among the most common techniques for fabricating either ceramic or polymeric nanofibers include template synthesis, phase separation, self-assembly, and electrospinning [1]. Within these techniques and due to new advances in nanotechnology, there has been an increasing interest in electrospinning [2].

The process of electrospinning consists of a high voltage source, a syringe holding the solution with a metallic needle as the spinneret, and a collector plate (grounded conductor). Generation of polymer fibers is achieved under the application of a high voltage between the needle and the collector, usually, in the range of 0 to 35 kV. With the electric potential, charges accumulate, promoting the formation of a drop in the tip of the needle, as intensity of the electric field increases, the drop elongates to create a conical shape known as the Taylor cone. This phenomenon is produced by the interaction between electrostatic repulsion forces between the surface charges and Coulombic forces exerted by the external electric field. Once the intensity of the electric field overcomes the cohesive forces of the solution, in most cases dominated by surface tension, a jet of polymer solution starts a journey from the tip of the Taylor cone to the collector plate; in its travel, the jet of polymer solution is elongated due to the electrostatic interactions between charges close to the same jet. Before reaching the collector, the solvent evaporates and finally, thin polymeric fibers solidify, laying randomly on the collector plate [3, 4]. The process described above is illustrated in Figure 1.

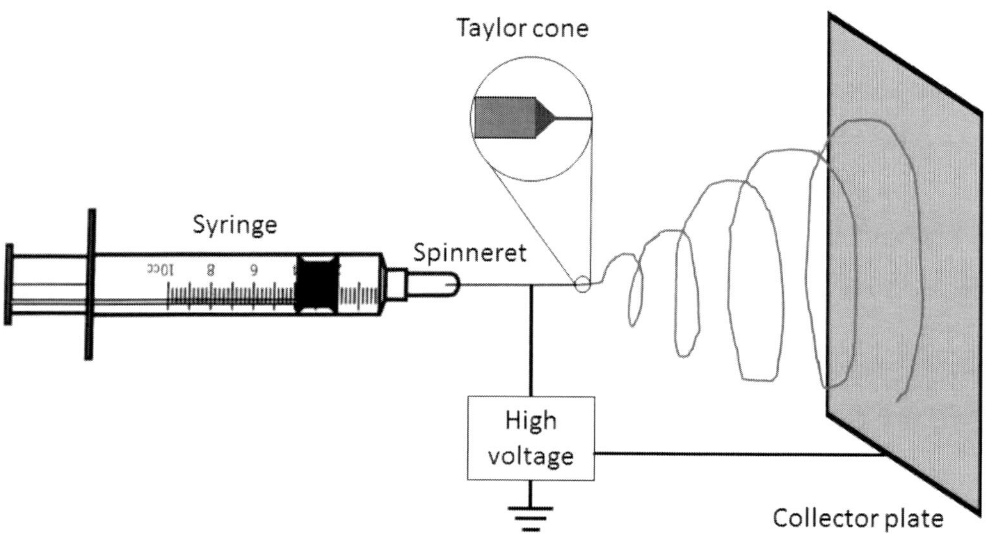

Figure 1. Schematic diagram of horizontal set up of electrospinning apparatus.

The diameter of the generated fibers is generally found in nanometric and micrometric ranges. Morphology of the fibers, such as size and porosity, is affected by parameters related to the process (distance between the tip of the needle to the collector and the applied voltage), the nature of the solution (concentration, viscosity and conductivity), and the ambient (temperature and humidity) [5, 6].

As electrospinning is technique that allows to change all those parameters in order to control the morphology of a membrane, it has recently attracted attention in a wide variety of areas, including biochemistry, biomedicine, energy, medicine, pharmaceutical industry, tissue engineering, among others. Some applications of electrospun membranes (ESMs) include solar cells, filtration systems, scaffolds, drug delivery, liquid crystal devices, sensors and biosensors [7].

Among the polymers that have been widely used recently in the electrospinning process are polyvinylidene fluoride (PVDF) and polylactic acid (PLA). Some features of these both polymers are described below.

Polylactic acid (PLA), is an aliphatic thermoplastic polyester commonly made from α hydroxy acids that presents some advantages among other polymers such as biocompatibility, renewability and energy saving [8]. This polymer is biodegradable, which make it suitable for biomedical applications like wound dressing/healing and scaffolds in tissue engineering [8, 9].

The method used to synthetize polylactic acid is by ring-opening polymerization (ROP) and the monomer used is lactide, a cyclic di-ester of lactic acid. As there are two lactic acid enantiomers (L(+) and D(-) lactic acid), lactide exists in three stereoisomeric forms: L-lactide, D-lactide and D,L-lactide, giving as a result, the production of poly-L-lactic acid (PLLA), poly-D-lactic acid (PDLA) and poly-D,L-lactic acid (PDLLA), respectively.

Commercial PLA is a blend of PLLA and PDLA. The ratio of L- and D-lactides serves to control the properties of the final polymer such as crystallinity, for example, if the content of PLLA is greater than 90 %, the final polymer tends to be crystalline, while with less optical purity, it becomes amorphous. The melting temperature (Tm), the glass transition temperature (Tg) and the crystallinity of the PLA decrease with decreasing amounts of PLLA. Properties such as thermal stability and impact resistance are inferior to those of conventional polymers for thermoplastic applications. In order to improve these properties and thus compete with other types of conventional polymers, copolymers of lactic acid and other monomers such as styrene, acrylate or poly (methylene oxide) derivatives can be obtained [8, 10, 11].

Many researches are based on developing modifications in PLA and its chemical structure (shown in Figure 2), besides, PLA has been used as a composite in order to obtain a polymer with higher properties.

Furthermore, polyvinylidene fluoride (PVDF) has received special attention over a wide variety of polymers due to its thermal and chemical stability, mechanical and ferroelectric properties, moreover, it is biocompatible, which makes it unique in the biomedical field [12-16].

Unlike other polymers, PVDF has three crystalline phases, namely α, β, and γ. The β phase is the most polar due to the polymer chains stacking and their respective polarizations aligned in the same direction, PVDF exhibits piezoelectric and pyroelectric properties because of β phase [17, 18]. Figure 3 shows the structures of a piezoelectric β-phase PVDF.

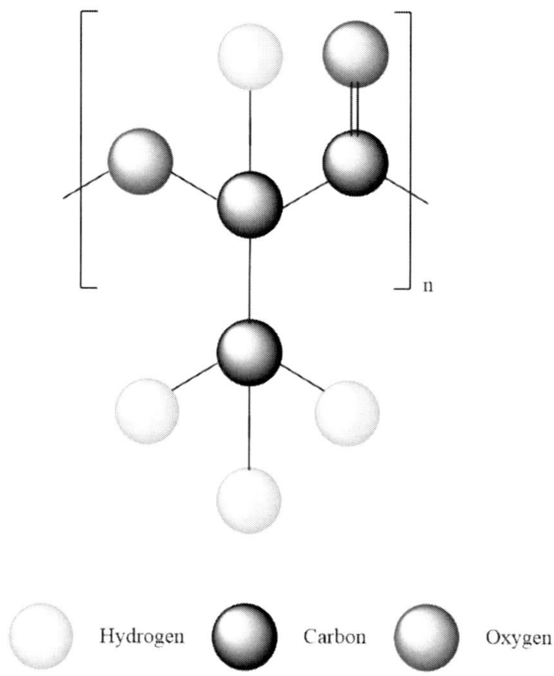

Figure 2. Chemical structure of polylactic acid (PLA).

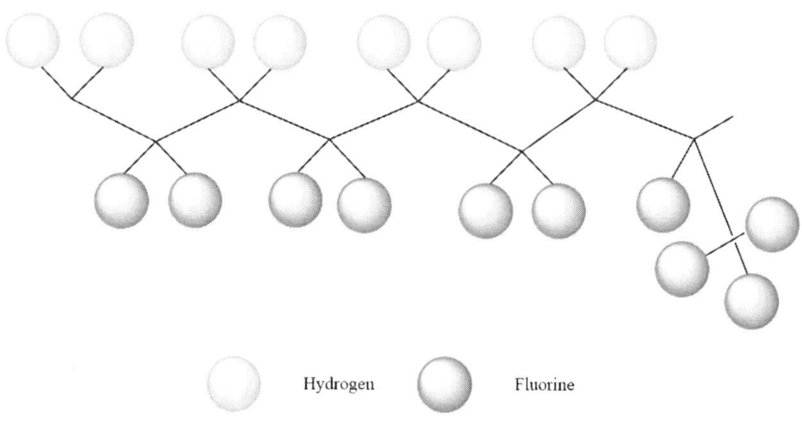

Figure 3. Chemical structure of β-phase polyvinylidene fluoride (PVDF).

The most common technique for obtaining the polar β phase from α phase involves first, mechanical extension at low temperatures and then electrical poling (plasma o corona poling). The technique can be observed in Figure 4 [17-19]. The development of PVDF fibers by electrospinning is another method to reach β phase directly from a polymer solution. As it was mentioned above, this technique involves solution casting and the application of a high electric field [19, 20].

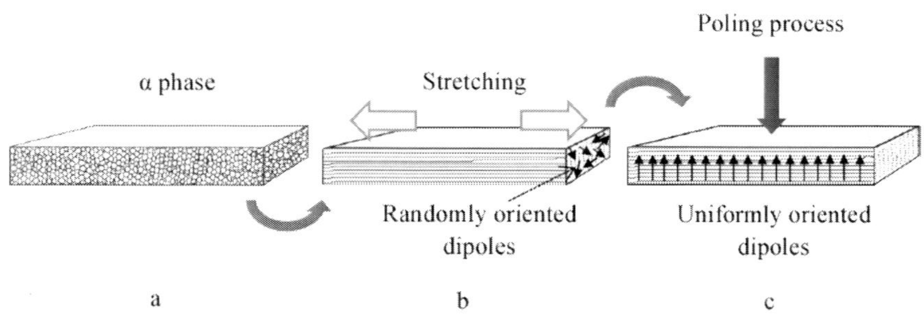

Figure 4. The process for obtaining the polar β phase from α phase: (a) α phase, (b) β phase uniaxially oriented and (c) β phase uniformly oriented of PVDF.

Ferroelectric properties of PVDF strongly depend on its crystallinity. Crystallinity is an important parameter which can significantly affect mechanical, chemical and thermal properties of a material. An important technique to know the crystallinity of a material is X-ray diffraction (XRD) analysis; this technique is based on constructive interference of monochromatic X-rays and a crystalline material. The diffraction patterns created when X-rays impact the sample can be used to determine the crystalline phases of the material.

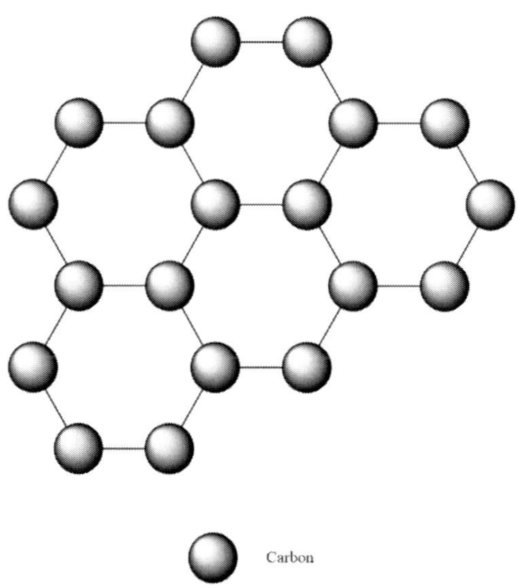

Figure 5. Chemical structure of graphene.

It is important to mention that the addition of carbon allotropes such as Graphene (G) improves the piezoelectric and pyroelectric properties of PVDF [21, 22]. G is the elementary structure of graphite, it is a two dimensional monoatomic thick sheet composed of carbon atoms arranged in a hexagonal lattice as illustrated in Figure 5. In recent years, there has been growing interest in G because of its electrical conductivity, mechanical strength and thermal conductivity [23, 24]. Accordingly, G-based materials are highly attractive in fields such as electronics, sensors, biosensors, prosthesis, energy and others [24, 25]. G has been used as an additive in a wide variety of materials in order to modify their electrical, mechanical, optical and thermal properties [25].

This chapter briefly discusses the electrospinning process and demonstrates the potentiality of this technique to fabricate PVDF, PVDF/PLA and PVDF/G membranes and applied them as temperature sensors by analyzing their dielectric behavior.

2. Experimental Section

2.1. Materials

Unless otherwise noted, all materials were obtained from commercial suppliers. Polylactic acid filament (PLA) was purchased from Makerbot, N, N-dimethylformamide (DMF) and polyvinylidene fluoride powder (PVDF), were purchased from Sigma-Aldrich (MO, USA). Ultra-high Concentration Dispersion of Graphene Nanoplatelets was purchased from Graphene Supermarket (NY, USA).

2.2. Equipment

All solutions were stirred using an ultrasonic dispersion machine AutoScience, AS3120B, AS3120B Ultrasonic Cleaner, micrographs of the membranes were acquired by a JSM-6360LV scanning electron microscope and XRD patterns were obtained using a Siemens-D5000 diffractometer. Membranes were heated using an oven from Carbolite, model ELF 11/6. A temperature meter from Amprobe, model TMD56 and a LCR bridge from Rohde & Schwarz, model HM8118 were also used. The apparatus for the electrospinning process was made in our laboratory (Mexican patent Mx/a/2014/006290). This technological development has made it possible for researchers to generate versatility and diversity in the electrospinning process.

2.3. Preparation of Solutions

PVDF Solution

In preparing the PVDF solution (33 wt %), 1 gr of PVDF powder were added to 3 ml of DMF. The mixture was heated and stirred in a boiling water bath for 30 minutes. Once the PVDF powder was completely dissolved, the resulting solution was stirred for 10 minutes using an ultrasonic dispersion machine. Figure 6 shows the process described above.

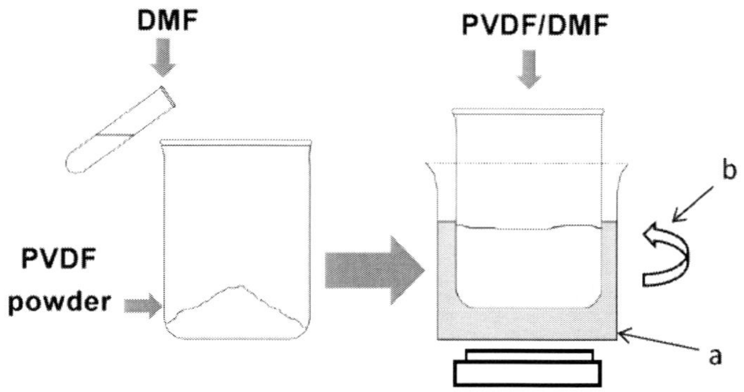

Figure 6. Fabrication process of PVDF/DMF solution: (a) Boling water bath and (b) Stirring.

PVDF/PLA Solution

Following the directions above, PVDF powder was dissolved in DMF to obtain a 33 wt % solution. PLA filament was cut into small pieces. 1 gr of PLA were added to 3 ml of DMF. This mixture was heated and stirred in a boiling water bath for 30 minutes in order to dissolve the PLA small pieces and ensure a homogeneous mixture. Then, both solutions, PVDF and PVDF/PLA were mixed and also, heated. Finally, the resulting solution was stirred for 10 minutes using an ultrasonic dispersion machine. Figure 7 shows the process described above.

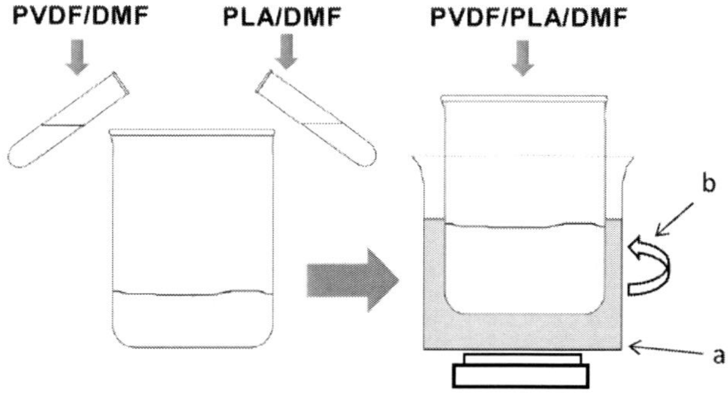

Figure 7. Fabrication process of PVDF/PLA solution: (a) Boling water bath and (b) Stirring.

PVDF/G Solution

PVDF powder and G were thoroughly weighted in order to obtain PVDF/G (99.5/0.5 wt %) membranes, this blend ratio was chosen based on the investigation about PVDF/G membranes [21]. Graphene was dispersed in DMF using an ultrasonic dispersion machine for three half hour sessions to get a homogenous solution. PVDF powder was dissolved in DMF to obtain a 20 wt % solution. Then, the solution was heated and stirred in a boiling water bath for 30 minutes in order to ensure a homogeneous mixture. PVDF/DMF and G/DMF solutions were mixed and then, stirred. Finally, PVDF/DMF/G solution was sonicated for two half hour sessions. Figure 8 shows the process described above.

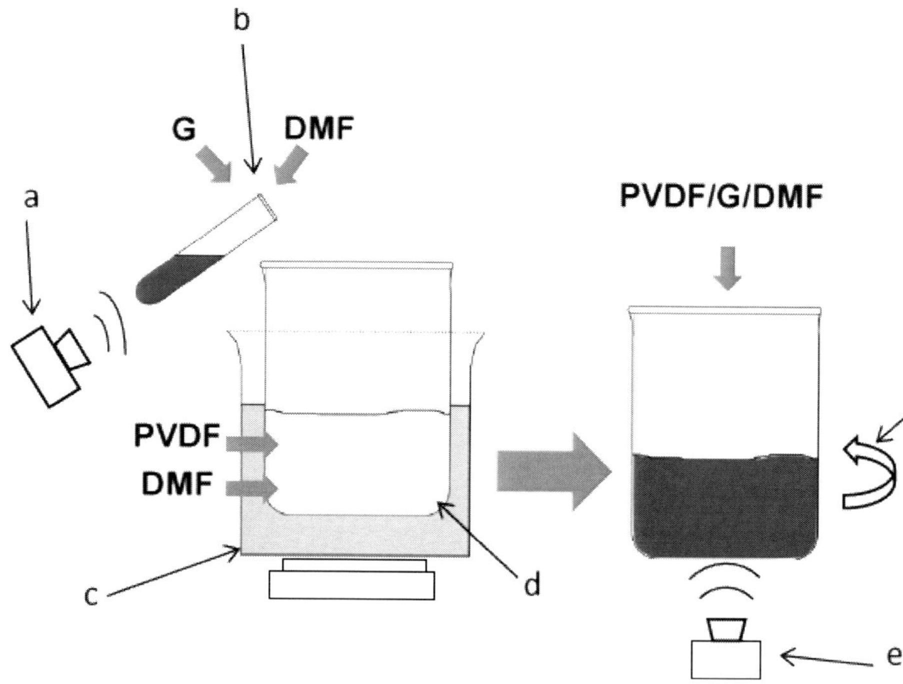

Figure 8. Fabrication process: (a) Sonication; (b) G/DMF solution; (c) Boling water bath; (d) PVDF/DMF; (e) Sonication and (f) Stirring.

2.4. Membranes Fabrication

Three milliliters of each solution mentioned above were used to fabricate ferroelectric membranes via electrospinning. The process was performed during 40 min at a feeding rate of 0.5 mL/h. The dimensions of the collector plate were 10x15 cm.

Table 1 shows the critical parameters used in the electrospinning process for each membrane.

Table 1. Critical parameters of electrospinning

Applied voltage	20 kV/cm
Tip to collector distance	15 cm
Feed rate	0.5 mL/h

The electrospinning process was performed as illustrated in Figure 9.

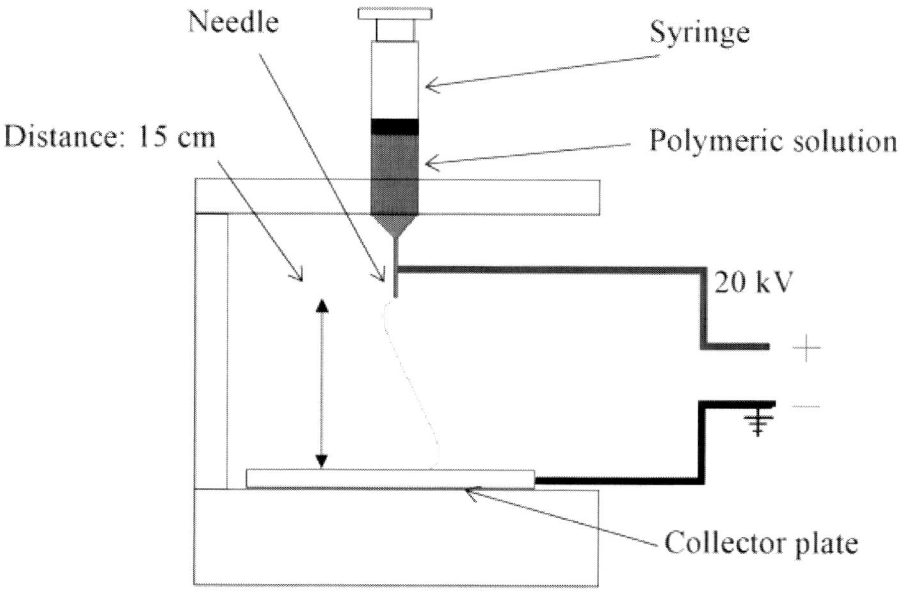

Figure 9. Schematic of electrospinning setup.

2.5. Characterization

2.5.1. Microscopy and Microanalysis

In order to obtain topographical, morphological and compositional information, samples were evaluated by scanning electron microscopy (SEM). Micrographs of the three membranes were acquired by a JSM-6360LV scanning electron microscope. Chemical composition was determined by energy dispersive X-ray spectroscopy (EDX) microanalysis.

2.5.2. Crystallographic Characterization

Although the development of PVDF membranes by electrospinning is a method used to obtain β phase and it is known that the addition of G improves the ferroelectric properties of PVDF, a crystallographic analysis was performed in order to get the crystalline phases of PVDF/G membrane. XRD patterns were obtained by means of a Siemens-D5000 diffractometer.

2.5.3. Temperature Response

Rectangles of the three membranes were cut out in order to test their dielectric behavior to controlled temperature changes. Rectangles were 1 cm long and 1 cm wide. The average thickness of the membranes was around 127 μm. Finally, copper tape electrodes were placed on both faces of the rectangular samples as shown in Figure 10.

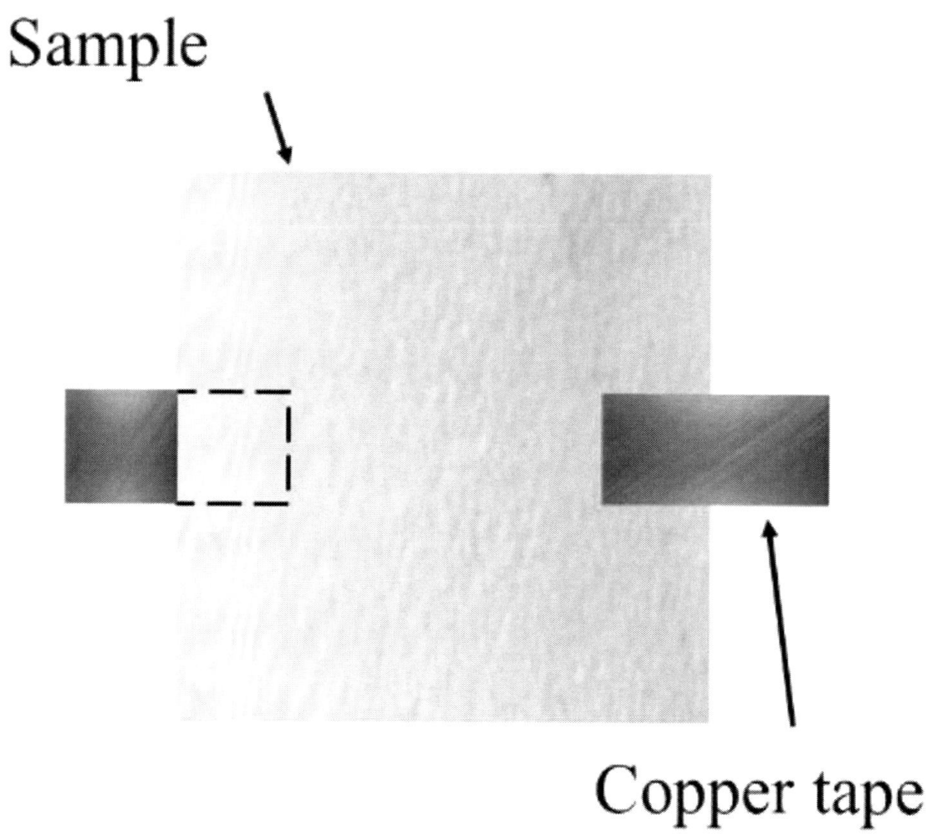

Figure 10. Copper electrodes placement.

Following this, samples were placed between two parallel copper plates in order to measure the temperature-dependent dielectric constant as shown in Figure 11. Samples were heated from 30° C to 90° C with a rate of 5° C/min, simultaneously, capacitive impedance was measured at 1 kHz.

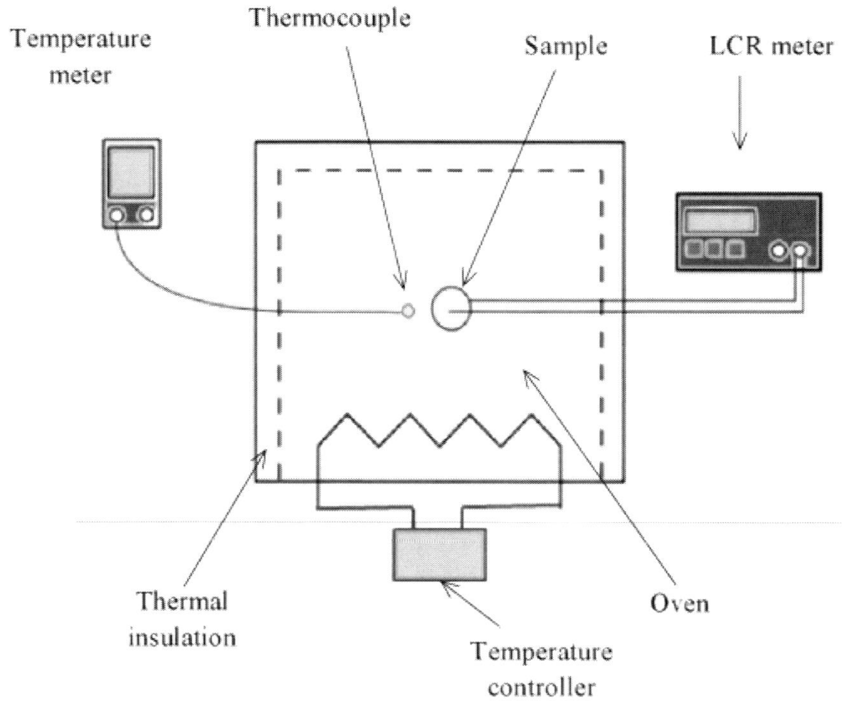

Figure 11. Diagram of temperature tests.

Then, dielectric constant (ε_r) of each membrane was calculated considering equation 1, where C is capacitance, d is distance between plates, A is the contact area and $\varepsilon_0 \left(8.854 \times 10^{-12} \frac{F}{M}\right)$ is the vacuum permittivity.

$$\varepsilon_r = \frac{C \times d}{\varepsilon_0 \times A} \tag{1}$$

3. Results

3.1. Microscopy and Microanalysis

PVDF Membrane

Micrographs of the PVDF membrane are exhibited in Figure 12. Electrospun PVDF nanofibers with diameters ranging from 50 nm to 700 nm were achieved.

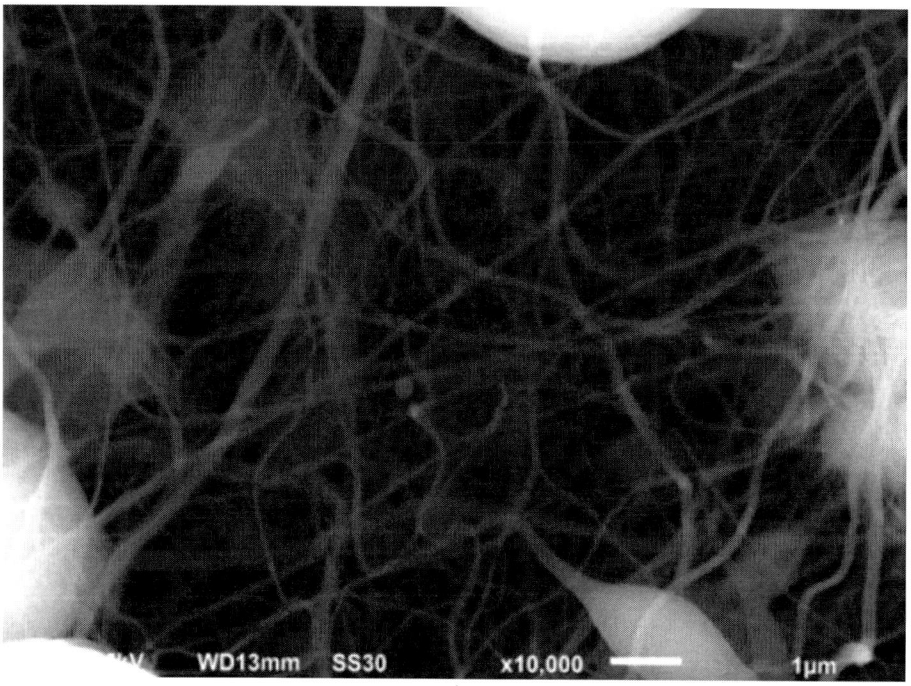

a)

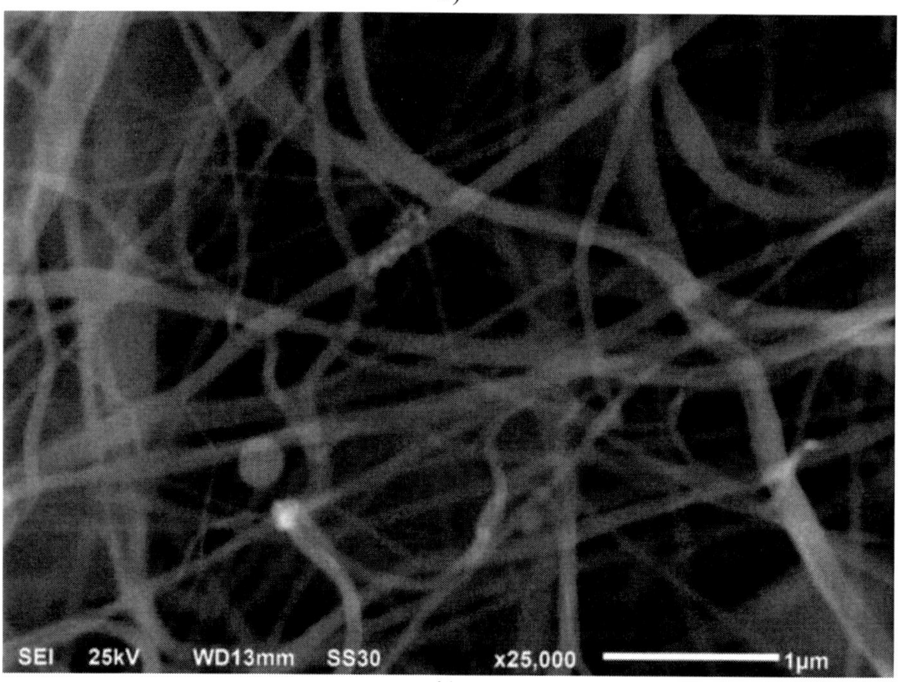

b)

Figure 12. Micrographs of the PVDF membrane at magnification: (a) 10000x, (b) 25000x.

Regarding the EDX spectrum, it can be observed in Figure 13 the presence of Carbon and Fluorine, both constituents of the PVDF membrane. However, microanalysis showed the presence of Oxygen, probably due to an incomplete evaporation of the solvent, DMF.

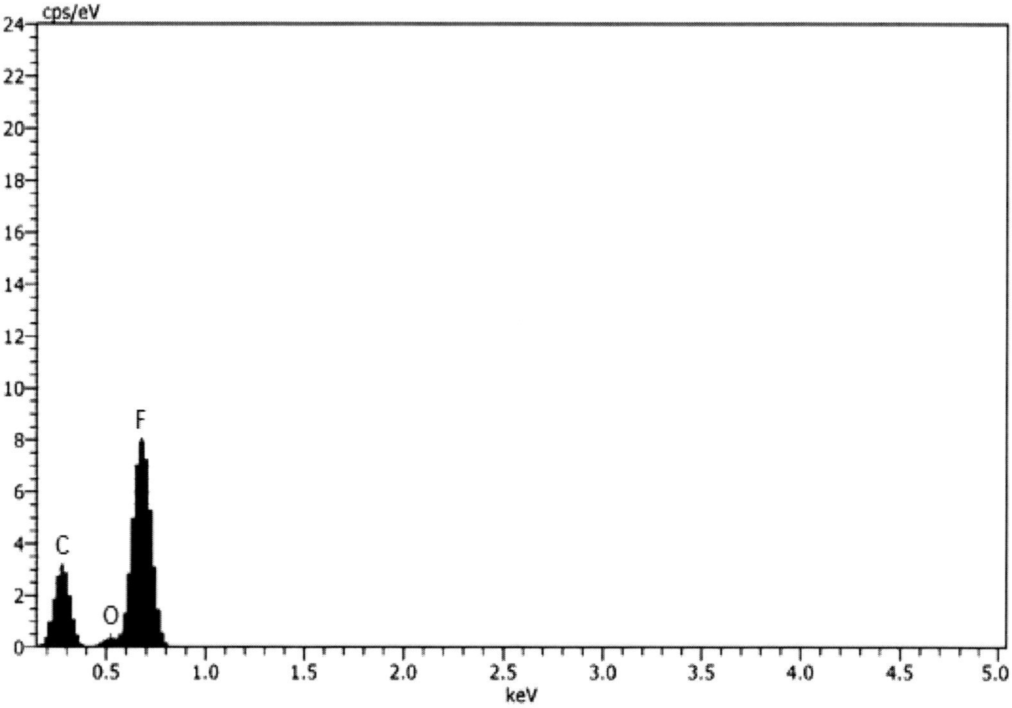

Figure 13. EDX microanalysis of PVDF membrane.

PVDF/PLA Membrane

Micrographs of the PVDF/PLA membrane are exhibited in Figure 14. Electrospun PVDF/PLA nanofibers with diameters ranging from 50 nm to 200 nm were achieved.

Figure 15 shows the EDX spectrum where it can be observed the presence of Carbon, Oxygen and Fluorine, all of them, constituents of the PVDF/PLA membrane.

PVDF/G Membrane

Micrographs of the PVDF/G membrane are exhibited in Figure 16. Electrospun PVDF/G nanofibers with diameters ranging from 130 nm to 600 nm were achieved. On the other hand, PVDF/G membrane tends to have a lower total porosity than PVDF membrane.

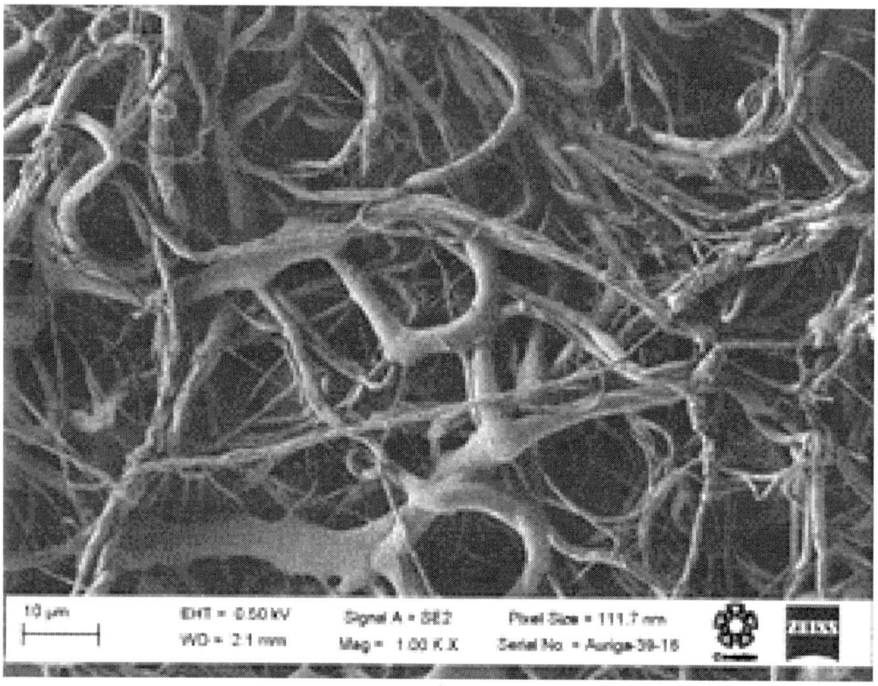

a)

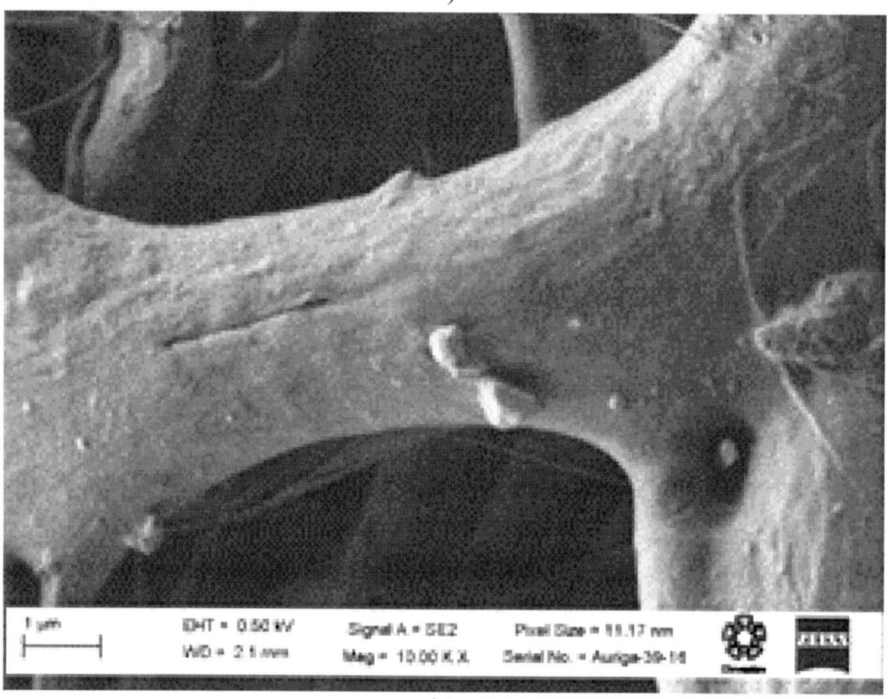

b)

Figure 14. Micrographs of the PVDF/PLA membrane at magnification: (a) 1000x, (b) 10000x.

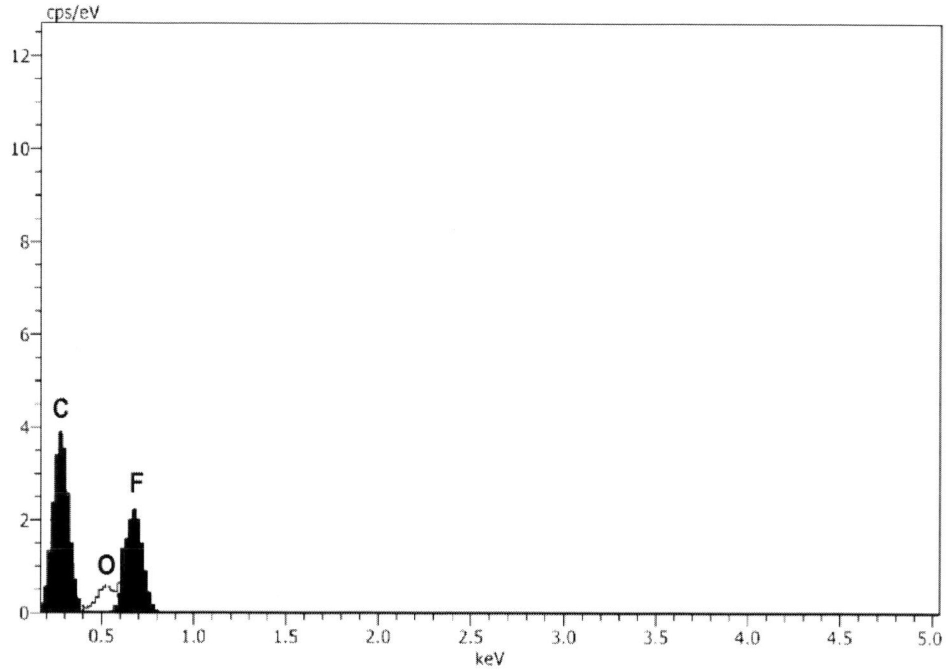

Figure 15. EDX microanalysis of PVDF/PLA membrane.

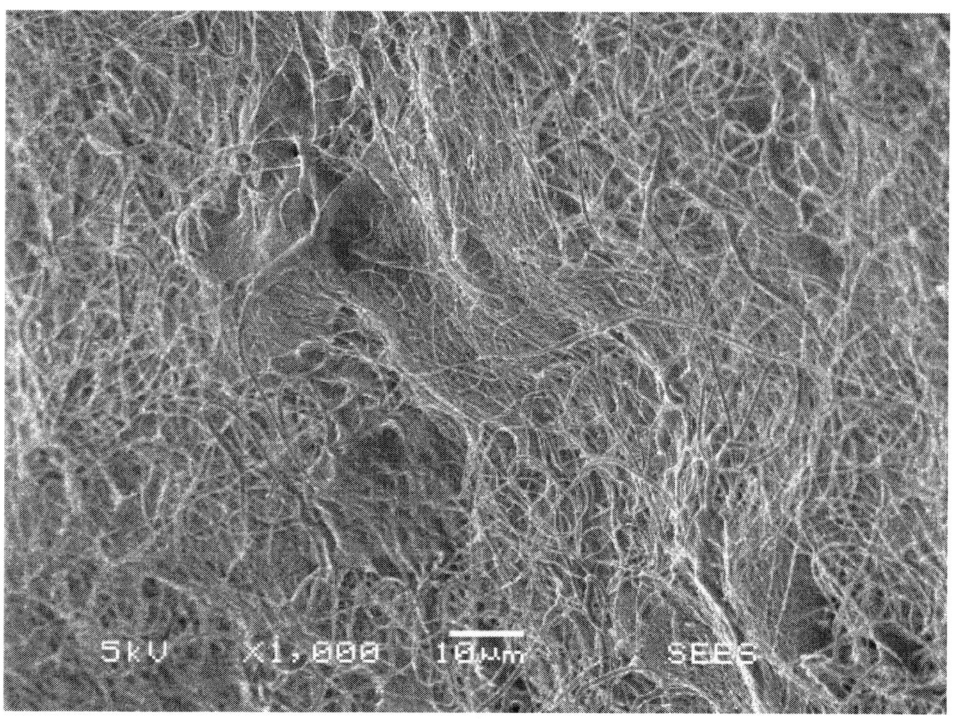

a)

Figure 16. (Continued)

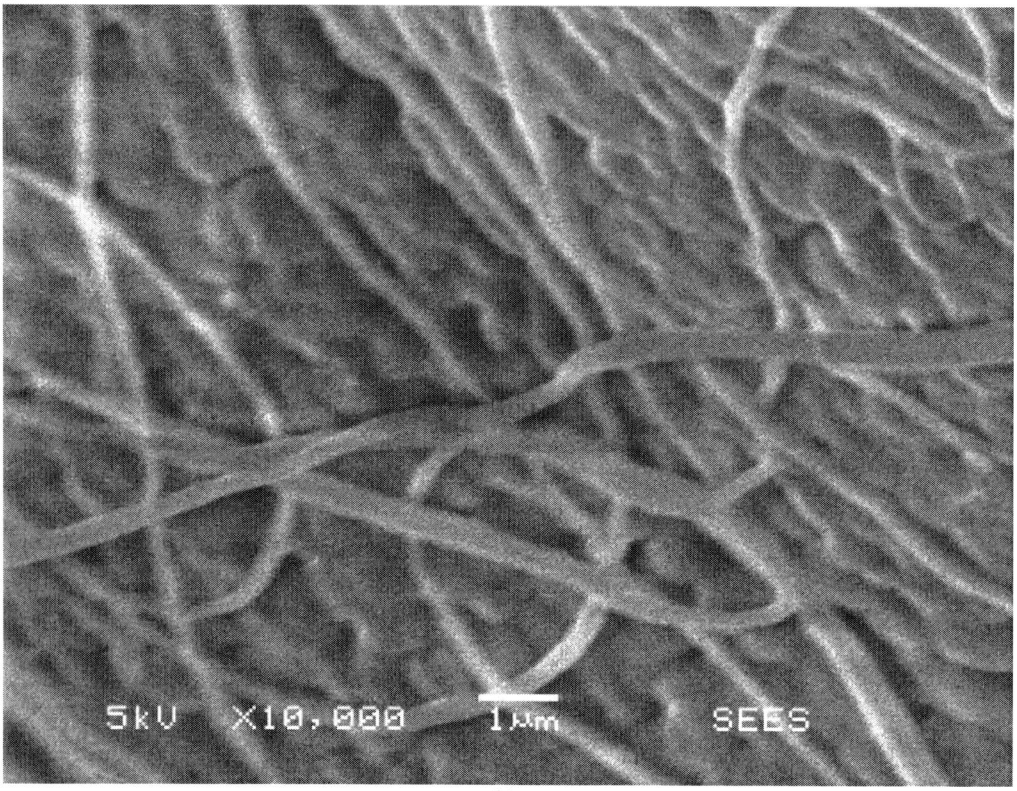

b)

Figure 16. Micrographs of the PVDF/G membrane at magnification: (a) 1000x, (b) 10000x.

The EDX spectrum shown in Figure 17 indicates the presence of Carbon and Fluorine, both constituents of the PVDF/G membrane.

3.2. Crystallographic Characterization

XRD patterns of PVDF/G samples were obtained at room temperature in the range of 2θ from 10° to 100°. Figure 18 shows the diffractogram of the PVDF/G membrane, where it can be observed the greater peak intensity at 2θ = 20.5°, which corresponds to the β phase [18-20, 26]. It can also be seen a minor peak at 2θ = 18.4° attributed to α phase [20, 26], however, β phase is predominant.

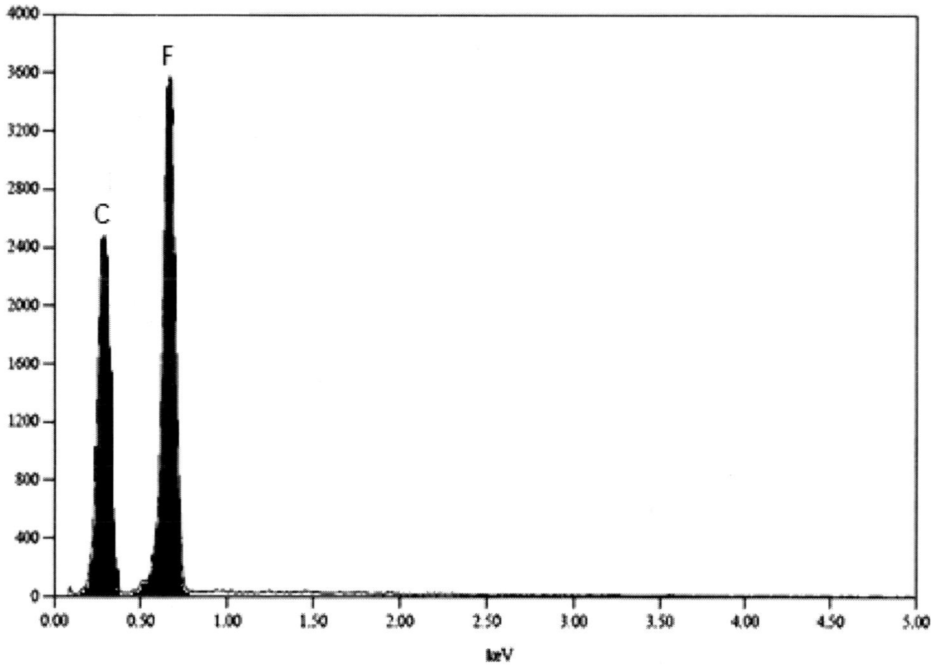

Figure 17. EDX microanalysis of PVDF/G membrane.

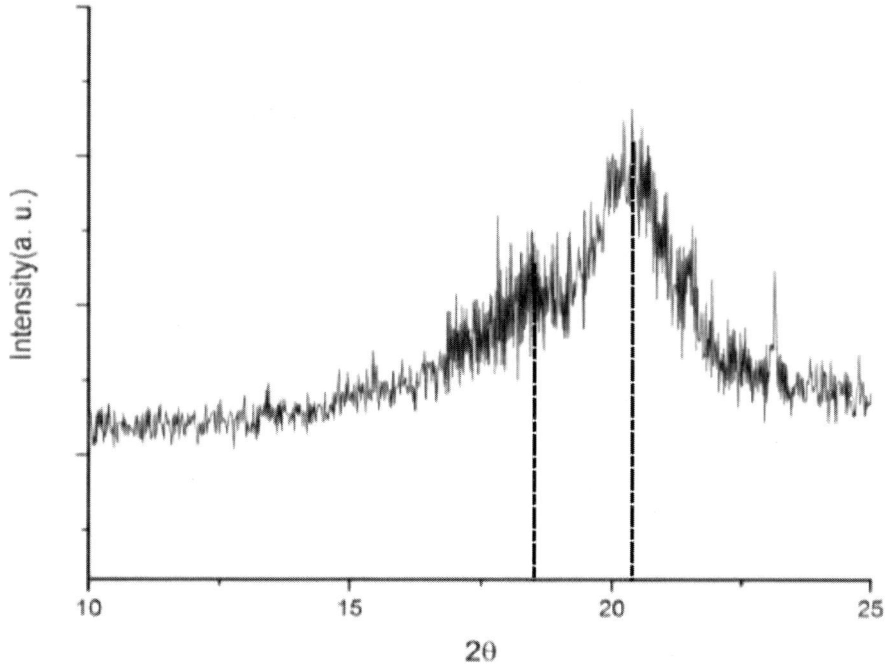

Figure 18. XRD patterns of PVDF/G membrane.

3.3. Temperature Response

Thermal behavior of each membrane is clearly illustrated in Figures 19, 20 and 21. Graphs show the capacitance response to temperature variations.

Dielectric constant of each membrane was calculated according equation (1), results can be observed in table 2.

Table 2. Dielectric constants of PVDF, PVDF/PLA, PVDF/G membranes (at room temperature)

Material	Dielectric constant (ε_r)
PVDF	7.31
PVDF/PLA	5.88
PVDF/G	6.05

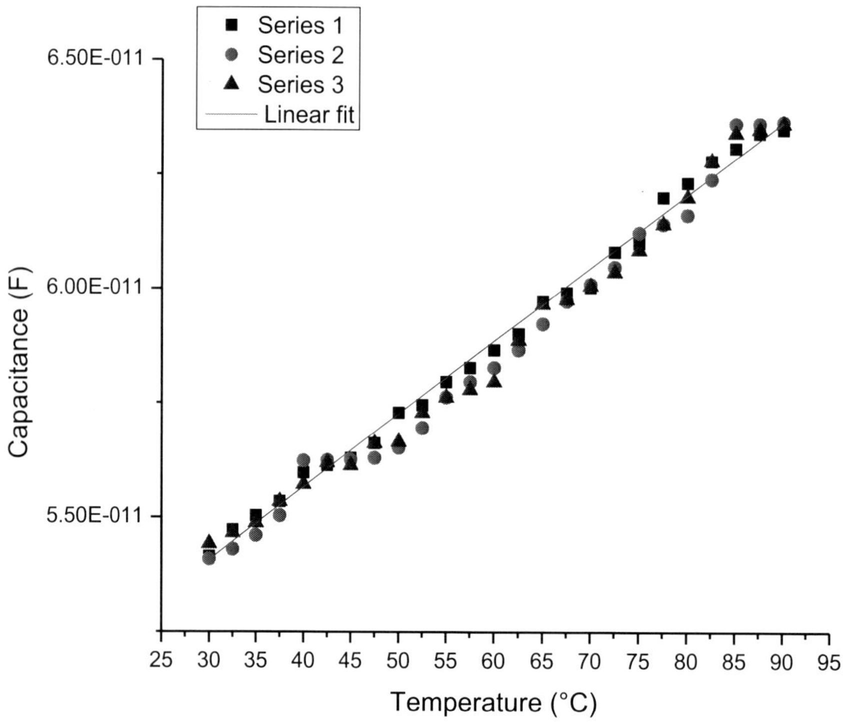

Figure 19. Dielectric behavior of PVDF membrane to controlled temperature changes.

The coefficient of determination, R2 is 0.9941.

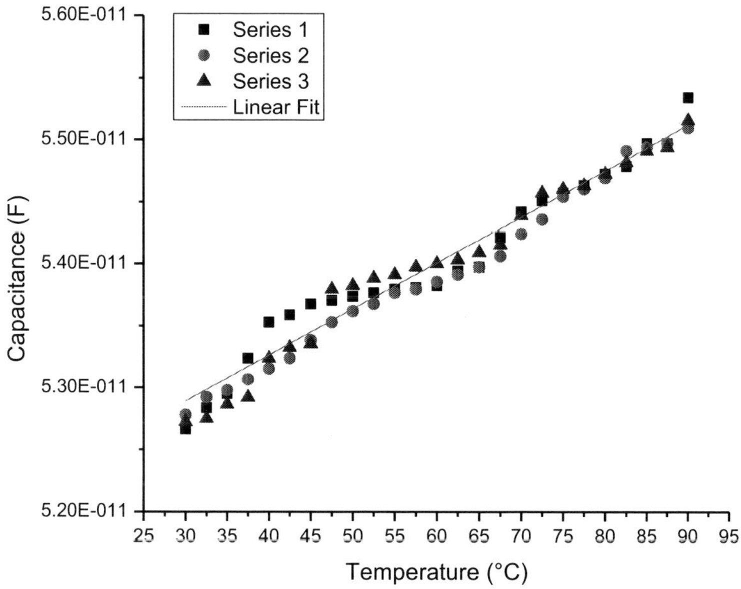

Figure 20. Dielectric behavior of PVDF/PLA membrane to controlled temperature changes.

The coefficient of determination, R^2 is 0.9559.

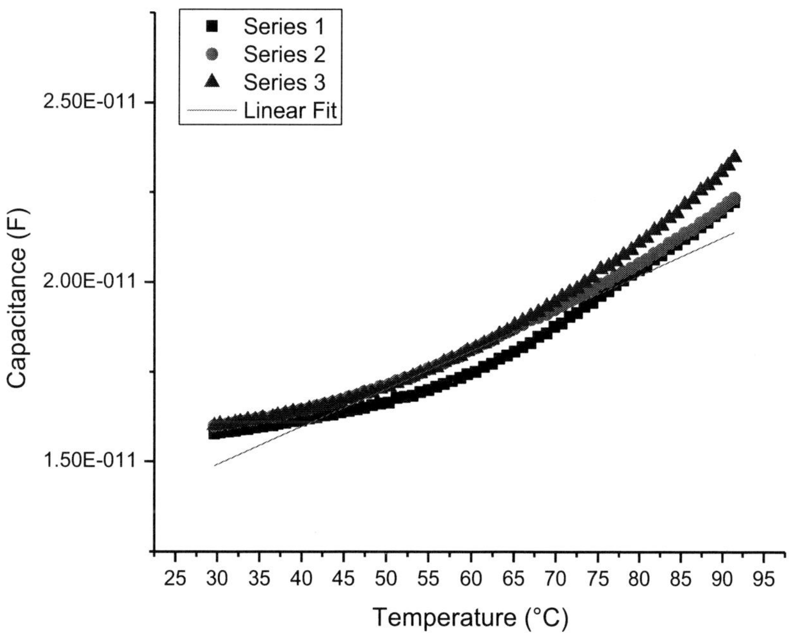

Figure 21. Dielectric behavior of PVDF/G membrane to controlled temperature changes.

The coefficient of determination, R2 is 0.9427.

4. Discussion

Analyzing the temperature responses of the three membranes, it can be clearly seen, that the PVDF membrane response is almost linear, the coefficient of determination was equal to 0.9941 which is very near to 1. By the other hand the PVDF/PLA and PVDF/G membranes are less linear, however, both membranes keep the same tendency.

It is important to note that although the PVDF/G membrane exhibited the least linear behavior, it presented similar responses to each test (repeatability) and lower noise in the acquired signals that the other two membranes.

By the other hand, dielectric constants could be obtained satisfactorily. As might be expected, PVDF had the highest dielectric constant value, and PVDF/PLA, the lowest. This situation is due to the fact that PVDF is a non-conductive polymer.

Regarding the crystallographic characterization, it can be observed that the β phase was predominant in the PVDF/G membranes. It could be caused by a widely variety of elements, however, it has been proven that the G improves the ferroelectric properties of PVDF and electrospinning is also a reliable method to form β phase [19, 22].

Separately, as seen in morphological analysis of PVDF, PVDF/PLA and PVDF/G membranes, fibers with diameters ranging from 50 nm to 700 nm were achieved. Nanofibers fabricated by electrospinning provide a rough and porous surface this way, modifying the mechanical properties and increasing hydrophobicity.

Conclusion

In this work, membranes made of PVDF, PVDF/PLA and PVDF/G were fabricated via electrospinning. Dielectric behaviour of the three membranes by applying an external stimulus, in this case, temperature, was tested. The characterization and mathematical models could be achieved satisfactorily. The typical response of the PVDF temperature sensors was found to be very reliable.

PVDF is well-know as it is widely used as sensor for a variety of applications [27], but, as temperature vs capacitance graphs shown, when PVDF is combined with a non-conductive nor piezoelectric polymer, in this case, polylactic acid (PLA), piezoelectric and pyroelectric properties decrease and responses are not as linear as PVDF response is.

By the other hand, although G is a conductive polymer, the temperature response was not linear either, however, PVDF/G blend has been widely studied in recent years and it has been proven that the G improves the ferroelectric properties of PVDF, moreover, electrospinning is a reliable method to get the β phase directly from a PVDF/DMF solution. In this paper, it was possible to apply a methodology to fabricate PVDF/G membranes by electrospinning and it was proven that β phase was predominant in these samples. This feature is particularly important because PVDF exhibits piezoelectric and pyroelectric properties because of the β phase.

It is also interesting to note, that all these membranes can work as temperature, humidity, light or pressure sensors due to its ferroelectrics properties [28-30]. Other possible applications could be filtration, growth of living tissues and the manufacture of orthosis or prosthesis where the rough and porous surface of these samples can be harnessed.

This way, PVDF, PVDF/PLA and PVDF/G membranes have great potentialities in electronics, robotics and bionics because of their sensibility, reliability, biocompatibility as well as flexibility [31].

References

[1] Ramakrishna, S.; Fujihara, K.; Teo, W.-E.; Lim, T.-C.; Ma, Z. An Introduction to Electrospinning and Nanofibers. *World Scientific*, 2005.

[2] Bhardwaj, N.; Kundu, S. C. Electrospinning: A fascinating fiber fabrication technique. *Biotechnology Advances,* 2010 28, 325-347.

[3] Li, D.; Xia, Y. Electrospinning of Nanofibers: Reinventing the Wheel? *Advanced Materials,* 2004 16, 1151-1170.

[4] Shamshina, J. L.; Zavgorodnya, O.; Bonner, J. R.; Gurau, G.; Di Nardo, T.; Rogers, R. D. "Practical" Electrospinning of Biopolymers in Ionic Liquids. *ChemSusChem,* 2017 10, 106-111.

[5] Ghelich, R.; Rad, M. K.; Youzbashi, A. A. Study on Morphology and Size Distribution of Electrospun NiO-GDC Composite Nanofibers. *J. Eng. Fiber Fabr.,* 2015 10, 12-19.

[6] Yarin, A. L.; Koombhongse, S.; Reneker, D. H. Bending instability in electrospinning of nanofibers. *Journal of Applied Physics,* 2001 89, 3018-3026.

[7] González, E.; Shepherd, L.; Saunders, L.; Frey, M. Surface Functional Poly(lactic Acid) Electrospun Nanofibers for Biosensor Applications. *Materials,* 2016 9, 47.

[8] Jamshidian, M.; Tehrany, E. A.; Imran, M.; Jacquot, M.; Desobry, S. Poly-Lactic Acid: Production, Applications, Nanocomposites, and Release Studies. *Comprehensive Reviews in Food Science and Food Safety,* 2010 9, 552-571.

[9] Alsaheb, R. A. A.; Aladdin, A.; Othman, N. Z.; Malek, R. A.; Leng, O. M.; Aziz, R.; Enshasy, H. A. E. Recent applications of polylactic acid in pharmaceutical and medical industries. *Journal of Chemical and Pharmaceutical Research,* 2015 7, 12.

[10] Dorgan, J. R.; Williams, J. S.; Lewis, D. N. Melt rheology of poly(lactic acid): Entanglement and chain architecture effects. *Journal of Rheology,* 1999 43, 1141-1155.

[11] Tabi, T.; Sajo, I. E.; Szabo, F.; Luyt, A. S.; Kovacs, J. G. Crystalline structure of annealed polylactic acid and its relation to processing. *Express Polymer Letters,* 2010 4, 659-668.

[12] Gu, H.; Zhao, Y.; Wang, M. L. A wireless smart PVDF sensor for structural health monitoring. *Struct Control Hlth,* 2005 12, 329-343.

[13] Moran, C. O. G.; Ballesteros, R. G.; Guzman, M. D. A. R.; Gomez, E. S. Polyvinylidene flouride polymer applied in an intraocular pressure sensor. *Jpn. J. Appl. Phys. 2,* 2005 44, L885-L887.

[14] Jayakumar, R.; Nair, S. V.; Beachley, V. Biomedical applications of polymeric nanofibers. In *Advances in polymer science,* Springer: Berlin, 2012.

[15] Suaste-Gomez, E.; Rodriguez-Roldan, G.; Reyes-Cruz, H.; Teran-Jimenez, O. Developing an Ear Prosthesis Fabricated in Polyvinylidene Fluoride by a 3D Printer with Sensory Intrinsic Properties of Pressure and Temperature. *Sensors-Basel,* 2016 16.

[16] Suaste-Gómez, E.; González-Morán, C. O. Materiales Inteligentes Piezocerámicos y Piezopolímeros. México:Innovación Editorial Lagares de México, 2013.

[17] Gregorio, J. R.; Ueno, E. M. Effect of crystalline phase, orientation and temperature on the dielectric properties of poly (vinylidene fluoride) (PVDF). *Journal of Materials Science,* 1999 34, 4489-4500.

[18] Benz, M.; Euler, W. B. Determination of the crystalline phases of poly(vinylidene fluoride) under different preparation conditions using differential scanning calorimetry and infrared spectroscopy. *Journal of Applied Polymer Science,* 2003 89, 1093-1100.

[19] Gregorio, R. Determination of the α, β, and γ crystalline phases of poly(vinylidene fluoride) films prepared at different conditions. *Journal of Applied Polymer Science,* 2006 100, 3272-3279.

[20] Liu, Z. H.; Pan, C. T.; Yen, C. K.; Lin, L. W.; Huang, J. C.; Ke, C. A. Crystallization and mechanical behavior of the ferroelectric polymer nonwoven fiber fabrics for highly durable wearable sensor applications. *Applied Surface Science,* 2015 346, 291-301.

[21] Alamusi; Xue, J. M.; Wu, L. K.; Hu, N.; Qiu, J. H.; Chang, C.; Atobe, S.; Fukunaga, H.; Watanabe, T.; Liu, Y. L.; Ning, H. M.; Li, J. H.; Li, Y.; Zhao, Y. H. Evaluation of piezoelectric property of reduced graphene oxide (rGO)-poly(vinylidene fluoride) nanocomposites. *Nanoscale,* 2012 4, 7250-7255.

[22] Hu, Y. C.; Hsu, W. L.; Wang, Y. T.; Ho, C. T.; Chang, P. Z. Enhance the Pyroelectricity of Polyvinylidene Fluoride by Graphene-Oxide Doping. *Sensors-Basel,* 2014 14, 6877-6890.

[23] Avouris, P.; Dimitrakopoulos, C. Graphene: synthesis and applications. *Mater Today,* 2012 15, 86-97.

[24] Pinto, A. M.; Goncalves, I. C.; Magalhaes, F. D. Graphene-based materials biocompatibility: A review. *Colloid Surface B,* 2013 111, 188-202.

[25] Yang, Y. Q.; Asiri, A. M.; Tang, Z. W.; Du, D.; Lin, Y. H. Graphene based materials for biomedical applications. *Mater Today,* 2013 16, 365-373.

[26] Mokhtari, F.; Latifi, M.; Shamshirsaz, M. Electrospinning/ electrospray of polyvinylidene fluoride (PVDF): piezoelectric nanofibers. *The Journal of The Textile Institute,* 2015, 1-19.

[27] Gallantree, H. R. Review of transducer applications of polyvinylidene fluoride. *IEE Proceedings I Solid State and Electron Devices,* 1983 130, 219.

[28] Ueberschlag, P. PVDF piezoelectric polymer. *Sensor Review,* 2001 21, 118-126.

[29] Klinge, U.; Klosterhalfen, B.; Öttinger, A. P.; Junge, K.; Schumpelick, V. PVDF as a new polymer for the construction of surgical meshes. *Biomaterials,* 2002 23, 3487-3493.

[30] González-Morán, C. O.; Pérez, G. A. Z.; Suaste-Gómez, E. System for Controlling the Moisture of the Soil Using Humidity Sensors from a Polyvinylidenefluoride Fiber Mats. *Advanced Science Letters,* 2013 19, 858-861.

[31] Xiao, L.; Wang, B.; Yang, G.; Gauthier, M. Poly (Lactic Acid)-Based Biomaterials: Synthesis, Modification and Applications. 2012.

In: Electrospinning and Electroplating
Editor: Toby Jacobs
ISBN: 978-1-53612-363-0

Chapter 6

ELECTRODEPOSITION OF ELECTROCATALYTIC AND PHOTOCATALYTIC Fe/TiO_2 COMPOSITE COATINGS USING METHANESULFONATE ELECTROLYTES

V. S. Protsenko**, E. A. Vasil'eva, A. V. Tsurkan and F. I. Danilov
Ukrainian State University of Chemical Technology, Dnipro, Ukraine

ABSTRACT

The chapter presents the main results of recent experimental investigation of the electrodeposition and characterization of Fe/TiO_2 composite coatings obtained from an environmentally friendly methanesulfonate iron plating bath containing colloidal TiO_2 particles. The effect of plating bath composition and electrolysis conditions on the content of titania particles in coatings has been investigated. The content of the TiO_2 particles in the electrodeposited composite coatings increases with an increase in titania concentrations in the suspension electrolyte and with a decrease in the current density. The kinetics of Fe/TiO_2 composites electrochemical deposition is shown to obey the improved Guglielmi's model. The inclusion of titania particles in the iron matrix results in an increase in microhardness of electrodeposits due to dispersion strengthening effect. The electrocatalytic properties of Fe/TiO_2 composites are studied by means of voltammetry, electrochemical impedance spectroscopy (EIS) and chronoamperometry methods. Iron/titania electrodeposited composite coatings exhibit enhanced electrocatalytic activity towards hydrogen and oxygen evolution reactions (HER and OER) in an alkaline solution. The electrocatalytic activity increases with an increase in TiO_2 content in iron matrix. The kinetic parameters are calculated on the basis of Tafel

---

* Address correspondence to: Vprotsenko7@gmail.com.

plots and EIS measurements and possible mechanisms of the HER and OER are considered. The chapter also reports the performance of Fe/TiO_2 electrodeposited composite coatings as heterogeneous photocatalysts for the decomposition of some organic contaminants. Although iron electrodeposited matrix is a cheap, available, nontoxic and easily repairable support for TiO_2 photocatalysts, it is not corrosion-resisting enough. In order to improve the corrosion stability, as-deposited Fe/TiO_2 composite coatings obtained from a methanesulfonate iron plating bath are modified by cathodic treatment in a solution containing cerium (III) methanesulfonate. As a result, a very thin layer of cerium oxides is formed on the surface of Fe matrix. The corrosion resistance of iron/titania coatings after their modification by ceria film is studied by means of voltammetry and electrochemical impedance spectroscopy. The surface modification of Fe/TiO_2 composites by ceria layer results in a marked improvement in their corrosion stability which allows their application as photocatalysts for wastewater treatment. The photocatalytic properties of TiO_2 particles immobilized on Fe/TiO_2 composite electrodeposits modified by ceria layers are tested in the reaction of photochemical degradation of methyl orange and methylene blue dyes in water under the action of UV radiation.

1. INTRODUCTION

Electrochemical synthesis and characterization of composite coatings have been particularly gaining considerable attention due to the superior physicochemical and service properties of electrodeposited composites as compared with "pure" metal coatings [1, 2]. The electrochemical embedding of finely dispersed nonmetallic phase in metallic matrices consists in electrolyzing a solution containing the dissolved metallic salt and the particles in suspension. This technique enables the controlled and flexible fabrication of composites with predictable composition and properties. Electrodeposition procedure is available, relatively simple and not expensive. In addition, the electrodeposition technique allows easily restoring worn layers.

To date, a great number of different kind of electrodeposited composite coatings have been synthesized and investigated. Among many metals used, copper and nickel have featured strongly [1]. As concerns dispersed particles incorporated into a metallic matrix, these include Al_2O_3, SiC, SiO_2, TiO_2, ZrO_2, Cr_2O_3, MoS_2, WC etc. [1-3].

The works dealing with composite electrodeposition are chiefly aimed to produce wear- and/or corrosion-resistant protective coatings, self-lubricating layers and dispersion strengthened coatings. However, a very important task is to synthesize deposits with some catalytic, electrocatalytic and photocatalytic properties [3]. In this context, it should be noted that searching for new and effective electrocatalysts for the hydrogen evolution reaction (HER) is very important in advanced industrial water electrolysis cells to produce hydrogen which is an environmentally clean and promising energy carrier for the so-called "Hydrogen Economy" [4].

It is known that various materials may be used as efficient and durable cathodic electrocatalysts for the HER [5]. Noble metals (Pt, Ru, etc.) seem to be the most active and stable materials, but their extremely high cost and limited natural abundance impede their wide industrial applications. Thus, non-platinum active metals such as Fe, Ni or Co as well as their alloys and composites have received great attention as electrocatalysts for the HER because of their relatively low prices and accessibility [5-18]. For instance, different types of steel electrodes were reported to be suitable as electrocatalytic materials for the HER [19-22].

Although there are various available methods of electrocatalysts fabrication, the electrodeposition technique is particularly attractive due to its simplicity, low cost and the possibility to influence easily on the structure, composition and properties of deposits obtained [5, 11].

It should be observed that the most studied electrodeposited electrocatalysts for the HER in alkaline media are based on Ni and Co alloys and composites. Nevertheless, electrocatalysts on the basis of electrodeposited iron also attract considerable attention, because Fe and its compounds are particularly cheap, available and low-toxic. For instance, Elezović N.R. et al. [13] studied the mechanism and kinetics of the HER in 1 M NaOH solution on Fe–Mo alloy prepared by electrodeposition. The real surface area of the electrodes was stated to increase with an increase in the molybdenum content. This factor was principally responsible for the increased electrocatalytic activity.

A suitable plating baths were developed to electroplate Fe–P, Fe–P–Pt and Fe–P–Ce amorphous alloys which act as electrocatalysts during alkaline water electrolysis [11]. The results of polarization measurements and electrochemical impedance spectroscopy showed that improved catalytic activity towards the HER was due to an increase in the effective surface area, the partial contribution of the Pt component, and the electrocatalytic synergism with Fe imposed by the Ce co-deposit.

The incorporation of colloidal particles into a metallic matrix (i.e., electrodeposition of composites) can also enhance electrocatalytic activity towards the hydrogen evolution reaction. Embedding the Fe_2O_3–TiO_2 mixed oxide in Ni–P matrix substantially reduces overpotential during the HER in NaOH solution [7]. The Ni/TiO_2 [23] and Ni/Co_3O_4 composite layers electrodeposited from a conventional Watts' electrolyte containing TiO_2 or Co_3O_4 powder, respectively, are characterized by enhanced electrochemical activity with respect to the HER in an alkaline electrolyte [24].

It is well-known that the composites containing titania particles have wide applications in photocatalytic degradation of organic pollutants, this technique being associated with promising and efficient advanced oxidation processes (AOPs) [25-27]. AOPs presuppose *in situ* generation of a powerful oxidizing agent (such as hydroxyl radicals •OH) and provide practically total mineralization of a great number of organic pollutants, including different organic dyes.

There are many types of treatment procedures that can produce •OH radicals, such as Fenton or photo-Fenton methods, peroxonation, H_2O_2 photolysis, O_3 photolysis and heterogeneous photocatalysis [25-27]. Among these types, the heterogeneous photocatalysis, AOPs chiefly based on the application of photo-excited semiconductor titanium dioxide, has been the object of a deep interest and tremendous development in the last decades. This is due to the fact that TiO_2 is close to being practically ideal photocatalyst for water/wastewater treatment [27-30].

Heterogeneous titania photocatalysts can be utilized either under dispersed form (powders or aqueous suspensions) or in thin film form (fixed immobilized TiO_2 catalytic layers) [25, 27]. Slurry systems show a number of advantages: they are easy to prepare and use, they provide a very high specific surface and can be easily aerated to prevent the recombining of electron-hole pairs and, therefore, to increase catalytic efficiency [27]. However, the suspensions of fine powdered TiO_2 are unstable and trend towards particles coarsening and sedimentation which reduces the photoreactor performances. In addition, slurry systems require a time consuming and costly process of TiO_2 post-treatment. Quite the contrary, there is no need to filtrate and separate catalytic particles for immobilized TiO_2 catalytic layers; such systems may be very stable and show high photocatalytic activity for a long time [31].

In order to anchor the titania photocatalyst particles, a great number of different types of supports have been developed: glasses, silica materials, activated carbon, polymers, zeolites, stainless steel, alumina clays, fibers and others [31, 32]. In this context, electrochemical deposition of composites containing dispersed particles of titania may be a very interesting approach to the development of new potential supports for TiO_2.

Spanou et al. [33] investigated the immobilization of titanium dioxide nano-particles in coatings with nickel matrix using the direct current electrodeposition method. The photocatalytic activity of the obtained composite coatings was studied under UVA illumination. Fine tuning of electrodeposition parameters was shown to facilitate the control of the nickel matrix structural and morphological characteristics and the titania nano-particles encapsulation on the films' surface. In this way, the photo-induced self-cleaning properties of the composite coatings (photocatalysis and hydrophilicity) can be simultaneously optimized.

Thus, the electrodeposited coatings with the embedded TiO_2 particles distinguished by both high electrocatalytic and photocatalytic properties. To obtain such coatings, Ni matrix is extremely often used for composite electrodeposition [1, 2]. We think that the replacement of the nickel electrodeposited matrix by an iron one can provide a number of advantages [34, 35]. Indeed, nickel and its salts are highly expensive and toxic. It is known that a skin contact with metallic nickel leads to a contact dermatitis. From this point of view, the development of electrodeposited composite Fe/TiO_2 coatings as versatile electrocatalysts and photocatalysts is very promising because iron and its salts are relatively cheap, available and low-toxic.

For iron matrix electrodeposition, we suggested a methanesulfonate plating bath [36, 37]. Methanesulfonate plating baths based on methanesulfonic acid CH_3SO_3H (MSA) are known to be an attractive alternative to common electroplating baths because MSA is considered as a "green acid" due to its environmental advantages [38]. MSA is far less corrosive and toxic than the usual mineral acids used in different branches of industry [39]. Methanesulfonates of various metals are highly soluble in water; the conductivity of the corresponding aqueous solutions is high. In addition, MSA is easily biodegradable [38]. Because of these advantages, electrochemical systems on the basis of MSA and its salts have been shown to be very promising for electroplating of different metals, alloys and composites [40-44]. Thus, the electrodeposition of Fe/TiO_2 films from a MSA based plating bath well agrees with the concept of "green chemistry."

This study was aimed (i) to characterize the main features of electrochemical deposition of Fe/TiO_2 composites from methanesulfonate electrolyte, (ii) to estimate the electrocatalytic properties of Fe/TiO_2 coatings towards the processes of hydrogen and oxygen evolution reactions, and (iii) to investigate the photocatalytic activity of Fe/TiO_2 composite layers towards the reactions of organic dyes degradation [34, 35, 45, 46].

2. Electrodeposition of Fe/TiO_2 Composite Coatings

2.1. Preparation of Fe/TiO_2 Electrodeposits

A methanesulfonate iron plating bath developed in our previous studies [34-37, 45, 46] was used to deposit Fe and Fe/TiO_2 layers. This plating bath allows obtaining nanocrystalline Fe coatings with a high current efficiency (ca. 95%) and a relatively high deposition rate (up to 2-4 $\mu m\ min^{-1}$).

All solutions were prepared using double distilled water and reagent grade chemicals. Iron (II) methanesulfonate was synthesized by the procedure reported in detail elsewhere [38]. The pH value of the plating bath was controlled through a common potentiometric method and adjusted to a required value by adding either Na_2CO_3 or MSA solutions. The concentration of Fe(II) ions in the electroplating bath was determined by the titrimetric analysis.

To obtain composite coatings, a weighed portion of TiO_2 nanopowder (Degussa P 25, Evonik; the average particle size 25 nm) was introduced directly into the electrodeposition bath. Degussa P 25 nanopowder represents a mixture of anatase and rutile (the ratio of anatase:rutile is about ≈80:20), as well as a slight amount of amorphous phase [47].

Before electrodeposition, the plating bath was stirred for 1 h by mechanical agitator and then ultrasonically treated with a UZDN-A ultrasonic disperser (1 h, 22.4 kHz, 340 W dm^{-3}) to reach uniform distribution of colloidal particles in the bath. The electrodeposition of Fe/TiO_2 composite coatings was performed under the conditions of a continuous bath agitation with a magnetic stirrer (ca. 60 rev min^{-1}).

Electrodeposition was performed at a steady current density in a usual thermostated glass cell (298 K) for 20 min. Iron and iron-titania films were deposited on the mild steel plates ($S = 1$ cm^2) fixed in a plastic holder. Prior to each experiment, the sample surface was treated with magnesium oxide, etched for several minutes in 1:1 (vol.) HCl solution and then thoroughly rinsed with double distilled water. The electrolysis was carried out with anodes made of mild steel.

The composition and operating parameters of the plating bath used for deposition of Fe/TiO_2 composite coatings in the present study are summarized in Table 1.

It is well-known that nanopowders of metal oxides in aqueous electrolyte tend to aggregate. Aggregation is due to compression of the double electric layer on the particle surface in the solution with comparatively high ionic force, which results in coagulation of lyophobic dispersed systems according to the DLVO (Derjaguin, Landau, Verwey, Overbeek) theory.

Table 1. Composition of Fe/TiO_2 plating bath and deposition parameters

$Fe(CH_3SO_3)_2$	1.25 mol dm^{-3}
TiO_2 nano-powder (Degussa P 25, Evonik)	1-12 g dm^{-3}
pH	1.3
Temperature	298 K
Current density	5-20 A dm^{-2}
Stirring	Magnetic stirrer, ~ 60 rev min^{-1}
Cathode	Mild steel
Anode	Mild steel

A Vibra HT-120 digital analytical balance (Shinko Denshi, Japan) was used for dispersion analysis of suspension electrolyte. The size of the particles was evaluated by the method of sedimentation in the gravitation field. The height of suspension column was 15 cm. As follows from the results of the sedimentation analysis of TiO_2 dispersion (Degussa P 25) in methanesulfonate electrolyte, the most probable radius of aggregates here is about 1 μm (Figure 1), which is almost the same as when TiO_2 (rutile) particles were used [45].

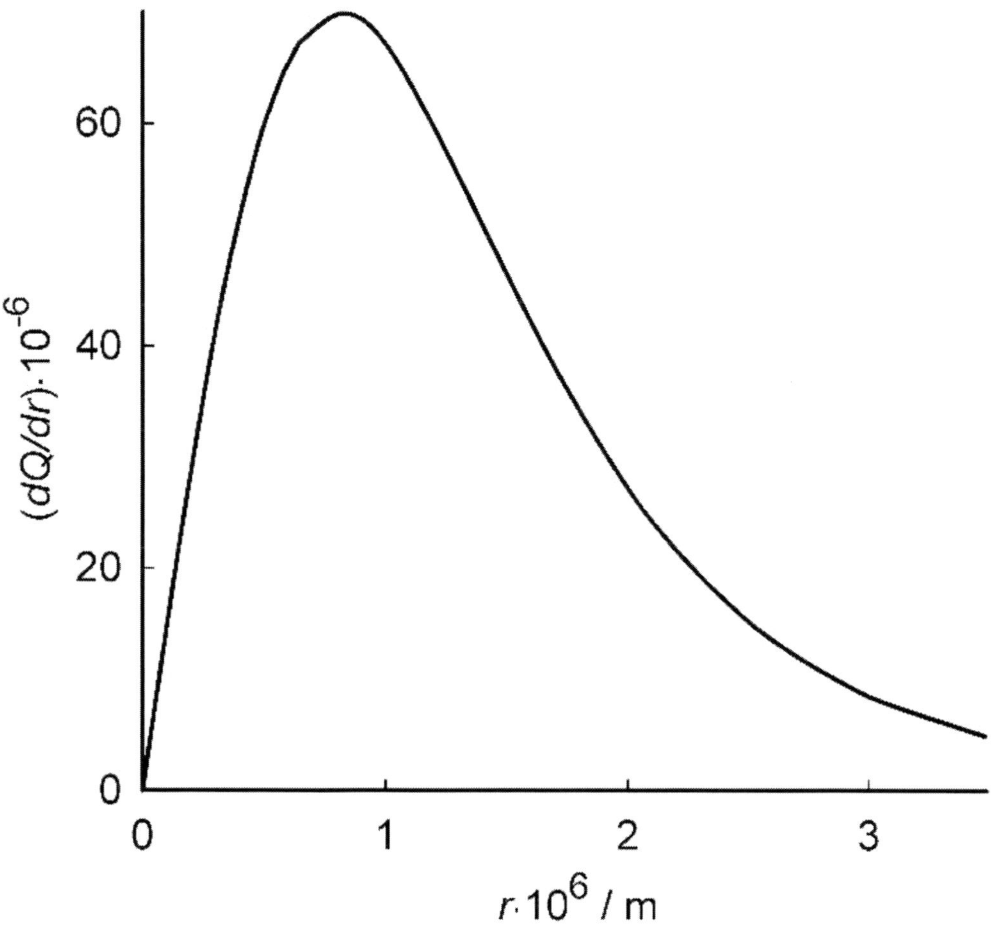

Figure 1. Differential curve of dispersed phase particle distribution in electrolyte containing 1.25 mol dm^{-3} $Fe(CH_3SO_3)_2$, 2 g dm^{-3} TiO_2 [46].

2.2. Kinetics and Mechanism of Fe/TiO_2 Composites Electrodeposition

Figure 2 shows the effect of TiO_2 concentration in the electroplating bath on the TiO_2 content in the deposits at various current densities. It is seen that the amount of the titania particles in the coatings increases with an increase in the TiO_2 concentrations in the electrolyte and with a decrease in the current density. Dependences of this kind are typical of electrochemical synthesis of different types of composite electrodeposited coatings [1].

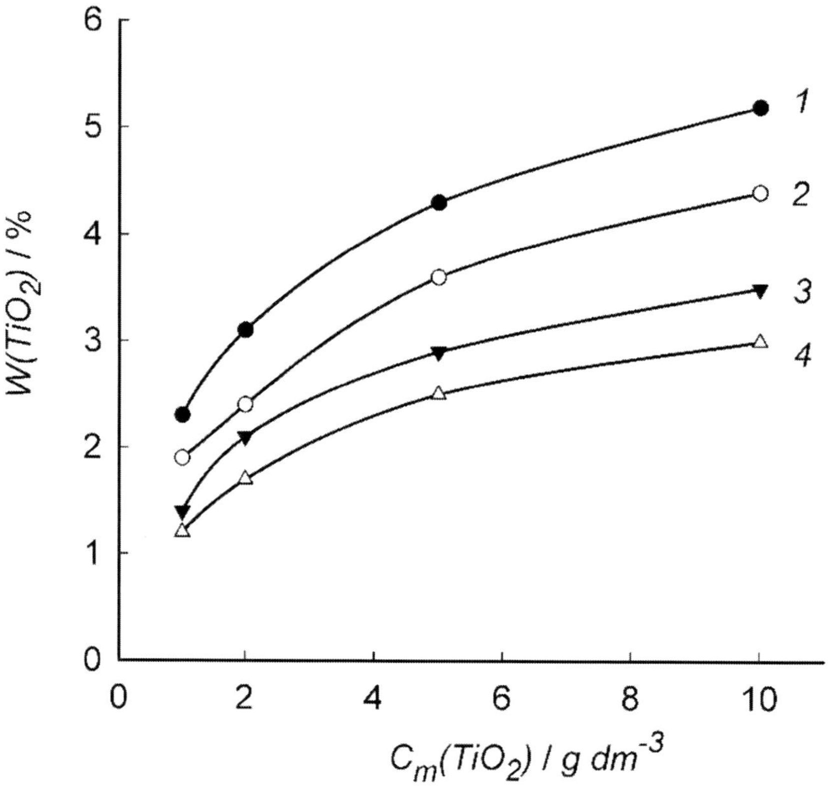

Figure 2. Dependences of titanium dioxide content in the composite coating on the concentration of TiO_2 in suspension at different current densities (A dm^{-2}): (*1*) 5, (*2*) 10, (*3*) 15, and (*4*) 20 [46].

The embedding of TiO_2 can be attributed to the adsorption of suspended particles on the electrode surface, as suggested by Guglielmi's two-step adsorption model [48]. This kinetic model is based on the assumption that dispersed phase particles are incorporated into the metallic matrix as a result of their adsorption on the electrode. It is proposed that adsorption of colloidal particles on the electrode surface is described by a Langmuir type equation. Here, adsorption of dispersed phase particles on the surface of the deposited metal occurs in two stages. The first stage, denoted by Guglielmi as "weak adsorption," has a physical nature; particles fixed on the electrode surface largely remain coated by adsorption-solvate shells. At the second stage of the so-called "strong adsorption," dispersed phased particles lose these shells and are firmly fixed on the metal surface. It is supposed that it is these dispersed phase particles that are strongly adsorbed on the metal surface; they are ultimately included into the structure of the forming composite electrodeposited coatings. The equation describing the kinetics of the codeposition of the dispersion phase and metallic matrix has the following form [48]:

$$\frac{C}{\alpha} = \frac{Mi_0}{nF\rho_m \upsilon_0} e^{(A-B)\eta} \left(\frac{1}{k} + C \right) \quad (1)$$

where C is the volume fraction (percentage) of particles in suspension, α is the volume fraction of particles in the composite coating, M is the atomic mass of the metal, i_0 is the exchange current of the metal deposition process, n is the number of electrons in the equation of the electrochemical reaction, F is the Faraday's number, ρ_m is the metal density, η is the overpotential of the electrochemical reaction of metal deposition, A is a constant in the kinetic equation of the electrochemical reaction $i = i_0 e^{A\eta}$, k is the adsorption coefficient (i.e., constant of adsorption equilibrium in the Langmuir-type equation), and B and υ_0 are the constants describing the kinetics of the process of inclusion of nonmetal phase particles into the composite coating and similar to the constants A and i_0 for the electrochemical process.

Obviously, if the kinetics of the electrodeposition of composite electrodeposited coatings is described by Eq. (1), then the dependences in the coordinates of $\frac{C}{\alpha} = f(C)$ obtained at different cathodic current densities will represent a family of straight lines in the plot that are extrapolated to the point on the x axis with the coordinate of $\left(-\frac{1}{k}\right)$.

However, the linear dependences in the coordinates of $\frac{C}{\alpha} = f(C)$ for iron codeposition with titanium dioxide Degussa P 25 are obviously not concurrent (Figure 3). Hence, Eq. (1) does not suitably describe the obtained experimental data.

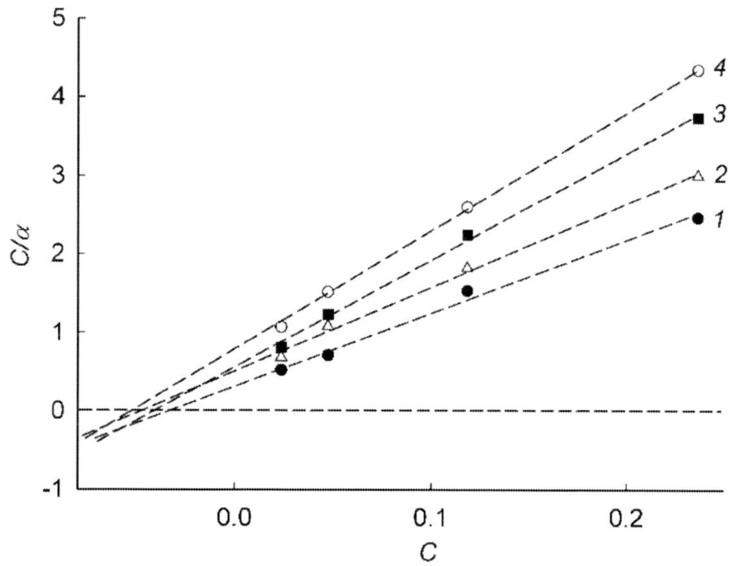

Figure 3. $\frac{C}{\alpha}, C$ - dependences for electrodeposition of Fe/TiO_2 composition coatings at different current densities (A dm^{-2}): (*1*) 5, (*2*) 10, (*3*) 15, and (*4*) 20 [46].

The kinetic model of composite coatings electrodeposition suggested by Guglielmi has been repeatedly elaborated and modified [1]. Thus, in derivation of the main equation (1) for simplification of the mathematics, Gugliemi neglected the content of dispersed phase particles in the metallic matrix. In other words, it was assumed in the corresponding algebraic manipulations that $1-\alpha \approx 1$. Taking into account that α is generally not a negligible quantity, Bahadormanesh and Dolati, based on the key propositions of the Guglielmi's theory, suggested an improved model [49], in which the main equation takes the following form:

$$\frac{C(1-\alpha)^{(2-B/A)}}{\alpha} = \frac{Mi_0^{B/A}}{nF\rho_m \upsilon_0} i^{(1-B/A)} \left(\frac{1}{k} + C\right) \tag{2}$$

Taking the logarithm of Eq. (2) yields the following expression:

$$\lg \frac{C(1-\alpha)}{\alpha} = \lg\left(\frac{Mi_0^{B/A}}{nF\rho_m \upsilon_0}\right) + \left(1-\frac{B}{A}\right)\lg\left(\frac{i}{1-\alpha}\right) + \lg\left(\frac{1}{k}+C\right) \tag{3}$$

According to Eq. (3), dependences plotted in the $\lg \frac{C(1-\alpha)}{\alpha}$, $\lg \frac{i}{1-\alpha}$ coordinates are linear; their slope allows calculating the value of $\frac{B}{A}$.

As can be easily seen (Figure 4), experimental data on deposition of Fe/TiO_2 composites are well linearized in the abovementioned coordinates. The obtained straight lines are parallel within the experimental error. This means that the $\frac{B}{A}$ ratio is independent of the suspension concentration and cathodic current density which may serve as a criterion confirming the adequacy of the improved Guglielmi's model to the obtained experimental data [49].

The calculated $\frac{B}{A}$ value is about 0.583; i.e., $B < A$. Such a ratio between B and A means that Fe(II) ions adsorbed on the surface of titanium dioxide particles are discharged more slowly than ions in the bulk of electrolyte [50]; this is typical of systems for which the value of α decreases at an increase in cathodic current density, which agrees with the obtained experimental data.

On the basis of the calculated $\frac{B}{A}$ value, one can plot $C(1-\alpha)^{(2-B/A)}/\alpha$ versus C for different values of deposition current density (Figure 5), which, according to Eq. (2), must correspond to a family of straight lines, extrapolation of which to the x axis will allow finding $\left(-\frac{1}{k}\right)$ [49].

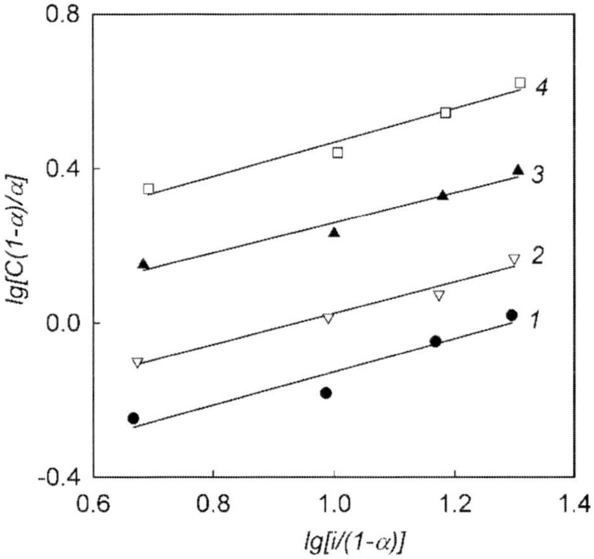

Figure 4. Plots of $\lg\frac{C(1-\alpha)}{\alpha}$, $\lg\frac{i}{1-\alpha}$ dependences for electrodeposition of Fe/TiO_2 composite coatings at various TiO_2 concentrations in the suspension (g dm^{-3}): (*1*) 1, (*2*) 2, (*3*) 5, and (*4*) 10 [46].

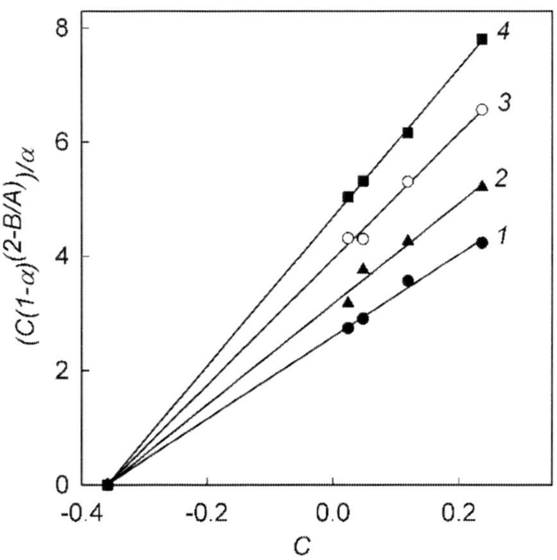

Figure 5. Plots of $C(1-\alpha)^{(2-B/A)}/\alpha, C$ dependences for electrodeposition of Fe/TiO_2 composite coatings at various current densities (A dm^{-2}): (*1*) 5, (*2*) 10, (*3*) 15, and (*4*) 20 [46].

The thus calculated adsorption coefficient proved to be $k = 2.8$. This is notably lower than the value found for adsorption of TiO_2 rutile on the surface of depositing iron from electrolyte of the same ionic composition ($k = 49.8$) [45]. Such significant differences appear to be due to noticeable dissimilarity of the colloid and chemical characteristics of anatase and rutile.

As follows from comparison of the data obtained in work [45] with the experimental results presented in this chapter, where the Degussa P 25 powder is used, the weight content of titanium dioxide particles proves to be much lower than in the case of introducing powder consisting solely of rutile into electrolyte (all other conditions being equal). Thus, for example, at the current density of 20 A dm^{-2} and mass concentration of suspension of 5 g dm^{-3}, TiO_2 content in the composite electrodeposited coating is 12.1% when rutile is used and only 2.5% in the case of Degussa P 25. This is obviously related to the discovered difference in the values of the corresponding adsorption coefficients.

On the basis of the calculated value of the adsorption coefficient k, one can calculate the surface coverage by dispersed phase particles due to weak adsorption. To this end, one should use the Langmuir equation written on the Guglielmi's suggestion in the following form [48, 49]:

$$\sigma = \frac{kC}{1+kC}(1-\theta) \tag{4}$$

where σ is the surface coverage due to weak adsorption and θ is the surface coverage due to strong adsorption.

In calculations, it is provisionally assumed [48, 49] that coverage by strongly adsorbed particles (θ) practically coincides with the volume fraction of particles in the composition coating (i.e., $\theta \approx \alpha$). The results of calculations for different current densities and suspension concentrations are presented in Table 2.

Table 2. Calculated values of surface coverage due to strong and weak adsorption at different concentrations of suspension and current densities [46]

C (%)	i (A dm^{-2})	σ (%)	θ (%)
0.024	5	5.93	4.20
	10	5.97	3.48
	15	6.02	2.57
	20	6.05	2.21
0.047	5	10.99	5.62
	10	11.14	4.37
	15	11.20	3.84
	20	11.28	3.12
0.118	5	22.87	7.71
	10	23.18	6.50
	15	23.48	5.26
	20	23.66	4.55
0.236	5	35.91	9.26
	10	36.59	7.89
	15	37.21	6.32
	20	37.60	5.44

The surface coverage by weakly adsorbed titanium dioxide particles is higher than by strongly adsorbed ones and grows at an increase in the dispersed phase concentration in the suspension. One can see that the electrode surface coverage by weakly adsorbed particles is noticeably lower than their fraction ultimately included in composite electrodeposited coatings. It follows from this that the process of incorporation of TiO_2 particles into the iron matrix is controlled by the rate of the transfer from weakly adsorbed particles to the strongly adsorbed state [48, 49, 51].

2.3. Surface Morphology and Microhardness of Fe/TiO_2 Composite Electrodeposits

The surface morphology of the Fe and Fe/TiO_2 electrodeposits with different TiO_2 content is shown in Figure 6 obtained by scanning electron microscopy (SEM). The SEM analysis of the surface morphology of "pure" iron reveals a number of small irregular grains growing out of the film (Figure 6A). The EDX analysis shows that the surface mainly consists of iron (ca. 97%), small amounts of oxygen and other elements have been also detected (Table 3).

Table 3. Chemical composition (wt.%) at points (1) and (2) in Figure 6C [34]

Point	Fe	Ti	O	Other elements
(1)	1.21	58.49	40.14	0.16
(2)	97.27	1.41	1.17	0.15

When the plating bath contains TiO_2 particles and composite coatings are obtained, flakelike particles of agglomerated TiO_2 with an average size of about several micrometers can be clearly seen on the surface (Figure 6B, 6C). The EDX analysis reveals that the surface regions, which correspond to flakelike particles in SEM images, consist essentially of titanium and oxygen (Table 3), the ratio of Ti to O being close to that typical of stoichiometric composition of TiO_2. The amount of these particles on the surface naturally increases with the concentration of titanium dioxide in the electrolyte.

The appearance of aggregated particles, which size sufficiently exceeds nanoscale, is associated with the aggregation process occurring in methanesulfonate solutions. As follows from the differential curves of particle size distribution (Figure 1), the colloidal system becomes polydispersed; the main fraction of the suspension contains aggregated particles with the average size of about several micrometers. The coarsening of the particles results in their enhanced sedimentation and subsequent phase separation. This is why the electrochemical synthesis of the Fe/TiO_2 composites was carried out under the conditions of a continuous bath agitation with a magnetic stirrer.

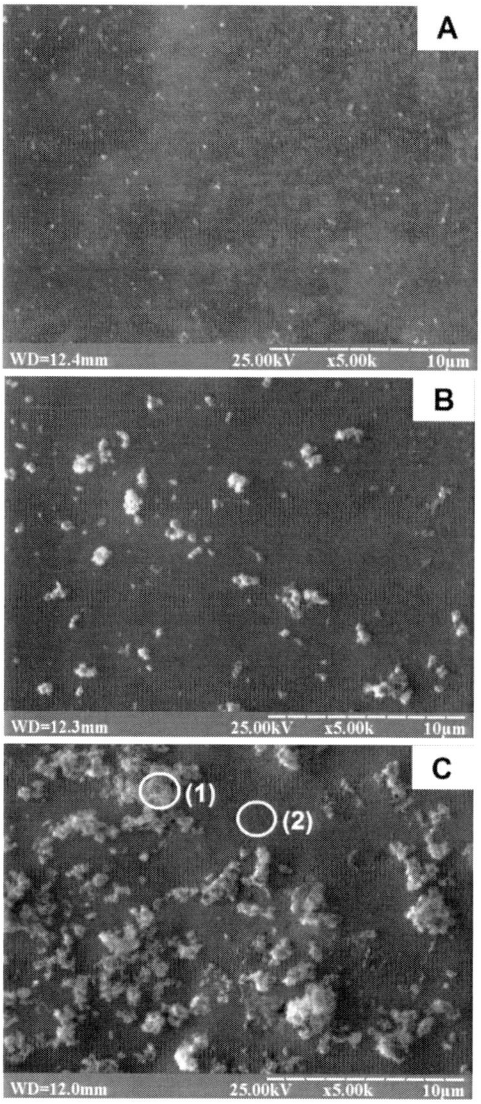

Figure 6. SEM images of (A) pure Fe, (B) Fe/TiO_2 (2% wt.), (C) Fe/TiO_2 (5% wt.) coatings deposited from methanesulfonate baths at 10 A dm^{-2} [34].

The EDX analysis indicates that a small amount of Ti (ca. 1%) can be detected on the surface areas that are free from the agglomerated titania particles entrapped. This means that some nanoparticles of TiO_2 are not aggregated and embedded in the bulk iron matrix.

The incorporation of TiO_2 particles into the iron matrix enhances the coatings microhardness (Figure 7). This may be associated with the so-called dispersion strengthening effect [52]. The dispersion strengthening effect is caused by a uniform distribution of dispersed phase particles in a metal matrix which prevents the dislocations migration and results in an increase in the material hardness. When compared to "pure" electrodeposited iron, the composite coatings are distinguished by an increased microhardness (i.e., enhanced mechanical strength), this feature is important in terms of their possible practical application.

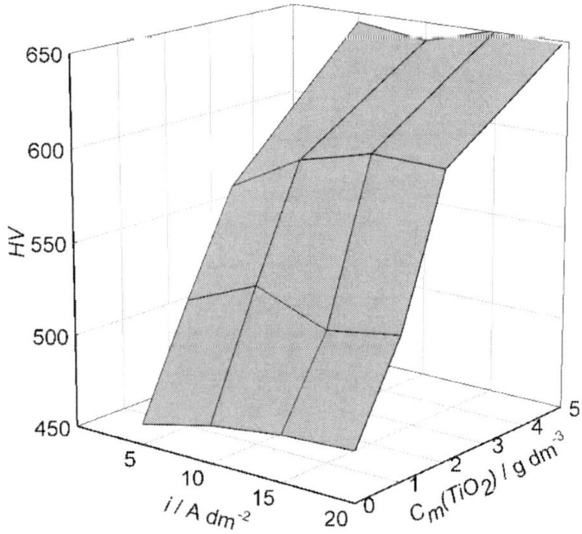

Figure 7. Dependence of microhardness of Fe/TiO_2 coatings on cathodic current density and TiO_2 concentration in suspension electrolyte [46].

3. Electrocatalytic Activity of Fe/TiO_2 Composite Electrodeposits

The study of electrocatalytic activity was performed by means of voltammetry, chronoamperometry and electrochemical impedance spectra techniques in 1 M NaOH solution at 298 K. All experiments were carried out using a Potentiostat/Galvanostat Reference 3000 (Gamry). The ohmic potential drop was measured and automatically compensated by means of the built-in iR-compensator of the potentiostat. A thermostated glass three-electrode cell with electrode compartments separated by a glass porous diaphragm was used. Dissolved atmospheric oxygen was removed by purging electrolytic hydrogen. The counter electrode was iron gauze, its surface area considerably exceeded the overall surface area of the working electrode. The potentials were measured with respect to the saturated Ag/AgCl-electrode and recalculated to the scale of standard hydrogen electrode.

The potential sweep rate in voltammetry study was 20 mV s^{-1}. The potential scan was initiated from the open circuit potential (OCP) in the negative direction. When the cathodic current of the HER was achieved, the scan direction was reversed.

Electrochemical impedance spectra were recorded in the potentiostatic mode both at open circuit potentials and at overpotentials of –100, –200, and –300 mV in the H_2 evolution region in the frequency range of 0.01 Hz to 100 kHz with a constant ac voltage amplitude of 10 mV. The data of electrochemical impedance spectroscopy were processed (development of electrical equivalent circuits and determination of quantitative parameters of their elements) using a computer system with the Gamry Elchem Analyst software package.

3.1. Electrocatalytic Activity towards Hydrogen Evolution Reaction

Electrochemical behavior of the Fe and Fe/TiO_2 deposits was preliminary evaluated by subjecting them to cyclic voltammetry study in 1 M NaOH (Figure 8). The current waves at $E < -1.2$ V and at $E > 0.7$ V correspond to hydrogen evolution reaction and oxygen evolution reaction, respectively.

A couple of ill-defined conjugate cathodic and anodic current peaks, characterized by irreversibility, are also observed at –0.8…–0.1 V and –0.8…0 V, correspondingly. Since the heights of these peaks are well correlated with the TiO_2 content in the deposits, these current peaks may be attributed to the reduction of surface Ti(IV) species and the re-oxidation of surface Ti(III) species [53].

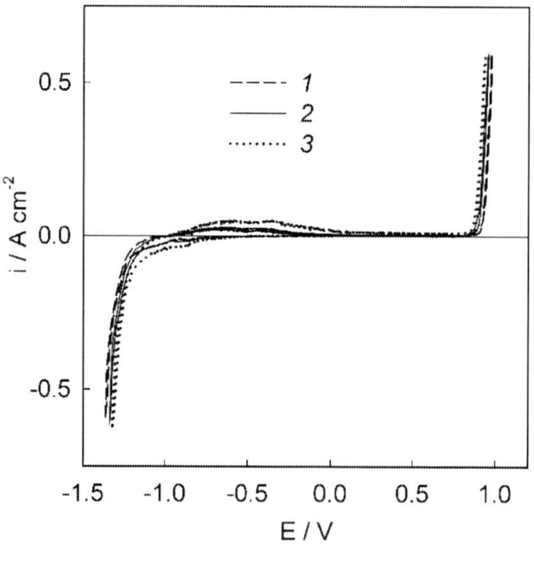

Figure 8. Cyclic voltammograms recorded on Fe (1), Fe/TiO_2 (2% wt.) (2) and Fe/TiO_2 (5% wt.) (3) electrodes in 1 M NaOH at 298 K. Scan rate 20 mV s^{-1} [34].

It is seen from the obtained cyclic voltammograms that the values of overpotential for both hydrogen evolution reaction and oxygen evolution reaction (OER) decrease with an increase in the TiO_2 content in the coatings. Hence, the incorporation of titania dispersed particles into an iron matrix enhances the electrocatalytic activities towards HER and OER.

The Tafel dependences for the HER occurring on Fe and Fe/TiO_2 coatings electrodeposited from methanesulfonate baths are given in Figure 9. The polarization curves well follow a typical linear Tafel behavior:

$$\eta = a + b\log|i| \tag{5}$$

where η is the overpotential, i is the current density (A cm^{-2}), a and b are the Tafel constants.

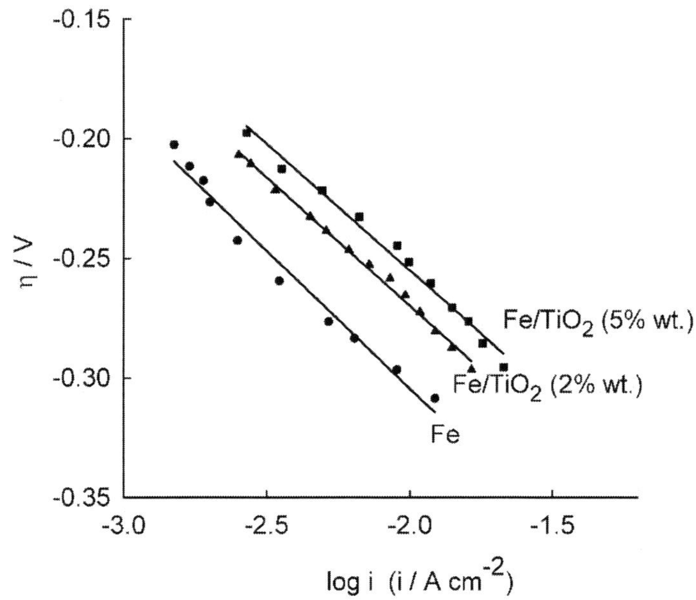

Figure 9. Tafel lines for the HER obtained on Fe and Fe/TiO_2 electrodes in 1 M NaOH solution at 298 K [34].

The exchange current density (i_0) and transfer coefficient (α) can be calculated by the following expressions:

$$\log i_0 = -\frac{a}{b} \tag{6}$$

$$\alpha = -\frac{2.303RT}{bF} \tag{7}$$

where R is the universal gas constant (8.314 J K^{-1} mol^{-1}), T is the thermodynamic temperature (K) and F is the Faraday constant (96487 A s mol^{-1}).

The kinetic parameters, a, b, i_0, α, and the overpotential at cathode current density of 250 mA cm^{-2} (η_{250}), for the selected electrodes are reported in Table 4.

Table 4. Kinetic parameters of the HER obtained from Tafel dependences recorded in 1 M NaOH solution at 298 K [34]

Electrode	a (V)	b (V dec^{-1})	i_0 (A cm^{-2})	α	η_{250} (V)
Fe	-0.528	-0.115	$2.56 \cdot 10^{-5}$	0.51	-0.52
Fe/TiO_2 (2% wt.)	-0.488	-0.108	$3.03 \cdot 10^{-5}$	0.55	-0.49
Fe/TiO_2 (5% wt.)	-0.467	-0.106	$3.93 \cdot 10^{-5}$	0.56	-0.47

It is well known that the HER mechanism in an alkaline solution generally involves three following steps [5, 7]:

(i) electroreduction of water molecule with the formation of an adsorbed hydrogen atom intermediate; Volmer reaction (Eq. (8)),

(ii) electrochemical hydrogen desorption; Heyrovsky reaction (Eq. (9)),

(iii) chemical desorption; Tafel reaction (Eq. (10)).

$$M + H_2O + e^- \Leftrightarrow MH_{ads} + OH^- \tag{8}$$

$$MH_{ads} + H_2O + e^- \Leftrightarrow H_2 + M + OH^- \tag{9}$$

$$MH_{ads} + MH_{ads} \Leftrightarrow H_2 + 2M \tag{10}$$

Here MH_{ads} denotes the hydrogen atom adsorbed on the metal surface.

As can be seen, the Tafel slopes are close to 120 mV dec^{-1}, i.e., the charge transfer coefficients are near to the value of 0.5. This may indicate that the mechanism of the HER on Fe and Fe/TiO_2 coatings under study is the combination of Volmer-Heyrovsky reactions [5, 7]. This means that the rate determining step of multistep hydrogen evolution reaction is the charge transfer (Eq. (8)) followed by the electrochemical desorption (Eq. (9)).

To get additional information on the electrocatalytic behavior of Fe and Fe/TiO_2 electrodeposits, chronoamperometry curves were recorded (Figure 10). This electrochemical method presupposes that the electrolysis is carried out at a constant value of electrode potential with respect to a selected reference electrode while the current flowing through the electrode is recorded as a function of time.

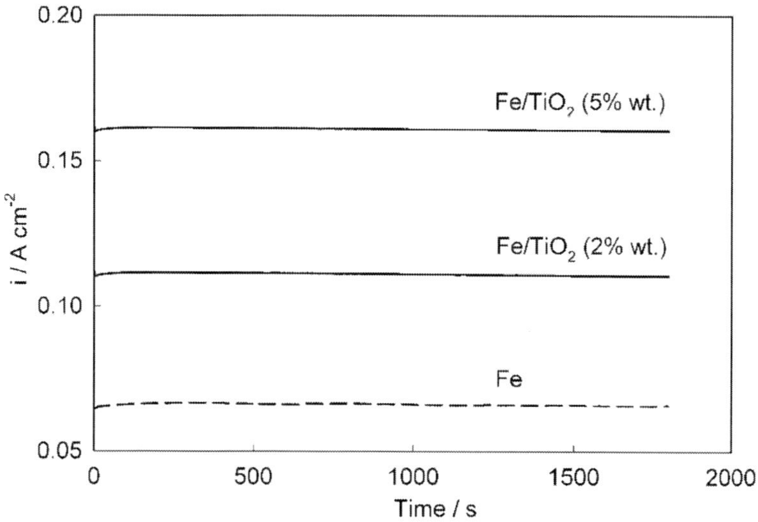

Figure 10. Chronoamperometry curves of the HER for Fe and Fe/TiO_2 composite electrodes with various TiO_2 content at electrode potential $E = -1.25$ V [34].

As can be seen, the current density of the HER increases in the following sequence Fe, Fe/TiO_2 (2%), and Fe/TiO_2 (5%) if the electrode potential is kept at a constant value. This confirms the conclusion that the introduction of titania colloidal particles into the iron matrix electrodeposited from methanesulfonate electrolyte leads to an increase in the electrocatalytic activity towards hydrogen evolution reaction. Additionally, the measured current density does not practically change with time which demonstrates a nearly constant electrocatalytic activity (good catalytic stability of the materials proposed) [12, 21].

In order to obtain more exhaustive data on the kinetics of the HER, the electrochemical impedance spectroscopy (EIS) method was used. EIS is a very sensitive and informative tool for studying electrode reactions [54, 55]. This powerful and non-destructive technique gives reliable and detailed data on the kinetics of various kinds of electrochemical processes. Earlier, EIS has been successfully used to study the electrocatalytic activity of electrodeposited metals, alloys and composites towards the HER [5, 7-13].

Nyquist plots (imaginary values Z_{imag} versus real values Z_{real}) were obtained both at the open circuit potential and at different overpotential values (-100, -200, and -300 mV) for the pure Fe coatings and Fe/TiO_2 electrodeposited composites (Figure 11).

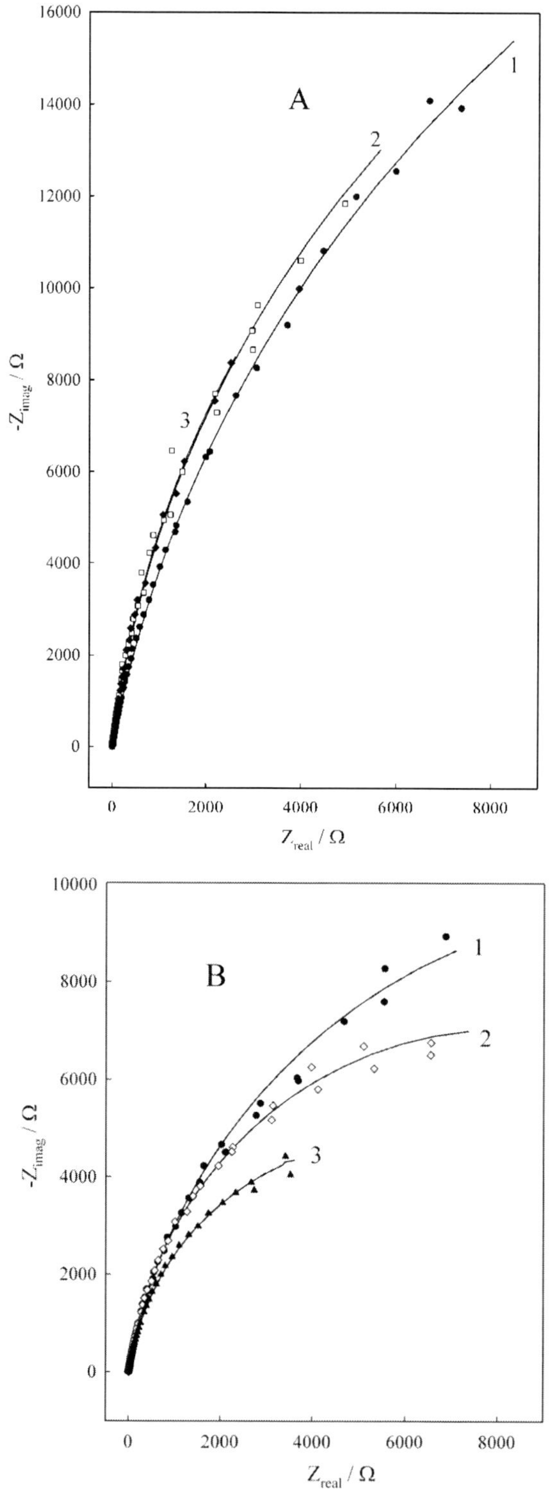

Figure 11. (Continued)

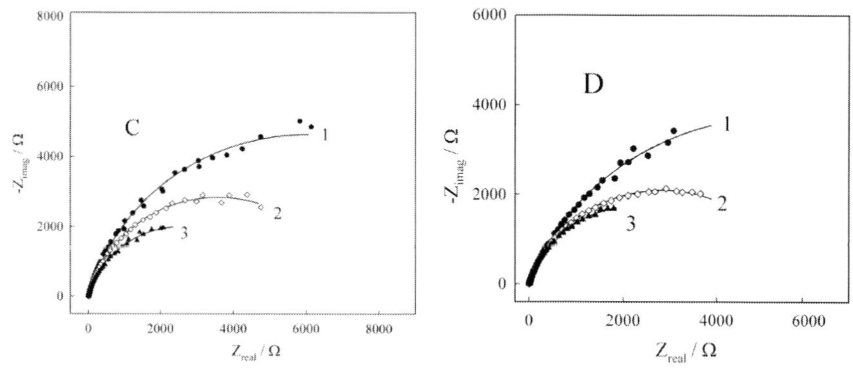

Figure 11. Nyquist plots of Fe (1), Fe/TiO_2 (2% wt.) (2) and Fe/TiO_2 (5% wt.) (3) electrodes in 1 M NaOH at 298 K at various values of overpotential: (A) $\eta = 0$ mV (OCP), (B) $\eta = -100$ mV, (C) $\eta = -200$ mV, (D) $\eta = -300$ mV. The symbols denote the measured (experimental) impedance spectra and solid lines represent fitted results [34].

The Nyquist plots look like depressed semicircles, which indicates that the HER is controlled by the charge transfer step [7]. With increasing overpotential value, the diameter of the semicircles diminishes; therefore, these semicircles are associated with the electrode kinetics [7]. A distorted, asymmetrical semicircle in complex-plane plots suggests inhomogeneity on the electrode surface. This phenomenon can be theoretically described with the so-called constant phase element (CPE) [56]. Taking into account all these considerations, we choose the electrical equivalent circuit (Figure 12) containing the following elements: polarization resistance of the electrochemical reaction (R_{ct}), constant phase element characterizing the interface of "solid electrode/solution" (*CPE*), and ohmic resistance of solution (R_s).

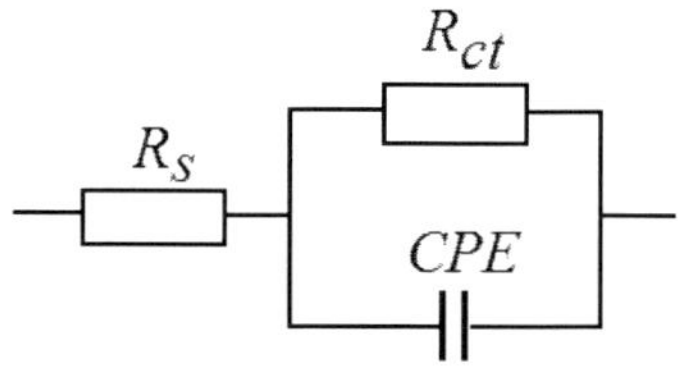

Figure 12. Electrical equivalent circuit modeling the solid electrode/solution interface.

The polarization resistance of the charge transfer process (R_{ct}) is determined as follows [54]:

$$R_{ct} = \lim_{\omega \to 0} R(Z_f) \tag{11}$$

where $R(Z_f)$ is the real part of complex faradaic impedance Z_f corresponding to zero frequency.

The impedance of the constant phase element can be given by the following formula [57]:

$$Z_{CPE} = \left[Q(j\omega)^n\right]^{-1} \qquad (12)$$

in which Q is a constant, $j = \sqrt{-1}$, $\omega = 2\pi f$ is the angular frequency in rad s^{-1}, where f is the frequency in Hertz, and n is the dimensionless empirical exponent corresponding to phase deviation.

The exponent n assumes its values in the range of from 0.5 (porous electrode) to 1 (ideally planar electrode, i.e., a perfect capacitor) [58]. The introduction of constant phase elements into the electrical equivalent circuits is related to the energy and geometric heterogeneity of the electrode surface [56, 57].

The experimental data in Figure 11 are presented as symbols and the continuous lines are obtained by curves fitting using the electrical equivalent circuit shown in Figure 12. The calculated kinetic parameters are summarized in Table 5.

Table 5. Calculated electrochemical impedance parameters of the HER for Fe and Fe/TiO_2 electrodes [34]

Electrode	Overpotential	R_s (Ω)	R_{ct} (kΩ cm^2)	Q (μ$Ω^{-1}$ s^n cm^{-2})	n
Fe	0 (OCP)	2.36	55.60	582.0	0.881
	-100 mV	2.20	23.03	803.2	0.880
	-200 mV	2.12	12.06	828.0	0.834
	-300 mV	2.37	10.52	1186.0	0.782
Fe/TiO_2 (2% wt.)	0 (OCP)	2.28	57.51	841.0	0.913
	-100 mV	2.28	16.18	853.6	0.911
	-200 mV	2.26	7.17	992.0	0.852
	-300 mV	2.26	5.67	1252.1	0.809
Fe/TiO_2 (5% wt.)	0 (OCP)	2.28	57.98	1417.3	0.916
	-100 mV	2.31	11.10	1425.0	0.895
	-200 mV	2.25	5.08	2253.5	0.846
	-300 mV	2.26	4.52	2789.2	0.832

It is interesting to note that the electrochemical impedance parameters measured at OCP for "pure" Fe and composite Fe/TiO_2 coatings with different titania content are very close (in the first approximation, the lines in Figure 11A overlap). However, the difference in the electrochemical behavior between iron and Fe/TiO_2 composites becomes quite evident when cathode current flows through the electrode, i.e., when $\eta \neq 0$ (Figure 11B, 11C and 11D).

The decreasing polarization resistance (R_{ct}) with overpotential can be related to a decrease in the activation energy of the charge transfer process [54]. Other conditions being equal, the R_{ct} value diminishes with an increase in TiO_2 content in electrodeposits. This convincingly confirms that the incorporation of TiO_2 into Fe matrix results in improvement in electrocatalytic properties towards hydrogen evolution reaction.

Q values are often associated with the surface area available for the cathodic reaction [58]. When comparing the *Q* values for iron and iron-titania composites, one could conclude that Fe/TiO_2 composites have more developed true surface area than pure iron coatings. However, it should be observed that the *Q* values are determined not only by average double layer capacitance but also by pseudo-capacitance, the latter may be much higher than the capacity in the double-layer region. Therefore, the determination of the real surface area of solid electrodes on the basis of *Q* measurements is a very difficult problem (see e.g., excellent discussion by Trasatti and Petrii [59]). Thus, it should be wary of estimating surface roughness based on *Q* values. Moreover, the values of parameter *n* increase with increasing TiO_2 content in electrodeposits (Table 5); this indicates diminishing the extent of fractal roughness of the electrode [56].

Summarizing the results of voltammetry and EIS studies, one canconclude that the emergence of surface active sites with enhanced catalytic properties should be the main factor influencing the TiO_2 composite electrode activity towards hydrogen evolution reaction. Earlier Gierlotka et al. [60] showed that the increase in the rate of hydrogen evolution reaction on the composite Ni-P-TiO_2 electrodeposited layer may be directly associated with the presence of TiO_2 and its protonated state or/and redox forms of $Ti_2O_3 \Leftrightarrow TiOOH$ which reinforces an electrocatalytic effect on the HER. The same mechanism of enhancement of the electrocatalytic effect can be also applicable to Fe/TiO_2 composite coatings. The growth of the concentration of surface active sites with increasing TiO_2 content in electrocatalysts leads to further improvement in electrocatalytic activity.

3.2. Electrocatalytic Activity towards Oxygen Evolution Reaction

It is worthwhile to estimate the electrocatalytic activity of the composites under consideration for OER. These data may be of interest for developing new bipolar electrolyzing materials for hydrogen and oxygen production.

The Tafel plots of the OER occurring on Fe and Fe/TiO_2 coatings look more complicated than those of the HER (Figure 13). The important feature evident in Figure 13 is the variation in the Tafel parameters with overpotential. Dual Tafel slopes are exhibited by all the electrocatalysts under study. The Tafel slope ca. 0.04 V dec^{-1} is observed at relatively low overpotentials, whereas the Tafel slope reaches ca. 0.12 V dec^{-}

[1] at higher overpotentials (Table 6). Two regions with different Tafel slopes are typical of oxygen evolution reaction on iron in alkaline media, analogous results were obtained in a number of papers [61-63].

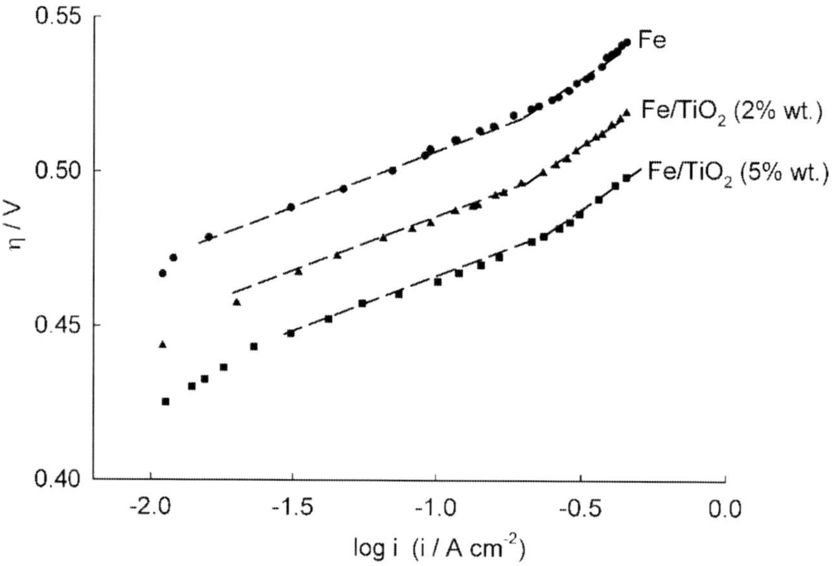

Figure 13. Tafel lines for the OER obtained on Fe and Fe/TiO_2 electrodes in 1 M NaOH solution at 298 K [34].

Table 6. Kinetic parameters of the OER obtained from Tafel dependences recorded in 1 M NaOH solution at 298 K [34]

Electrode	Low overpotentials region			High overpotentials region				
	a (V)	b (V dec^{-1})	i_0 (A cm^{-2})	a (V)	b (V dec^{-1})	β	i_0 (A cm^{-2})	η_{250} (V)
Fe	0.549	0.042	$0.64\cdot10^{-13}$	0.584	0.119	0.49	$1.30\cdot10^{-5}$	0.52
Fe/TiO_2 (2% wt.)	0.525	0.041	$1.09\cdot10^{-13}$	0.562	0.118	0.50	$1.84\cdot10^{-5}$	0.50
Fe/TiO_2 (5% wt.)	0.504	0.039	$1.02\cdot10^{-13}$	0.540	0.116	0.51	$2.29\cdot10^{-5}$	0.48

According to the modern concepts developed in studies [61, 62], the mechanism of the OER on iron electrodes in basic electrolyte is described by the following reaction sequence:

$$SOH_2 + OH^- \rightarrow SOH^- + H_2O \quad (13)$$

$$SOH^- \rightarrow SOH + e^- \quad (14)$$

$$SOH + OH^- \rightarrow SO^- + H_2O \quad (15)$$

$$SO^{-} \rightarrow SO + e^{-} \quad (16)$$

$$SO + OH^{-} \rightarrow SOOH + e^{-} \quad (17)$$

$$SOOH + OH^{-} \rightarrow SO_2 + H_2O + e^{-} \quad (18)$$

$$SO_2 + OH^{-} \rightarrow SOH^{-} + O_2 \quad (19)$$

were *S* represents a surface aquo-group attached to the hydrous oxide surface by bridging oxygen ligands. These groups act as surface catalytic sites [61, 62].

It was earlier shown [61-63] that the step in Eq. (17) may be rate determining at low anodic overpotentials, and then the Tafel slope should be close to 0.04 V dec^{-1}. At higher overpotentials, the formation of surface complexes *SO* (Eq. (16)) becomes rate determining step and the Tafel slope increases to 0.12 V dec^{-1}. It is evident that the experimental findings given above are in good agreement with literature data.

The obtained results show that the calculated values of charge transfer coefficients for the OER (β) do not change when TiO_2 particles are introduced into the iron matrix. This indicates that the mechanism of the electrochemical reaction remains unchanged.

The values of exchange current increase with increasing TiO_2 content in composite coating; hence, the electrocatalytic activity towards oxygen evolution reaction in NaOH solution grows in the following sequence: Fe, Fe/TiO_2 (2%), and Fe/TiO_2 (5%).

The increase in the rate of the OER on Fe/TiO_2 composite electrodes may be connected with the evolution of the surface active sites and resulted from the emergence of the redox couple $TiO_2 \Leftrightarrow Ti_2O_3 \Leftrightarrow$ TiOOH [60]. Indeed, Trasatti [64] pointed out that the electrocatalytic activity of oxide electrodes in different anodic processes is generally governed by the redox behavior of the surface active sites.

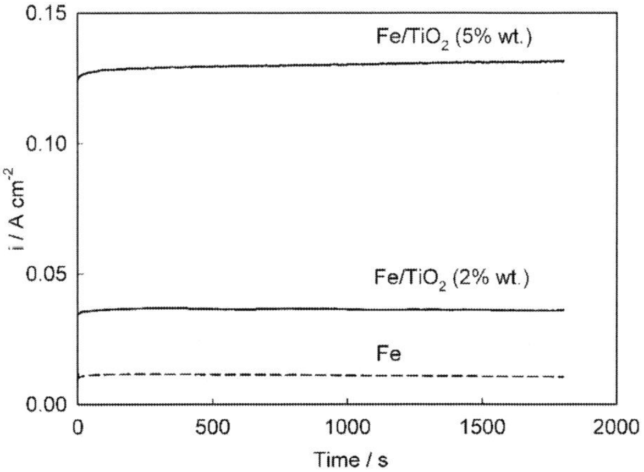

Figure 14. Chronoamperometry curves of the OER for Fe and Fe/TiO_2 composite electrodes with various TiO_2 content at electrode potential E = + 0.9 V [34].

The results of chronoamperometry study (Figure 14) demonstrate that the anodic current density does not practically change with time when the value of overpotential is kept constant. Thus, the electrocatalysts under consideration show good catalytic stability.

4. Photocatalytic Activity of Fe/TiO_2 Composite Electrodeposits Modified by Ceria Layer

Previous publications [45, 46] reported that Fe/TiO_2 composite coatings deposited from methanesulfonate baths showed a high photocatalytic activity towards the reaction of methyl orange dye destruction in aqueous solutions under exposure to UV radiation. However, all data on photocatalytic activity of Fe/TiO_2 composite coatings were obtained for a relatively concentrated alkaline solution (0.1 M NaOH) that is far from the compositions of real wastewaters. The choice of an alkaline solution was due to a fast corrosion of iron matrix in weak-acid or neutral aqueous solutions. Hence, it is necessary to reliably protect iron matrix in Fe/TiO_2 composites against corrosion damage before using them as photocatalysts for wastewater treatment.

In order to improve the corrosion resistance of Fe matrix, cerium oxide layers can be electrodeposited on the metal surface. It is known that ceria films are successfully used for the corrosion protection of iron and steel [65-74]. They are considered as a very promising alternative to the chromate coatings which are extremely dangerous to human health and environment [65, 66].

Ceria layers can be obtained from various types of electrolytes: chloride [65-70], nitrate [71-73], acetate [74]. The application of methanesulfonate systems for ceria electrodeposition was reported for the first time in work [35]; thereby entirely environmentally friendly corrosion inhibitors for iron and its composites have been proposed. An important task was to estimate the effects of protective ceria layers on the photocatalytic performance of immobilized TiO_2 particles.

4.1. Electrodeposition of Cerium Oxide Films on the Surface of Fe/TiO_2 Composites

A methanesulfonate electrolyte was used to deposit ceria layer on the surface of Fe and Fe/TiO_2 coatings [35]. Cerium (III) methanesulfonate solution was synthesized by chemical interaction between concentrated MSA solution and powdered cerium (III) carbonate. The electrolyte for ceria cathodic synthesis contained 0.5 M $Ce(CH_3SO_3)_3$, its pH value was adjusted to 1.3. The electrodeposition was carried out in a galvanostatic mode by means of Potentiostat/Galvanostat Reference 3000 (Gamry). The ohmic potential drop was measured and automatically compensated using the built-in iR-compensator of the potentiostat. All potentials were measured with respect to the saturated Ag/AgCl-electrode and recalculated to the standard hydrogen electrode. The temperature of $Ce(CH_3SO_3)_3$ solution was maintained at 298 K during the electrochemical synthesis of ceria films.

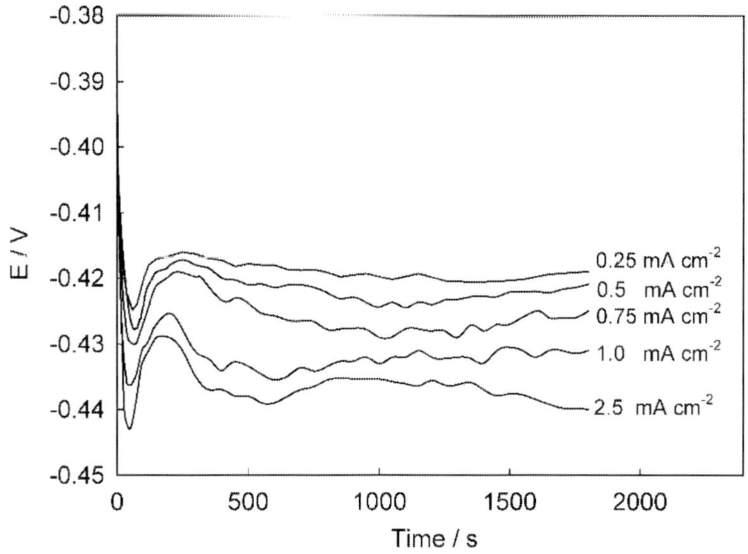

Figure 15. Evolution of electrode potential with deposition time for different applied current densities in 0.5 M $Ce(CH_3SO_3)_3$ solution; pH 1.3; temperature 298 K [35].

The cerium oxide layers were deposited on fresh deposited Fe/TiO_2 composites, the counter electrode was made of platinum sheet. After ceria layer electrodeposition, the samples were rinsed in double distilled water and dried in a hot air jet (ca. 80 °C) for 3 min.

Figure 15 presents the variation of electrode potential versus time during cathodic treatment of as-deposited Fe/TiO_2 composite coatings at different current densities. As can be seen, an abrupt growth of cathode polarization is observed during ca. 50 seconds after turning on the electric current. Then the electrode potential reaches a minimum value and begins to increase. Finally, after about 300-400 seconds, the electrode potential again decreases slightly and stabilizes showing small oscillations. Other conditions being equal, an increase in cathode current density results in a decrease in electrode potential.

This complex behavior of electrode potential with time can be related to diverse electrochemical and chemical reactions occurring on the electrode surface. First of all, hydrogen evolution reaction and electroreduction of oxygen dissolved in solution take place on the electrode in an aqueous medium [71]:

$$2H_2O + 2e^- \rightarrow H_2 + 2OH^- \tag{20}$$

$$2H_3O^+ + 2e^- \rightarrow H_2 + 2H_2O \tag{21}$$

$$O_2 + 2H_2O + 4e^- \rightarrow 4OH^- \tag{22}$$

$$O_2 + 2H_2O + 2e^- \rightarrow 2OH^- + H_2O_2 \tag{23}$$

All these reactions are accompanied by an increase in pH value in the near electrode solution layer because MSA is a very strong acid [38] and its solutions do not show any pronounced buffering effect. As a result, the following reactions of Ce(III) hydroxides and hydroxo-complexes formation can occur on the electrode [71]:

$$Ce^{3+} + 3OH^- \rightarrow Ce(OH)_3 \tag{24}$$

$$4Ce^{3+} + O_2 + 4OH^- + 2H_2O \rightarrow 4[Ce(OH)]_2^{2+} \tag{25}$$

In addition, the further oxidation of Ce(III) with the formation of Ce(IV) complex ions and cerium (IV) oxide layer becomes possible:

$$2Ce^{3+} + 2OH^- + H_2O_2 \rightarrow 2[Ce(OH)]_2^{2+} \tag{26}$$

$$Ce(OH)_3 + O_2 \rightarrow 4CeO_2 + 6H_2O \tag{27}$$

$$[Ce(OH)]_2^{2+} \rightarrow CeO_2 + 2H_2O \tag{28}$$

It is evident that in the initial stage of deposition (first several tens seconds) the nucleation and the growth of nuclei of new solid phase CeO_2 occur on the electrode surface [71]. The formation of some blocking surface layer on Fe matrix hinders both the HER and other electrochemical processes. This causes shifting the electrode potential towards more negative values.

It should be noted that the potential range under consideration (-0.4 … -0.45 V) corresponds to the redox activity of TiO_{2-x} [53, 75]. For the sake of convenience, the cathode reaction of Ti(IV) reduction can be written in the following simplified form:

$$Ti(IV) + e^- \rightarrow Ti(III) \tag{29}$$

This solid-phase process proceeds on the cathode simultaneously with the reactions of Eqs. (20)-(28). It has been stated that the presence of TiO_2, its protonated states and/or redox forms of $Ti_2O_3 \Leftrightarrow TiOOH$ reinforces an electrocatalytic effect towards the HER [60]. The redox activity of titanium dioxide causes enhanced electrocatalytic properties of Fe/TiO_2 composites obtained from methanesulfonate electrolytes. The growth of the concentration of surface active sites may result in some disinhibition of the HER and a decrease in cathodic overpotential which is observed after the reaching of a potential minimum (see Figure 15).

If the current density exceeded the value of about 3 mA cm^{-2}, the electrodeposition experiments showed the formation of a brownish spongy deposit of CeO_2 practically without any adhesion to the substrate. Therefore, the electrochemical synthesis of ceria layer was performed in all further experiments at current densities less than 3 mA cm^{-2}.

The cathodic treatment of Fe/TiO_2 coatings in methanesulfonate electrolyte leads to the change in their visible surface appearance. If before treating they are light grey, they become greyish-blue with a sheen resembling temper colors on oxidized steel surface after the formation of ceria films. At the same time, the SEM images of Fe and Fe/TiO_2 electrodeposits presented in Figure 16 do not show any noticeable differences between electrodeposits with and without ceria films. Indeed, similarly to the SEM images given above (see Figure 6), there is a superficial network of cracks on the surface of "pure" iron (Figure 16A). In case of Fe/TiO_2 electroplating, the SEM analysis reveals a number of agglomerated flakelike TiO_2 particles entrapped by iron matrix (Figure 16B). Thus, no visible specific features of surface morphology appear in SEM images after the cathodic treatment of samples with Fe and Fe/TiO_2 coatings in methanesulfonate electrolytes. This behavior may be connected with a very small thickness of the obtained ceria layer. The gravimetric measurements do not show any weight gain of the samples even after 30 minutes of electrochemical treatment in methanesulfonate solutions. If we take into account the sensitivity of the utilized analytical balance ($\Delta m = 5 \cdot 10^{-5}$ g), the density of CeO_2 ($\rho = 7.65$ g cm^{-3} [76]) and the surface area of the sample (S = 1 cm^2), then we can easily estimate the upper limit of the thickness of cerium oxide layer (δ) by means of the following formulae:

$$\delta = \frac{\Delta m}{\rho \cdot S} \tag{30}$$

The calculated value of the thickness proved to be close to 60-70 nm. Earlier the deposition of nanometer-thick ceria films has been reported in a number of publications [74, 77].

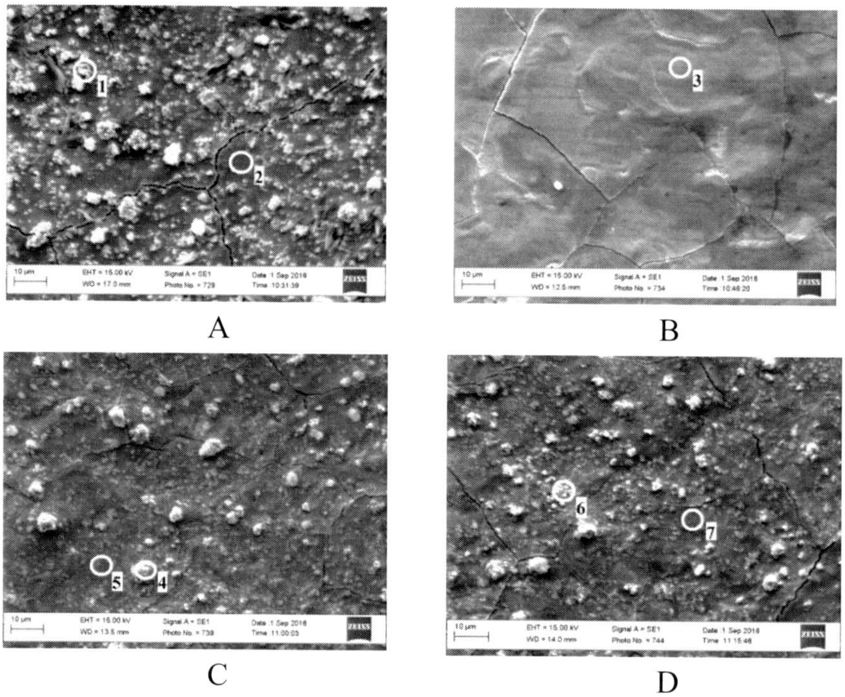

Figure 16. SEM images of (A) Fe/TiO_2 composite coating, (B) Fe coating with electrodeposited ceria layer, (C) Fe/TiO_2 composite coating with electrodeposited ceria layer (0.25 mA cm^{-2}, 1800 s), (D) Fe/TiO_2 composite coating with electrodeposited ceria layer (1 mA cm^{-2}, 1800 s). The results of EDX analysis for the marked points are given in Table 7 [35].

Although the SEM images did not show any changes in the surface morphology of Fe and Fe/TiO_2 coatings after cathodic treatment in methanesulfonate electrolyte, the EDX investigations clearly revealed the presence of cerium oxides on the surface. Table 7 summarizes the typical results of local EDX analysis performed at several points over the surface which are marked in Figure 16.

Table 7. Chemical composition at points marked in Figure 16 [35]

Elements	Content (at.%)						
	1	2	3	4	5	6	7
O	64.92	11.77	16.64	61.16	14.04	65.51	12.20
Ti	6.04	0.54	-	12.87	1.52	7.55	1.01
Fe	29.04	87.69	82.79	25.33	83.14	26.32	85.53
Ce	-	-	0.57	0.64	1.30	0.62	1.26

The EDX analysis indicated the presence of Fe, O, Ti (only for Fe/TiO_2 composites) and Ce (only for the coatings treated in $Ce(CH_3SO_3)_3$ solution). No other elements have been detected.

As stated above, the flakelike particles with an average size of about several micrometers that can be clearly seen on the surface in SEM images are associated with agglomerated TiO_2. According to EDX data, the surface in these regions consists essentially of titanium, oxygen and iron.

The surface of Fe/TiO_2 electrodeposits in the regions which are free from the flakelike agglomerated particles mainly consists of iron and oxygen and also contains a small amount of titanium. The detection of oxygen in the regions that are free from the incorporated dispersed TiO_2 particles can be explained by easy oxidation of fresh deposited iron surface resulted from contacting with atmospheric oxygen and moist air.

The electrodeposited cerium (in the form of its oxide) is for the most part concentrated in the zones without TiO_2 agglomerates (i.e., on the segmental surfaces corresponding to the "free" iron matrix). The variation of current density has no considerable effect on the cerium content on the surface.

Despite a relative small thickness of the synthesized cerium oxide layers, their adhesion to the substrate seems to be satisfactory. At least, according to the obtained EDX data, these ceria films cannot be removed from the surface after rinsing by water.

4.2. Corrosion-Electrochemical Behavior of Fe/TiO_2 Composites Modified by Cerium Oxide Films

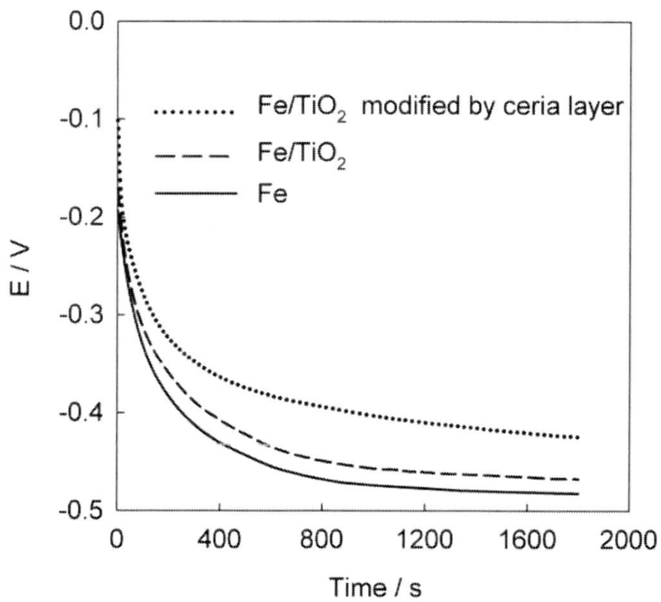

Figure 17. Variation of open circuit potential (OCP) with time for Fe coating and Fe/TiO_2 composite coatings without and with electrodeposited ceria films in 3% NaCl solution at 298 K. Cathodic treatment in 0.5 M $Ce(CH_3SO_3)_3$ was performed at 1 mA cm^{-2} during 1800 s [35].

The open circuit potential (OCP) vs. time curves, as depicted in Figure 17, were recorded for Fe coating and Fe/TiO_2 composite coatings without and with electrodeposited ceria films in an aggressive environment containing 3% NaCl. The obtained results show a decrease of OCP during a short transition period; then the OCP value reaches practically a steady-state condition.

The introduction of titania particles into the Fe matrix (i.e., electrodeposition of composite coatings) results in an increase of OCP indicating an enhancement of corrosion stability. An increase in OCP means that the improvement in corrosion resistance is provided not only by the formation of a protective physical barrier, which partially blocks the electrode surface and is composed of "inert" TiO_2 particles, but also by the formation of corrosion micro-cells in which TiO_2 acts as cathode and Fe matrix as anode.

A further shift of corrosion potentials to nobler values is observed when cerium oxide layers have been deposited on the composite surface. An increase of OCP of the samples, modified by ceria film, is attributed to the occurrence of another cathodic process in addition to the oxygen and Ti(IV) electroreduction reactions and the hydrogen evolution reaction. Indeed, the reduction of CeO_2 as a very effective depolarization process can occur at the corrosion potentials according to the following reactions [66]:

$$CeO_2 + 2H^+ \rightarrow Ce(OH)_2^{2+} \tag{31}$$

$$2Ce(OH)_2^{2+} + 2e^- \rightarrow Ce_2O_3 + H_2O + 2H^+ \tag{32}$$

The released Ce(III) compounds can be again oxidized to Ce(IV) which provides the so-called self-healing properties of ceria thin films [78, 79].

Figure 18 represents typical potentiodynamic polarization curves obtained during the first scanning in 3% NaCl solution for the studied electrodeposits. The current wave corresponding to the anodic dissolution of iron shifts towards more positive potentials in the following sequence: Fe, Fe/TiO_2, and Fe/TiO_2 modified by ceria layer. This suggests the inhibition of iron dissolution rate in case of TiO_2 particles incorporation and, especially, after the cathode treatment in electrolyte containing cerium (III) methanesulfonate. The anodic segments of the obtained voltammograms are well linearized in coordinates E vs. log i (Figure 19) which allows calculating the Tafel slopes (b_a) and corrosion currents (Table 8). The degree of inhibition efficiency, Z, has been calculated by the following equation:

$$Z(\%) = \frac{i_{corr,o} - i_{corr}}{i_{corr,0}} \times 100\% \tag{33}$$

where $i_{corr,0}$ and i_{corr} are the corrosion currents of "pure" iron coatings and iron-titania composites (with or without modification by ceria layer), respectively.

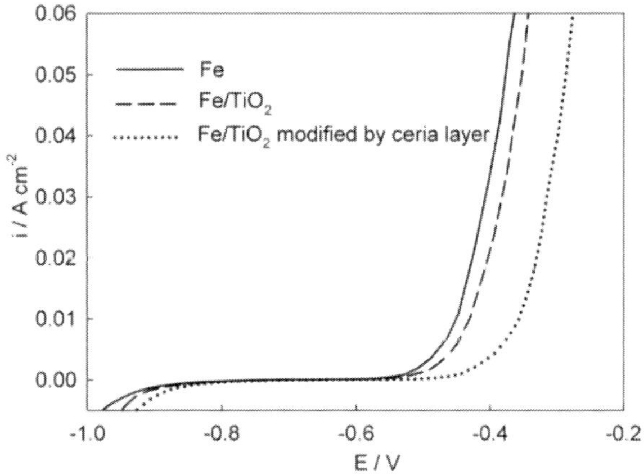

Figure 18. Polarization curves of Fe coating and Fe/TiO_2 composite coatings without and with electrodeposited ceria films in 3% NaCl solution at 298 K (scanning rate 5 mV s^{-1}). Cathodic treatment in 0.5 M $Ce(CH_3SO_3)_3$ was performed at 1 mA cm^{-2} during 1800 s [35].

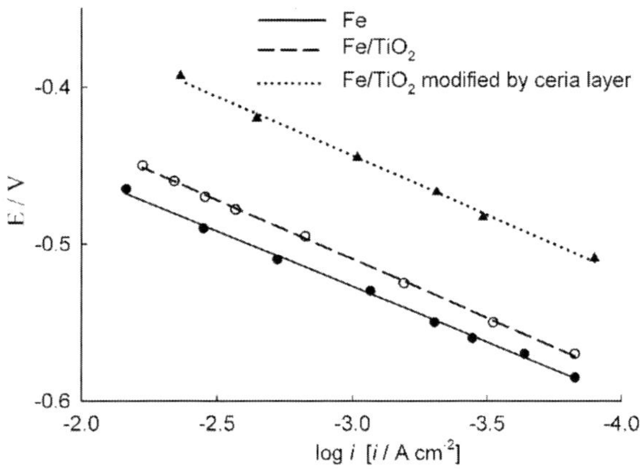

Figure 19. Plots of *E* vs. log *i* for the anodic segments of voltammograms presented in Figure 18 [35].

Table 8. Electrochemical parameters characterizing the corrosion behavior of coatings in 3% NaCl solution at 298 K according to potentiodynamic polarization measurements [35]

Coating	b_a (V dec^{-1})	E_{corr} (V)	i_{corr} (mA cm^{-2})	Z (%)
Fe	0.071	-0.455	10.47	-
Fe/TiO_2 (5% wt. of titania)	0.075	-0.435	10.09	3.6
Fe/TiO_2 (5% wt. of titania) modified by ceria layer	0.075	-0.387	5.89	43.7

It can be clearly seen in Table 8 that the calculated Tafel slopes for all coatings under study are practically identical which indicates that the mechanism of anodic process (electrochemical dissolution of Fe matrix) remains unchanged. The inclusion of titania particles in electrodeposited iron matrix causes only a slight increase in corrosion resistance (Z = 3.6%). At the same time, the modification of composites surface by ceria layer results in a significant increase in the corrosion stability and the degree of inhibition efficiency increases to Z = 43.7%, although does not approaches 100%. Nevertheless, these data suggest that the corrosion resistance of the modified coatings will be satisfactory in media containing no such aggressive environment as sodium chloride solution (for instance, wastewater containing organic pollutants with pH near to neutral values).

In order to obtain more comprehensive data on the kinetics of corrosion process, the electrochemical impedance spectroscopy method was used. Nyquist plots (imaginary values Z_{imag} versus real values Z_{real}) were obtained at the OCP for the "pure" Fe coatings and Fe/TiO_2 electrodeposited composites with and without ceria layer on their surface (Figure 20). Nyquist plots of as-deposited iron and iron/titania composite coatings without CeO_2 film look like conventional depressed semicircles which indicates that the electrochemical reaction is controlled by the charge transfer step and occurs on inhomogeneous surface [56].

Nyquist plots obtained for iron and iron/titania composite coatings with electrodeposited film of cerium oxide are more complicated. In addition to capacitive loop at higher frequencies, the electrochemical impedance spectra show diffusion behavior at lower frequencies indicating Warburg impedance [80]. Thus one can conclude that the impedance values measured at the high-frequencies range only responded to the surface characteristics of the corroded Fe matrix, whereas the precipitation of CeO_2 films forms a thin passive barrier layer which is responsible for diffusion behavior resulted in Warburg resistance at lower frequencies [80].

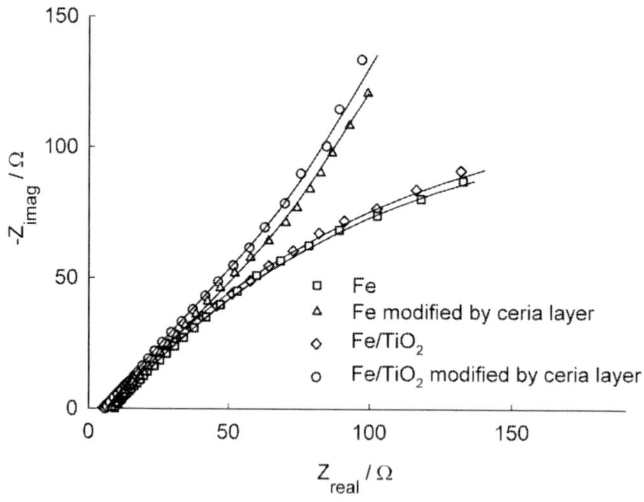

Figure 20. Nyquist plots of Fe and Fe/TiO_2 composite coatings with and without modification by ceria layer in 3% NaCl solution at OCP and temperature of 298 K. Cathodic treatment in 0.5 M $Ce(CH_3SO_3)_3$ was performed at 1 mA cm^{-2} during 1800 s. The symbols denote the measured (experimental) impedance spectra and solid lines represent fitted results [35].

Taking into account the above arguments, two typical electrical equivalent circuits were used to fit experimental data as shown in Figure 21. The first equivalent circuit (Figure 21A) fully coincides with that presented in Figure 12 and is duplicated here for the sake of convenience. This equivalent circuit contains polarization resistance of the electrochemical reaction (R_{ct}), constant phase element (*CPE*), and ohmic resistance of solution (R_{sol}). The polarization resistance of the charge transfer process (R_{ct}) is determined by expression (11). The impedance of the constant phase element can be given by formula (12). The first electrical equivalent circuit shown in Fig. 21A was employed for the description of the corrosion behavior of as-deposited coatings without surface ceria modification.

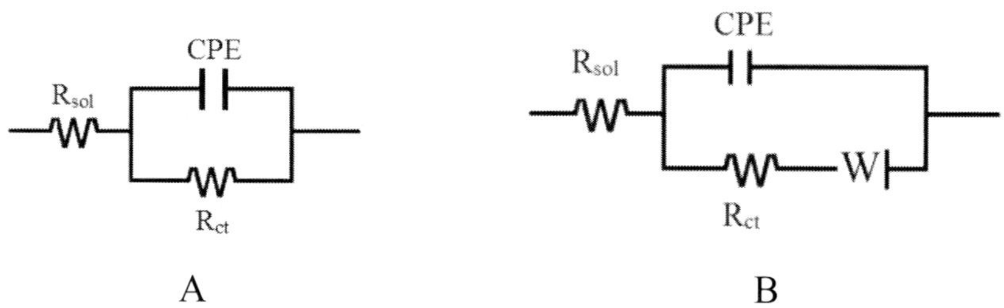

Figure 21. Electrical equivalent circuits modeling the solid electrode/solution interface: (A) for as-deposited coatings without surface ceria modification, and (B) for coatings modified by ceria layer [35].

The second equivalent circuit (Figure 21B), used for the modeling of electrochemical impedance spectra recorded for the corrosion of the coatings with CeO_2 layer, additionally contains the so-called finite Warburg impedance which is given by the following equation [81]:

$$W_c = \left[Y_W (j\omega)^{1/2}\right]^{-1} \coth\left[B(j\omega)^{1/2}\right] \tag{34}$$

where Y_W is the proportionality factor, $B = \delta / D^{1/2}$, δ is the diffusion-layer thickness, and D is the diffusion coefficient.

The experimental data in Fig. 20 are presented as symbols and the continuous lines are obtained by curves fitting using the electrical equivalent circuits shown in Fig. 21. The calculated kinetic parameters are summarized in Table 9.

As can be seen in Table 9, the values of parameter n are appreciably less than unity. This means a relatively high extent of fractal roughness of the electrode [57] and, in the general case, could be favorable to catalytic performance.

Table 9. Calculated electrochemical impedance parameters [35]

Electrode	R_{sol} (Ω)	R_{ct} (Ω cm^2)	$Q\cdot10^3$ (Ω^{-1} s^n cm^{-2})	n	$Y_W\cdot10^3$ (Ω^{-1} s$^{1/2}$)	$B\cdot10^3$ (s$^{1/2}$)
Fe coating	9.74	354.1	25.6	0.603	-	-
Fe coating modified by CeO_2	8.01	587.9	24.7	0.583	284.4	52.7-
Fe/TiO_2 coating	5.43	443.6	21.38	0.569	-	-
Fe/TiO_2 coating modified by CeO_2	6.31	611.6	27.15	0.605	224.1	80.3

In the adopted electrical equivalent circuits, the value of R_{ct} can be considered as a parameter which can define the corrosion resistance of a coating in a general way. It is clear that the introduction of TiO_2 particles into the iron matrix results in some improvement in the corrosion stability. However, the electrodeposition of ceria layers has a far greater influence on the values of R_{ct} both for "pure" iron coatings and for Fe/TiO_2 ones. All these results are in full agreement with those obtained from voltammetric studies and OCP measurements (see above) and indicate that the modification of the deposits surface by cerium oxide films considerably enhances the corrosion stability.

4.3. Photocatalytic Activity of Fe/TiO_2 Composites

The photocatalytic activity of TiO_2 particles immobilized on composite electrodeposits was evaluated for the reactions of photochemical degradation of methyl orange (MO) and methylene blue (MB) dyes in water [82-84]. The initial concentration of MO dye was $6.11\cdot10^{-6}$ mol dm^{-3} (i.e., $2\cdot10^{-3}$ g dm^{-3}). The initial concentrations of MB were $2.5\cdot10^{-5}$, $5\cdot10^{-5}$ and $1\cdot10^{-4}$ mol dm^{-3}. The investigations were conducted both in aqueous solutions with natural pH and in 0.1 M NaOH as a supporting electrolyte. The decolorization kinetics was studied during 75-90 min at the temperature of 298 K.

The photocatalytic activity of the catalysts was tested using an in-house fabricated reactor (Figure 22). A DKB 9 UV lamp with an effective spectral range of 180–275 nm was used as the irradiation source. The intensity of UV irradiation was measured to be ca. 3 mW cm^{-2}. The lamp was arranged over the dye solution at a distance of 10 cm from its surface. In the course of photocatalytic decomposition, the dye solution with working volume of 20 cm^3 was continuously stirred with a magnetic agitator. Steel plate with the electrodeposited composite catalyst (3 cm^2) was placed at a depth of 2 mm in the solution parallel to its surface (i.e., at the angle of 90° to the UV radiation beam). The content of a dye in the solution was determined as a function of irradiation time from the absorbance change at wavelengths of 490 nm and 670 nm for MO and MB solutions, respectively.

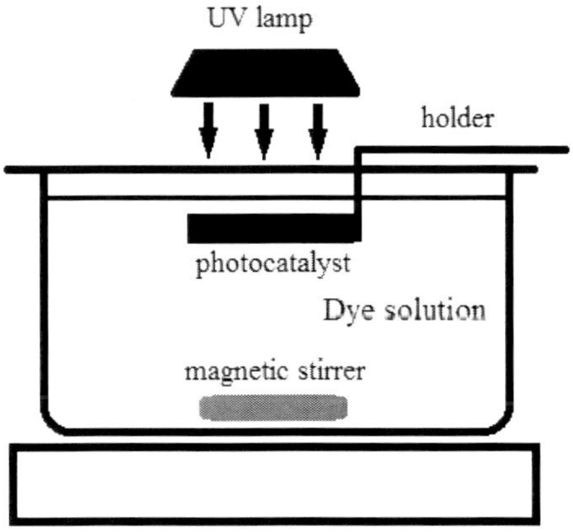

Figure 22. Schematic diagram of reactor for photochemical decomposition of organic dyes [35].

The kinetic curves for the process of MO decolorization are given in Figure 23. First of all, it should be stressed that MO does not undergo spontaneous decomposition in the dark (without UV illumination) both in the presence of the Fe/TiO_2 composite immersed in the dye solution and in its absence. In addition, no photocatalytic properties of Fe coatings modified by ceria layers were observed under the condition of UV radiation. The destruction of MO molecules occurs in solutions exposed to UV radiation, this process considerably accelerates in the presence of the Fe/TiO_2 composite catalyst (see Figure 23).

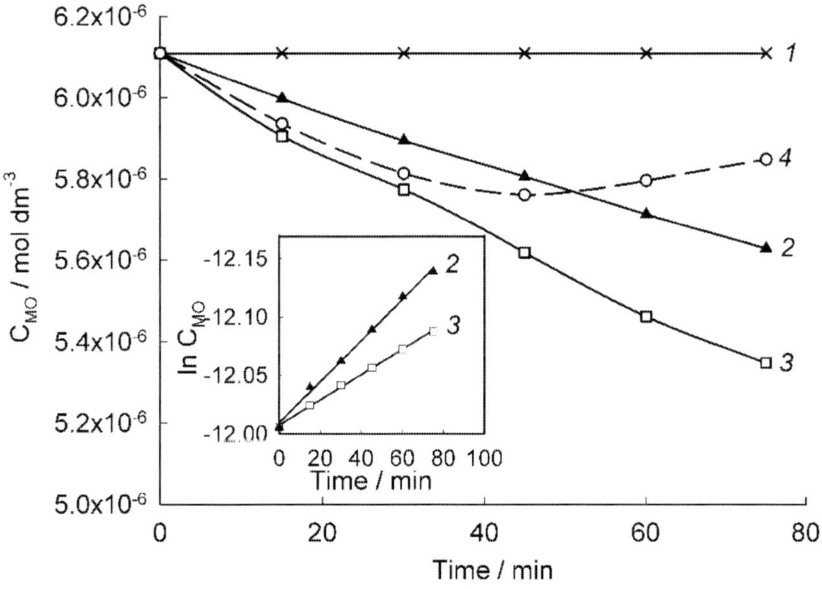

Figure 23. Kinetic curves of the degradation of MO dye in aqueous solution: (1) in the dark, (2) under UV irradiation without photocatalyst, (3) under UV irradiation with Fe/TiO_2 modified by ceria layer, and (4) under UV irradiation with Fe/TiO_2 (not modified). In the insert: first-order linear transforms $lnC = f(\tau)$ [35].

The decay in dyes concentration during their photodegradation often obeys the pseudo-first order kinetics [82]. To ascertain the kinetic model describing the reaction of MO destruction, the plots following the first order model were obtained according to the following equation:

$$\ln C = \ln C_0 - k\tau \tag{35}$$

where C is the concentration of dye at time τ; C_0 is the initial concentration of dye (at $\tau = 0$), and k is the apparent rate constant.

Kinetic curves linearized in the coordinates of "logarithm of the MO concentration *versus* time" (see the insert in Figure 23) do indicate the pseudo-first reaction order. The slopes of these lines give the apparent rate constants which are equal to 0.0011 and 0.0018 min^{-1} for the dye destruction without catalyst (photolysis) and in the presence of the Fe/TiO_2 photocatalyst, respectively.

A kinetic curve was recorded that characterizes the photocatalytic MO destruction in the presence of Fe/TiO_2 composite catalyst without its cathode treatment in cerium (III) based electrolyte (Figure 23, curve 4). It turned out that the obtained kinetic curve has a minimum, the occurrence of which is somewhat unexpected. In order to elucidate this behavior, we measured the time dependences of absorbance of water and MO solutions contacting with Fe/TiO_2 coatings in the dark (Figure 24).

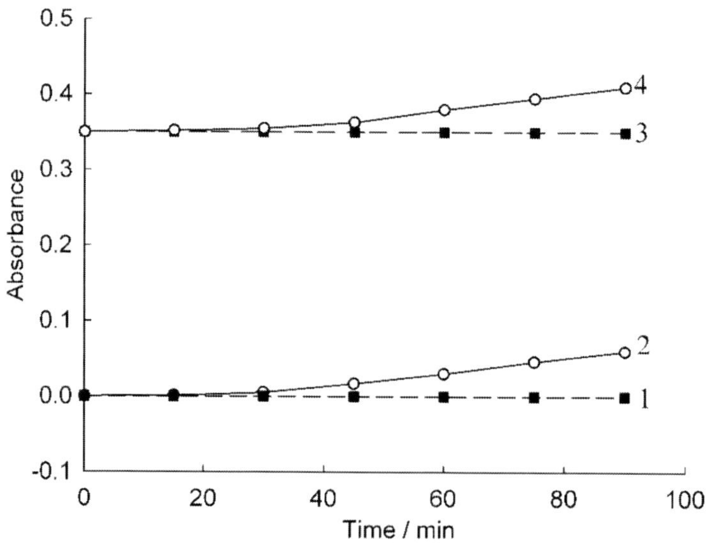

Figure 24. Variation of absorbance with time for (1), (2) pure water and (3), (4) for aqueous solution of $6.11 \cdot 10^{-6}$ mol dm^{-3} MO in which Fe/TiO_2 coatings (2), (4) without any surface modification and (1), (3) modified by CeO_2 were immersed. Wavelength $\lambda = 490$ nm, absorption layer thickness $l = 30$ mm [35].

As can be seen, absorbance does not change with time in cases of the Fe/TiO_2 composites modified by CeO_2 both in water and in a neutral solution of methyl orange dye. However, as-deposited Fe/TiO_2 coating without cathode treatment shows a growth in measured absorbance about 15 min after the beginning of experiment. This phenomenon is due to a rapid corrosion damage of unprotected iron matrix in water. The corrosion products in the form of a yellowish iron hydroxide sol are accumulated in liquid which is also easily visible to the unaided eye. Evidently, the absorbance associated with the presence of iron hydroxide sol distorts the results of the spectral determination of dye content and causes an observed increase in light absorption.

Taking into account these observations, one can conclude that the appearance of an ascending segment of curve 4 in Figure 23 (after reaching a minimum) is caused by the accumulation of Fe matrix corrosion products in a solution rather than by the actual changes in dye concentration.

In addition, the data presented in Figure 24 confirm that the modification of Fe/TiO_2 composites surface by ceria layer provides a good protection against corrosion destruction, whereas composites without protective films rapidly corrode in aqueous medium even at pH close to neutral values.

It should be observed that the kinetic curves recorded for the Fe/TiO_2 composite photocatalysts, which were modified by ceria layers electrodeposited at different current densities (0.25 and 1 mA cm^{-2}), coincide with each other.

If we compare the initial segments in curves 2 and 4 in Figure 23 where corrosion products of unmodified Fe/TiO_2 surface do not strongly distort the results of the spectral measurements, then we can easily see that these segments of the curves practically coincide. This means that the cathode treatment in cerium (III) methanesulfonate solutions does not affect the photocatalytic activity.

It was interesting to establish the effect of the modification by ceria layer upon the photocatalytic activity of Fe/TiO_2 composites in an alkaline solution where iron does not corrode and, hence, the corrosion products will not interfere with spectral measurements. Figure 25 presents the kinetic curves of the degradation of methyl orange dye under UV irradiation in 0.1 M NaOH solution in the presence of the Fe/TiO_2 photocatalysts with and without modification by CeO_2 film. The lines are given in the coordinates of ln C vs. time. As can be seen, these lines practically coincide. The corresponding apparent rate constant was calculated to be 0.0128 min^{-1}. The results for the photolysis of MO (i.e., in the absence of Fe/TiO_2 composite) are shown for comparison. The apparent rate constant of photolysis is equal to 0.0054 min^{-1}.

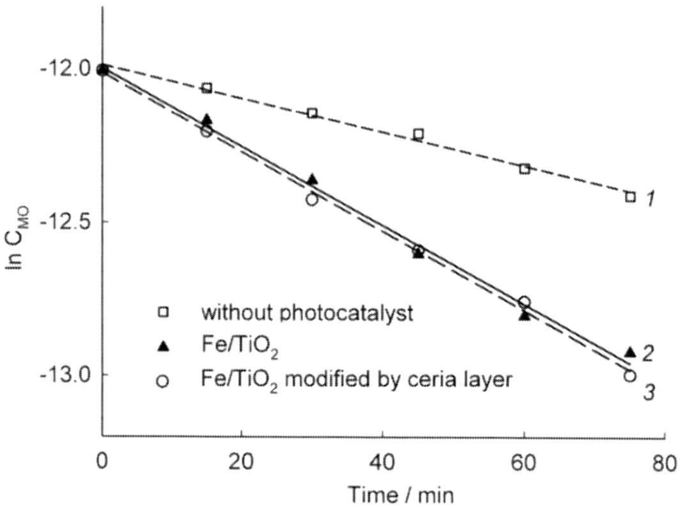

Figure 25. Kinetic curves of the degradation of MO dye in 0.1 M NaOH: (1) under UV irradiation without photocatalyst,(2) under UV irradiation with Fe/TiO_2 (not modified), and (3) under UV irradiation with Fe/TiO_2 modified by ceria layer. The data are presented as first-order linear transforms $lnC = f(\tau)$ [35].

Two conclusions can be drawn on the basis of these findings. Firstly, the rates of photolysis and photocatalytic destruction increase with higher pH's, other conditions being equal. According to ref. [85], an enhanced photocatalytic efficiency of TiO_2 at basic pH is mainly attributed to an increase in the surface density of TiO^- adsorption sites rather than to an increase in the generation of more •OH radicals formed by the reaction of OH^- with positive holes in semiconductor. Secondly, the electrodeposition of a cerium oxide film on the surface of Fe/TiO_2 composites has no effect on the photocatalytic performance both in alkaline solutions and in solutions with pH's close to neutral values.

At the same time, it is well-known that the efficiency of TiO_2 photocatalytic materials can be improved by their doping with other elements, including cerium [29]. However, neither the occurrence of photocatalytic activity in the visible light region nor the improvement of UV light-induced photocatalytic properties after electrochemical treating the composites in electrolytes containing Ce(III) ions have been detected. Probably, the adopted procedure of cathodic treatment does not lead to the doping of TiO_2 because the electrodeposition of ceria films is performed after the synthesis of titania particles and, therefore, cannot change the chemical composition, crystal and electronic structures which are crucial issues in TiO_2 doping [29].

The plot of change in the concentration of methylene blue dye with the time of irradiation is shown in Figure 26. Experiments were also made in the absence of Fe/TiO_2 composites (neat photochemical regime, not shown). The results suggested that the photolysis of MB could be neglected with respect to the photocatalysis. The kinetics of MB photodegradation followed the pseudo-first reaction order. The calculated value of the apparent rate constant was stated to be 0.0056 min^{-1} and independent of the initial concentration of the dye that is typical of the first reaction order [86].

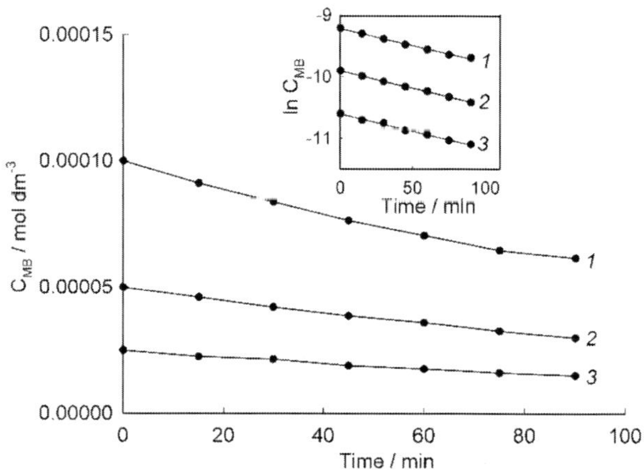

Figure 26. Kinetic curves of the photocatalytic degradation at various initial concentrations of MB dye in solution. In the insert: first-order linear transforms
$lnC = f(\tau)$ [35].

In order to contextualize the obtained data on MO and MB dyes photodegradation by using the composite Fe/TiO_2 photocatalyst, the calculated values of apparent rate constant and half-life of organic dyes are summarized in Table 10. The half-life, $\tau_{1/2}$, for the processes of the pseudo-first reaction order was evaluated by the following expression [86]:

$$\tau_{1/2} = \frac{\ln 2}{k} \quad (36)$$

Table 10. Calculated values of apparent constant and half-life for the reaction of methyl orange and methylene blue dyes degradation on Fe/TiO_2 photocatalyst under UV irradiation [35]

System	k (min^{-1})	$\tau_{1/2}$ (min)
MO in aqueous solution (at natural pH)	0.0018	385.1
MO in 0.1 M NaOH aqueous solution	0.0128	54.2
MB in aqueous solution (at natural pH)	0.0056	123.8

As follows from the obtained data, Fe/TiO_2 composite coatings can be considered as a relatively efficient photocatalyst with respect to the reaction of destruction of the MO and MB dyes in aqueous solutions under exposure to UV radiation.

As concerns the mechanism of heterogeneous photocatalysis taking place at the surface of TiO_2 particles immobilized on iron matrix, it evidently satisfies the recognized basic mechanism which involves the steps of the absorption of a photon, the excitation of an electron with simultaneous generation of a positive hole, the further oxidation of water molecules with the formation of •OH radicals, and the reduction of molecular oxygen with the formation of superoxide radical anions, hydroperoxyl radicals and hydrogen peroxide [28, 29]. All these reactive oxygen-containing species can contribute to the oxidative pathways such as the degradation of organic pollutants. It is known that TiO_2/UV-based photocatalysis provides practically total mineralization of organic dyes (such as MO and MB) and their final oxidation into CO_2, SO_4^{2-}, NO_3^- and H_2O [83, 84, 87].

CONCLUSION

Fe/TiO_2 composite coatings with titania content up to 5% wt. are synthesized by electrodeposition method from an environmentally friendly methanesulfonate iron plating bath containing titania nanopowder. The TiO_2 nano-particles are shown to tend to aggregate in the methanesulfonate electrolyte.

The amount of the TiO_2 particles in the electrodeposited composite coatings increases with an increase in the TiO_2 concentrations in the suspension electrolyte and with a decrease in the current density. The kinetics of Fe and TiO_2 codeposition is adequately described by the improved Guglielmi's model. The values of the surface coverage due to strong and weak adsorption at different concentrations of suspension have been calculated and the adsorption coefficient of TiO_2 has been determined. The inclusion of titania particles in the iron matrix results in an increase in microhardness of electrodeposits.

The Fe/TiO_2 composites exhibit enhanced electrocatalytic activity towards hydrogen and oxygen evolution reactions in 1 M NaOH solution. The kinetic parameters of the HER and OER are calculated from Tafel plots and the results of EIS investigations; possible mechanisms of electrode processes are discussed. A higher catalytic activity of Fe/TiO_2 composites towards hydrogen and oxygen evolution reactions may be associated with the growth of the concentration of the surface active sites and the presence of the redox couple containing titanium compounds in different valence states. The results of chronoamperometry study confirm good catalytic stability of the Fe/TiO_2 electrocatalysts, which makes them promising for alkaline electrolyzers to produce hydrogen and oxygen.

The synthesized Fe-TiO_2 composite coatings manifest high photocatalytic activity with respect to the reactions of the destruction of some organic dyes in aqueous solutions under exposure to UV radiation.

Although iron matrix seems to be a cheap, available, and environmentally safe anchor for TiO_2 particles and possesses satisfactory mechanical properties, its corrosion resistivity is not satisfactory enough. To enhance the corrosion stability, the modification of the surface of Fe/TiO_2 composite coatings by CeO_2 film is suggested via electrodeposition technique using a methanesulfonate electrolyte containing Ce(III) ions.

A specific feature of the ceria deposits obtained from MSA-based electrolytes is their relatively small thickness. This may be regarded as an advantage of the proposed procedure, because otherwise thicker layers of cerium oxides would block the active surface of TiO_2 aggregates embedded in iron matrix and reduce the photocatalytic activity.

A detailed study of corrosion-electrochemical behavior by means of voltammetry method and electrochemical impedance spectroscopy revealed that the electrodeposition of ceria film on the surface of Fe matrix improves the corrosion resistance. This creates favorable conditions for the practical application of such photocatalysts for the degradation of organic pollutants in aqueous media with natural pH (i.e., close to neutral values). Without protective cerium oxide films, the composite Fe/TiO_2 coatings undergo fast corrosion damage.

The Fe/TiO_2 composites modified by CeO_2 layers have been successfully passed the test in the reactions of the photochemical degradation of methyl orange and methylene blue dyes in water under the action of UV irradiation. Apparently, the modification of Fe/TiO_2 composites surface by cerium oxide layers has no effect on their photocatalytic performance in the reaction of MO and MB dyes destruction.

REFERENCES

[1] Low, C. T. J., Wills, R. G. A., Walsh F. C. (2006). Electrodeposition of composite coatings containing nanoparticles in a metal deposit. *Surface and Coatings Technology, 201*, 371-383.

[2] Walsh, F. C., Ponce de Leon, C. (2014) A review of the electrodeposition of metal matrix composite coatings by inclusion of particles in a metal layer: an established and diversifying technology. *Transactions of the Institute of Metal Finishing, 92*, 83-98.

[3] Musiani, M. (2000). Electrodeposition of composites: an expanding subject in electrochemical materials science. *Electrochimica Acta, 45*, 3397-3402.

[4] Bockris, J. O'M. (2002). The origin of ideas on a Hydrogen Economy and its solution to the decay of the environment. *International Journal of Hydrogen Energy, 27*, 731-740.

[5] Safizadeh, F., Ghali, E., Houlachi, G. (2015). Electrocatalysis developments for hydrogen evolution reaction in alkaline solutions – A review. *International Journal of Hydrogen Energy, 40*, 256-274.

[6] Ullal, Y., Hegde, A. C. (2014). Electrodeposition and electro-catalytic study of nanocrystalline Ni–Fe alloy. *International Journal of Hydrogen Energy, 39*, 10485-10492.

[7] Shibli, S. M. A., Sebeelamol, J. N. (2013). Development of Fe_2O_3–TiO_2 mixed oxide incorporated Ni–P coating for electrocatalytic hydrogen evolution reaction. *International Journal of Hydrogen Energy, 38*, 2271-2282.

[8] Shibli, S. M. A., Dilimon, V. S. (2008). Development of TiO_2-supported nano-RuO_2-incorporated catalytic nickel coating for hydrogen evolution reaction. *International Journal of Hydrogen Energy, 33*, 1104-1111.

[9] Shibli, S. M. A., Dilimon, V. S. (2007). Effect of phosphorous content and TiO_2-reinforcement on Ni–P electroless plates for hydrogen evolution reaction. *International Journal of Hydrogen Energy, 32*, 1694-1700.

[10] Solmaz, R., Kardaş, G. (2009). Electrochemical deposition and characterization of NiFe coatings as electrocatalytic materials for alkaline water electrolysis. *Electrochimica Acta, 54*, 3726-3734.

[11] Sequeira, C. A. C., Santos, D. M. F., Brito, P. S. D. (2011). Electrocatalytic activity of simple and modified Fe–P electrodeposits for hydrogen evolution from alkaline media. *Energy, 36*, 847-853.

[12] Shervedani, R. K., Madram, A. R. (2007). Kinetics of hydrogen evolution reaction on nanocrystalline electrodeposited Ni62Fe35C3 cathode in alkaline solution by electrochemical impedance spectroscopy. *Electrochimica Acta, 53*, 426-433.

[13] Elezović, N. R., Jović, V. D. Krstajić, N. V. (2005). Kinetics of the hydrogen evolution reaction on Fe–Mo film deposited on mild steel support in alkaline solution. *Electrochimica Acta, 50*, 5594-5601.

[14] Song, L. J., Meng, H. M. (2010). Effect of carbon content on Ni–Fe–C electrodes for hydrogen evolution reaction in seawater. *International Journal of Hydrogen Energy, 35*, 10060-10066.

[15] Arul Raj, I., Vasu, K. I. (1990). Transition metal-based hydrogen electrodes in alkaline solution – electrocatalysis on nickel based binary alloy coatings. *Journal of Applied Electrochemistry, 20*, 32-38.

[16] Krstajić, N. V., Gajić-Krstajić, L., Lačnjevac, U., Jović, B.M., Mora, S., Jović, V. D. (2011). Non-noble metal composite cathodes for hydrogen evolution. Part I: the Ni–MoO_x coatings electrodeposited from Watt's type bath containing MoO_3 powder particles. *International Journal of Hydrogen Energy, 36*, 6441-6449.

[17] Krstajić, N. V., Lačnjevac, U., Jović, B. M., Mora, S., Jović, V. D. (2011). Non-noble metal composite cathodes for hydrogen evolution. Part II: the Ni–MoO_2 coatings electrodeposited from nickel chloride–ammonium chloride bath containing MoO_2 powder particles. *International Journal of Hydrogen Energy, 36*, 6450-6461.

[18] Müller, C. I., Rauscher, T., Schmidt, A., Schubert, T., Weißgärber, T., Kieback, B., Röntzsch, L. (2014). Electrochemical investigations on amorphous Fe-base alloys for alkaline water electrolysis. *International Journal of Hydrogen Energy, 39*, 8926-8937.

[19] Olivares-Ramírez, J. M., Campos-Cornelio, M. L., Uribe Godínez, J., Borja-Arco, E., Castellanos, R.H. (2007). Studies on the hydrogen evolution reaction on different stainless steels. *International Journal of Hydrogen Energy, 32*, 3170-3173.

[20] El-Meligi, A. A., Ismail, N. (2009). Hydrogen evolution reaction of low carbon steel electrode in hydrochloric acid as a source for hydrogen production. *International Journal of Hydrogen Energy, 34*, 91-97.

[21] De Silva Muñoz, L., Bergel, A., Féron, D., Basséguy, R. (2010). Hydrogen production by electrolysis of a phosphate solution on a stainless steel cathode. *International Journal of Hydrogen Energy, 35*, 8561-8568.

[22] Fekry, A. M., Ameer, M. A. (2011). Electrochemical investigation on the corrosion and hydrogen evolution rate of mild steel in sulphuric acid solution. *International Journal of Hydrogen Energy, 36*, 11207-11215.

[23] Mirkova, L., Monev, M., Petkova, N. (2009). Hydrogen evolution, diffusion and solution in Ni/based composite electrodeposits. *ECS Transactions, 19*, 105-112.

[24] Mirkova, L., Pashova, V. Monev, M. (2011). Study of hydrogen evolution reaction on Ni/Co_3O_4 composite electrode in alkaline solution. *ECS Transactions, 35*, 77-84.

[25] Ahmad, R., Ahmad, Z., Khan, A. U., Mastoi, N.R., Aslam, M., Kim, J. (2016). Photocatalytic systems as an advanced environmental remediation: Recent developments, limitations and new avenues for applications. *Journal of Environmental Chemical Engineering, 4*, 4143-4164.

[26] Nasirian, M., Mehrvar, M. (2016). Modification of TiO_2 to enhance photocatalytic degradation of organics in aqueous solutions. *Journal of Environmental Chemical Engineering, 4*, 4072-4082.

[27] Oturan, M. A., Aaron, J.-J. (2014). Advanced oxidation processes in water/wastewater treatment: Principles and applications. A review. *Critical Reviews in Environmental Science and Technology, 44*, 2577-2641.

[28] Pelaez, M., Nolan, N. T., Pillai, S. C., Seery, M. K., Falaras, P., Kontos, A. G., Dunlop, P. S. M., Hamilton, J. W. J., Byme, J. A., O'Shea, K., Entezari, M.H., Dionisiou, D.D. (2012). A review on the visible light active titanium dioxide photocatalysts for environmental applications. *Applied Catalysis, B: Environmental, 125*, 331-349.

[29] Chen, X., Mao, S.S. (2007). Titanium dioxide nanomaterials: Synthesis, properties, modifications, and applications. *Chemical Reviews, 107*, 2891-2959.

[30] Diebold, U. (2003). The surface science of titanium dioxide. *Surface Science Reports, 48*, 53-229.

[31] Shan, A. Y., Ghazi, T. I. M., Rashid, S. A. (2010). Immobilisation of titanium dioxide onto supporting materials in heterogeneous photocatalysis: A review. *Applied Catalysis A: General, 389*, 1-8.

[32] Pozzo, R. L., Baltanás, M.A., Cassano, A.E. (1997). Supported titanium oxide as photocatalyst in water decontamination: State of the art. *Catalysis Today, 39*, 219-231.

[33] Spanou, S., Kontos, A. I., Siokou, A., Kontos, A.G., Vaenas, N., Falaras, P., Pavlatou, E.A. (2013). Self-cleaning behaviour of Ni/nano-TiO_2 metal matrix composites. *Electrochimica Acta, 105*, 324-332.

[34] Danilov, F. I., Tsurkan, A. V., Vasil'eva, E. A., Protsenko, V. S. (2016). Electrocatalytic activity of composite Fe/TiO_2 electrodeposits for hydrogen evolution reaction in alkaline solutions. *International Journal of Hydrogen Energy, 41*, 7363-7372.

[35] Protsenko, V. S., Vasil'eva, E.A., Tsurkan, A. V., Kityk, A. A., Korniy, S. A., Danilov, F. I. (2017). Fe/TiO_2 composite coatings modified by ceria layer: Electrochemical synthesis using environmentally friendly methanesulfonate electrolytes and application as photocatalysts for organic dyes degradation. *Journal of Environmental Chemical Engineering, 5*, 136-146.

[36] Vasil'eva, E. A., Smenova, I. V., Protsenko, V. S., Konstantinova, T. E., Danilov, F. I. (2013). Electrodeposition of hard iron–zirconia dioxide composite coatings from a methanesulfonate electrolyte. *Russian Journal of Applied Chemistry, 86*, 1735-1740.

[37] Protsenko, V. S., Vasil'eva, E. A., Smenova, I. V., Baskevich, A. S., Danilenko, I.A., Konstantinova, T.E., Danilov, F.I. (2015). Electrodeposition of Fe and composite Fe/ZrO_2 coatings from a methanesulfonate bath. *Surface Engineering and Applied Electrochemistry, 51*, 65-75.

[38] Gernon, M. D., Wu, M., Buszta, T., Janney, P. (1999). Environmental benefits of methanesulfonic acid: comparative properties and advantages. *Green Chemistry, 1*, 127-140.

[39] Finšgar, M., Milošev, I. (2010). Corrosion behaviour of stainless steels in aqueous solutions of methanesulfonic acid. *Corrosion Science, 52*, 2430-2438.

[40] Walsh, F. C., Ponce de León, C. (2014). Versatile electrochemical coatings and surface layers from aqueous methanesulfonic acid. *Surface and Coatings Technology, 259*, 676-697.

[41] Low, C. T. J., Walsh, F. C. (2008). Electrodeposition of tin, copper and tin-copper alloys from a methanesulfonic acid electrolyte containing a perfluorinated cationic surfactant. *Surface and Coatings Technology, 202*, 1339-1349.

[42] Pewnim, N., Roy, S. (2013). Electrodeposition of tin-rich Cu–Sn alloys from a methanesulfonic acid electrolyte. *Electrochimica Acta, 90*, 498-506.

[43] Danilov, F. I., Protsenko, V. S., Vasil'eva, E. A., Kabat, O. S. (2011). Antifriction coatings of Pb-Sn-Cu alloy electrodeposited from methanesulphonate bath. *Transactions of the Institute of Metal Finishing, 89*, 151-154.

[44] Protsenko, V. S., Kityk, A. A., Danilov, F. I. (2014). Kinetics and mechanism of chromium electrodeposition from methanesulfonate solutions of Cr(III) salts. *Surface Engineering and Applied Electrochemistry, 50*, 384-389.

[45] Protsenko, V. S., Vasil'eva, E.A., Smenova, I. V., Danilov, F. I. (2014). Electrodeposition of iron/titania composite coatings from methanesulfonate electrolyte. *Russian Journal of Applied Chemistry, 87*, 283-288.

[46] Vasil'eva, E. A., Tsurkan, A. V., Protsenko, V. S., Danilov, F. I. (2016). Electrodeposition of composite Fe–TiO_2 coatings from methanesulfonate electrolyte. *Protection of Metals and Physical Chemistry of Surfaces, 52*, 532-537.

[47] Ohtani, B., Prieto-Mahaney, O. O., Li, D., Abe, R. (2010). What is Degussa (Evonik) P25? Crystalline composition analysis, reconstruction from isolated pure particles and photocatalytic activity test. *Journal of Photochemistry and Photobiology A: Chemistry, 216*, 179-182.

[48] Guglielmi, N. (1972). Kinetics of the deposition of inert particles from electrolytic baths. *Journal of the Electrochemical Society, 119*, 1009-1012.

[49] Bahadormanesh, B., Dolati, A. (2010). The kinetics of Ni-Co/SiC composite coatings electrodeposition. *Journal of Alloys and Compounds, 504*, 514-518.

[50] Berçot, P., Peña-Muñoz, E., Pagetti, J. (2002). Electrolytic composite Ni-PTFE coatings: an adaptation of Guglielmi's model for the phenomena of incorporation. *Surface and Coatings Technology, 157*, 282-289.

[51] Wang, S.-C., Wei, W.-C. J. (2003). Kinetics of electroplating process of nano-sized ceramic particle/Ni composite. *Materials Chemistry and Physics, 78*, 574-580.

[52] Hou, F., Wang, W., Guo, H. (2006). Effect of the dispersibility of ZrO_2 nanoparticles in Ni–ZrO_2 electroplated nanocomposite coatings on the mechanical properties of nanocomposite coatings. *Applied Surface Science, 252*, 3812-3817.

[53] Baez, V. B., Graves, J. E., Pletcher, D. (1992). The reduction of oxygen on titanium oxide electrodes. *Journal of Electroanalytical Chemistry, 340*, 273-286.

[54] Macdonald, D. D. (1990). Review of mechanistic analysis by electrochemical impedance spectroscopy. *Electrochimica Acta, 35*, 1509-1525.

[55] Chang, B.-Y., Park, S.-M. (2010). Electrochemical impedance spectroscopy. *Annual Review of Analytical Chemistry, 3*, 207-229.

[56] Mulder, W. H., Sluyters, J. H. (1988). An explanation of depressed semi-circular arcs in impedance plots for irreversible electrode reactions. *Electrochimica Acta, 33*, 303-310.

[57] Rammelt, U., Reinhard, G. (1990). On the applicability of a constant phase element (CPE) to the estimation of roughness of solid metal electrodes. *Electrochimica Acta, 35*, 1045-1049.

[58] Najafi Sayar, P., Bahrololoom, M. E. (2009). Comparison of anodic dissolution, surface brightness and surface roughness of nanocrystalline nickel coatings with conventional decorative chromium coatings. *Journal of Applied Electrochemistry, 39*, 2489-2496.

[59] Trasatti, S., Petrii, O. A. (1991). Real surface area measurements in electrochemistry. *Pure and Applied Chemistry, 63*, 711-734.

[60] Gierlotka, D., Rowinski, E., Budniok, A., Lagiewka, E. (1997). Production and properties of electrolytic Ni-P-TiO_2 composite layers. *Journal of Applied Electrochemistry, 27*, 1349-1354.

[61] Doyle, R. L., Lyons, M. E. G. (2013). Kinetics and mechanistic aspects of the oxygen evolution reaction at hydrous iron oxide films in base. *Journal of the Electrochemical Society, 160*, H142-H154.

[62] Lyons, M. E. G., Doyle, R.L. (2012). Oxygen evolution at oxidised iron electrodes: a tale of two slopes. *International Journal of Electrochemical Science, 7*, 9488-9501.

[63] Lyons, M. E. G., Brandon, M.P. (2010). A comparative study of the oxygen evolution reaction on oxidised nickel, cobalt and iron electrodes in base. *Journal of Electroanalytical Chemistry, 641*, 119-130.

[64] Trasatti, S. (1991). Physical electrochemistry of ceramic oxides. *Electrochimica Acta, 36*, 225-241.

[65] Aldykiewicz, A. J., Davenport, A. J., Isaacs, H. S. (1996). Studies of the formation of cerium-rich protective folims using X-ray absorption near-edge spectroscopy and rotating disk electrode methods. *Journal of Electrochemical Society, 143*, 147-154.

[66] Stoychev, D. (2013). Corrosion protective ability of electrodeposited ceria layers. *Journal of Solid State Electrochemistry, 17*, 497-509.

[67] Yang, L., Pang, X., Fox-Rabinovich, G., Veldhuis, S., Zhitomirsky, I. (2011). Electrodeposition of cerium oxide films and composite. *Surface and Coatings Technology, 206*, 1-7.

[68] Arenas, M.A., de Damborenea, J.J. (2003). Growth mechanisms of cerium layers on galvanised steel. *Electrochimica Acta, 48*, 3693-3698.

[69] Nickolova, D., Stoyanova, E., Stoychev, D., Avramova, I., Stefanov, P. (2008). Protective effect in sulfuric acid media of alumina and ceria oxide layers electrodeposited on stainless steel. *Surface and Coatings Technology, 202*, 1876-1888.

[70] Creus, J., Brezault, F., Rebere, C., Gadouleau, M. (2006). Synthesis and characterisation of thin cerium oxide coatings elaborated by cathodic electrolytic deposition on steel substrate. *Surface and Coatings Technology, 200*, 4636-4645.

[71] Hamlaoui, Y., Pedraza, F., Remazeilles, C., Cohendoz, S., Rebere, C., Tifouti, L., Creus, J. (2009). Cathodic electrodeposition of cerium-based oxides on carbon steel from concentrated cerium nitrate solutions. Part I. Electrochemical and analytical characterisation. *Materials Chemistry and Physics, 113*, 650-657.

[72] Hamlaoui, Y., Tifouti, L., Remazeilles, C., Pedraza, F. (2010). Cathodic electrodeposition of cerium based oxides on carbon steel from concentrated cerium nitrate. Part II: Influence of electrodeposition parameters and of the addition of PEG. *Materials Chemistry and Physics, 120*, 172-180.

[73] Arurault, L., Monsang, P., Salley, J., Bes, R.S. (2004). Electrochemical preparation of adherent ceria coatings on ferritic stainless steel. *Thin Solid Films, 466*, 75-80.

[74] Kulp, E. A., Limmer, S. J., Bohannan, E. W., Switzer, J. A. (2007). Electrodeposition of nanometer-thick ceria films by oxidation of cerium(III)–acetate. *Solid State Ionics, 178*, 749-757.

[75] Hayden, B. E., Malevich, D. V., Pletcher, D. (2001). Electrode coatings from sprayed titanium dioxide nanoparticles – behaviour in NaOH solutions. *Electrochemistry Communications, 3*, 390-394.

[76] Lide, D. R. (2003-2004). *CRC Handbook of Chemistry and Physics*, *84th Edition*. CRC Press.

[77] Edington, J., O'Keefe, M. J., O'Keefe, T. J. (2006). Development of a spontaneous immersion process for deposition of cerium oxide coatings on copper substrates. *Surface and Coatings Technology, 200*, 5733-5737.

[78] Guergova, D., Stoyanova, E., Stoychev, D., Avramova, I., Stefanov, P. (2015). Self-healing effect of ceria electrodeposited thin films on stainless steel in aggressive 0.5 mol/L NaCl aqueous solution. *Journal of Rare Earths, 33*, 1212-1227.

[79] Girčienė, O., Gudavičiūtė, L., Selskis, A., Jasulaitienė, V., Šakirzanovas, S., Ramanauskas, R. (2015). The self-healing ability of cerium oxide films on carbon steel. *Chemija, 26(3)*, 175-183.

[80] Zhou, X., Shen, Y. (2013). Beneficial effects of CeO_2 addition on microstructure and corrosion behavior of electrodeposited Ni nanocrystalline coatings. *Surface and Coatings Technology, 235*, 433-446.

[81] Danilov, F. I., Protsenko, V.S., Kityk, A. A. (2014). Estimation of the protective ability of chromium coatings deposited from sulfate and methanesulfonate electrolytes based on Cr(III). *Protection of Metals and Physical Chemistry of Surfaces, 50*, 672-678.

[82] Han, F., Kambala, V. S. R., Srinivasan, M., Rajarathnam, D., Naidu, R. (2009). Tailored titanium dioxide photocatalysts for the degradation of organic dyes in wastewater treatment: A review. *Applied Catalysis A: General, 359*, 25-40.

[83] Lachheb, H., Puzenat, E., Houas, A., Ksibi, M., Elaloui, E., Guillard, C., Herrmann, J.-M. (2002). Photocatalytic degradation of various types of dyes (Alizarin S, Crocein Orange G, Methyl Red, Congo Red, Methylene Blue) in water by UV-irradiated titania. *Applied Catalysis B: Environmental, 39*, 75-90.

[84] Sonawane, R. S., Kale, B. B., Dongare, M. K. (2004). Preparation of photo-catalytic activity of Fe–TiO_2 thin films prepared by sol–gel dip coatings. *Materials Chemistry and Physics, 85*, 52-57.

[85] Guillard, C., Puzenat, E., Lachheb, H., Houas, A., Herrmann, J.-M. (2005). Why inorganic salts decrease the TiO_2 photocatalytic efficiency. *International Journal of Photoenergy, 7*, 1-9.

[86] Atkins, P., Paula, J. (2005). *Physical Chemistry*. New York, Oxford University Press.

[87] Houas, A., Lachheb, H., Ksibi, M., Elaloui, E., Guillard, C., Herrmann, J.-M. (2001). Photocatalytic degradation pathway of methylene blue in water. *Applied Catalysis B: Environmental, 31*, 145-157.

INDEX

#

A

B

C

D

E

L

M

N

O

P

Q

R

S